NUTRITIONAL GUIDELINES FOR ATHLETIC PERFORMANCE

THE TRAINING TABLE

NUTRITIONAL GUIDELINES FOR ATHLETIC PERFORMANCE

THE TRAINING TABLE

Edited By
LEMUEL W. TAYLOR IV

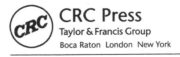

CRC Press
Taylor & Francis Group
Boca Raton London New York

CRC Press is an imprint of the
Taylor & Francis Group, an **informa** business

CRC Press
Taylor & Francis Group
6000 Broken Sound Parkway NW, Suite 300
Boca Raton, FL 33487-2742

First issued in paperback 2019

© 2012 by Taylor & Francis Group, LLC
CRC Press is an imprint of Taylor & Francis Group, an Informa business

No claim to original U.S. Government works

ISBN-13: 978-1-4398-3936-2 (hbk)
ISBN-13: 978-0-367-38154-7 (pbk)

Visit the Taylor & Francis Web site at
http://www.taylorandfrancis.com

and the CRC Press Web site at
http://www.crcpress.com

To the most important people in my life:
my wife Vanessa, my parents Maria and Lem Taylor III,
and all the rest of my family and close friends
who have supported me over the years

Contents

SECTION I   Caloric Demands of Sport

SECTION II   Role of Individual Nutrients

SECTION III   Other Training Table Considerations

Preface

The idea and origination of this project came during a phone conversation with Dr. Ira Wolinsky, who read a previous book chapter that I had authored. After a couple more conversations and e-mail exchanges, the idea for this book developed.

The concept of the "Training Table" became the primary interest and direction of this book for various reasons. The practice known as the "training table," which is defined as a table where athletes in a training program eat planned meals to help in their conditioning/training, leads ultimately to improved adaptation and enhanced performance.

Even though many factors contribute to athletic performance, the role of proper nutrition cannot be emphasized enough. The importance of proper daily nutrition has several implications on overall health and proper homeostatic functioning of the body, but that can be said for any person, whether sedentary or an elite-level athlete. We do know that when an individual goes from a sedentary to an active lifestyle, their daily nutrient needs change. If we extrapolate that to an elite athlete who is training a minimum of 15–20 hours per week, but in some cases as many as 40–60 hours per week, these nutrient requirements grow in proportion to this level of activity. Knowing this, it is vital for athletes and for the individuals who train these athletes to know the proper nutritional requirements that are appropriate for a particular sport, body size, gender, set of goals, etc.

This book addresses these needs for athletes on a comprehensive basis from a training table perspective and provides practical recommendations along the way to include the most significant parts of a training table. The book focuses on the key nutritional guidelines for the macronutrients, basic calorie needs, and macronutrient-specific needs for various types of athletes.

During the editorial process and upon reviewing all of the up-to-date research presented in the text, it became clear to me that knowing these basic requirements and combining them with proper training are the two most important factors in maximizing training adaptations and performance. The world of sports nutrition has evolved immensely over the last 10–15 years, and it will continue to evolve as the field moves forward. I hope this book will contribute to the field by presenting practical information based on up-to-date research.

Lem W. Taylor IV, PhD, FISSN, CISSN
Assistant Professor
University of Mary Hardin-Baylor

Acknowledgments

I am most grateful to the various contributors who played a vital role in completing this book. They are experts in all aspects of the exercise science and sport nutrition fields, and their willingness to contribute to this book cannot go unnoticed.

I thank Dr. Ira Wolinsky, who sought me out as the editor of this book and provided great insight during this process. Additionally, I thank the various staff at the Taylor & Francis Group for their guidance and support during the completion of this book.

Finally, I thank my mentor and friend, Dr. Darryn Willoughby, and other mentors—Dr. Curt Dickson, Dr. Joel Mitchell, Dr. Richard Kreider—for all of their personal and educational guidance over the years, which has helped me to develop into the person I am as well as the scientist I have become. These individuals, who introduced me to and taught me the field of exercise science and sports nutrition, are the reason I am able to work in a field that I love, and for this I will always be grateful.

Lem W. Taylor IV

Editor

Lem W. Taylor IV, PhD, FISSN, CISSN, is currently an assistant professor of exercise physiology and director of the exercise biochemistry lab at the University of Mary Hardin-Baylor in Belton, Texas. He received his BS degree in exercise physiology from Abilene Christian University, his MS in exercise physiology from Texas Christian University, and a PhD in exercise, nutrition, and preventive health from Baylor University. He is also a fellow (FISSN) and a certified sports nutritionist (CISSN) under the International Society of Sports Nutrition.

Dr. Taylor is a member of the Texas Chapter of the American College of Sports Medicine (ACSM), the International Society of Sports Nutrition (ISSN), and the National Strength and Conditioning Association (NSCA), as well as other organizations. Currently, he serves as president (2011–2014) of the International Society of Sports Nutrition. Additionally, he is serving his second stint on the board of directors for the TACSM as a non-medicine representative, and he served as the student representative during his studies at Baylor University. He also held other service roles within these organizations over the last eight years.

Dr. Taylor has participated in numerous clinical studies investigating the effects of various sports supplements and nutritional interventions and their effects on body composition and performance. This research involvement has led to several presentations at ISSN, ACSM, and NSCA annual meetings as well as numerous publications in various research journals, published abstracts, and authored chapters in both mainstream and reference books in areas of exercise physiology and sports nutrition. He also serves as a journal reviewer and/or is a member of the editorial boards for various journals concerning exercise science and sports nutrition.

Contributors

Jose Antonio, PhD, FACSM, FNSCA, FISSN
International Society of Sports Nutrition
Deerfield Beach, Florida

Thomas W. Buford, PhD
Department of Aging and Geriatric Research
University of Florida College of Medicine
Gainesville, Florida

Amanda Carlson-Phillips, MS, RD, CSSD
Athletes' Performance, Inc.
Phoenix, Arizona

Matthew B. Cooke, BSc(Hons), PhD
School of Biomedical and Health Sciences
Faculty of Health, Engineering, and Science
Victoria University
Melbourne, Victoria, Australia

Vincent J. Dalbo, PhD
Medical and Applied Sciences
Institute for Health and Social Science Research
Central Queensland University
Rockhampton, Queensland, Australia

Justin P. Dobson, MS
Department of Health and Kinesiology
Texas A&M University
College Station, Texas

Fanny Dufour, MS, CISSN, CSCS, NASM-CPT
Department of Exercise and Sport Science
University of Mary Hardin-Baylor
Belton, Texas

Kristin Dugan, MS, SPT
Department of Exercise and Sport Science
University of Mary Hardin-Baylor
Belton, Texas

David H. Fukuda, MS, CSCS
Department of Health and Exercise Science
University of Oklahoma
Norman, Oklahoma

Jean L. Gutierrez PhD, RD
Department of Exercise Science
The George Washington University
Washington, DC

Chad Kerksick, PhD, ATC, CSCS*D, NSCA-CPT*D
Health and Exercise Science Department
University of Oklahoma
Norman, Oklahoma

Julie Kresta, PhD
Health and Kinesiology Department
Texas A&M University
College Station, Texas

Paul M. La Bounty, PhD, MPT, CSCS
Department of Health, Human Performance, and Recreation
Baylor University
Waco, Texas

Michelle A. Mardock, MS, RD
Department of Health and Kinesiology
Texas A&M University
College Station, Texas

**Ronald W. Mendel, PhD, FISSN,
  CISSN**
Department of Human Performance and
  Sport Business
University of Mount Union
Alliance, Ohio

Jonathan M. Oliver, MEd
Department of Health and Kinesiology
Texas A&M University
College Station, Texas

Chris N. Poole, MS, CSCS
Health and Exercise Science Department
University of Oklahoma
Norman, Oklahoma

**Christopher J. Rasmussen, MS,
  CSCS**
Department of Health and Kinesiology
Texas A&M University
College Station, Texas

Michael D. Roberts, PhD
Department of Biomedical Science
University of Missouri-Columbia
Columbia, Missouri

Kara A. Sample, RD
Weld County School District 6
Greeley, Colorado

Brian D. Shelmadine, PhD
Department of Health, Human
  Performance, and Recreation
Baylor University
Waco, Texas

**Abbie E. Smith, PhD, CSCS*D,
  CISSN**
Department of Exercise and Sports
  Science
University of North Carolina Chapel
  Hill
Chapel Hill, North Carolina

**Lem W. Taylor IV, PhD, FISSN,
  CISSN**
Department of Exercise and Sport
  Science
University of Mary Hardin-Baylor
Belton, Texas

**Colin D. Wilborn, PhD, FISSN,
  CSCS, ATC**
Department of Exercise and Sport
  Science
University of Mary Hardin-Baylor
Belton, Texas

1 Introduction
The Role of the Training Table

Michael D. Roberts and Lem W. Taylor IV

CONTENTS

1.1 SPORTS NUTRITION: A HISTORICAL PERSPECTIVE

Sports nutrition is a science that has existed for thousands of years. In this regard, the Greek philosopher Pythagoras of Samos (who lived from 580 to 500 BCE) has been touted as the first person to train athletes on a meat diet because he realized the need for extraneous protein consumption to support the demands of athletic participation (Grivetti and Applegate 1997). Furthermore, Greek athletes who preceded Pythagoras were known for consuming a diet consisting of dry figs, moist cheese, and wheat in order to support the increased demands imposed by training. Nearly two and one-half millennia later, scientist Paul Schenk observed the diets of Olympic athletes participating in the Berlin Games of 1936. Interestingly, Schenk reported that the typical pre-event meals of endurance athletes consisted of high-carbohydrate foods including porridge, shredded wheat, corn flakes, and pasta, and that athletes averaged macronutrient intakes of 320 g of protein, 270 g of fat, and 850 g of carbohydrates per day (Grivetti and Applegate 1997), although these dietary patterns were left to the discretion of the athletes.

According to a recent publication describing advances in the sports nutrition field, the dining hall of the athlete's village at the Sydney 2000 Olympic Games contained menus that were developed and informed by focus groups, scientific literature reviews, and food-preference surveys of athletes; all of this was spurred by the notion that nutritional adequacy for athletes during the games was a prominent concern (Pelly et al. 2009). In regards to current-day efforts, molecular biologists in the sports nutrition field are unveiling how ingesting various macronutrients interacts with the genome in order to promote optimal recovery and optimize training adaptations, for example, how post-exercise protein ingestion increases anabolic gene expression patterns in skeletal muscle (Hulmi et al. 2009).

1

In a scientific paper describing this research trend, scientist Amy Heck and colleagues (Heck et al. 2004) indicate that the DNA in skeletal muscle transcribes genes that encode signalers (interleukin-6 as an example) to help replenish glycogen following a prolonged exercise bout. In some instances, these signalers can be catabolic in that they lead to muscle protein breakdown in order to favor gluconeogenesis, or new glucose formation. However, when an athlete minimizes the loss of muscle glycogen through nutritional adequacy (i.e., proper nutrition prior to, during, and after exercise), this aforementioned process is diminished, an effect that optimizes not only performance but also muscle recovery. Hence, it is evident that the sports nutrition field has rapidly evolved over thousands of years, and these trends emphasize the importance of nutritional adequacy in athletes.

1.2   TRAINING TABLES: INNOVATIVE TREND OR IVORY TOWER?

It is now common knowledge that implementing a sound diet for athletes is an integral phase of training that undoubtedly optimizes sports performance. According to an *NBC Sports* online periodical, the Notre Dame football program recently implemented a training table for the 2009–2010 season that provided specialized dinner items with the intent of optimizing performance. In describing this undertaking, journalist Keith Arnold states (Arnold 2010):

> Most people don't drop 200 grand on a Ferrari only to fill it up with low-grade gasoline. With this new meal plan and performance program, it's clear that the Irish are intent on fixing both the macro and micro issues.

This movement is one of the many current-day examples of how collegiate and professional sports organizations are adopting nutritional practices that ensure that their athletes are sustaining nutritional adequacy during mealtime.

So much attention on nutrition is placed on what an athlete eats right before and during most exercise/competition/events, but what we now know from the backing of scientific research is that optimal performance will only be achieved if daily nutrition is optimized from the time an athlete wakes up in the morning until he goes to bed. However, a discouraging yet evident current-day tendency exists: athletes who do not have the luxuries of training tables, sports nutritionists, etc., typically possess a poor knowledge base in regards to various nutritional concepts. Such examples include the following:

- Approximately 65% of high school athletes in a recent survey supplemented with protein powders, providing reasons such as "athletes should take protein supplements" and indicating that they take supplements "to gain as much muscle as possible" (Duellman et al. 2008, p. 1124).
- In a broad spectrum of Brazilian adolescent athletes: 1) females engaged in strength/power sports did not ingest adequate carbohydrates; 2) all survey athletes typically consumed inadequate intakes of thiamin, vitamin E, folate, magnesium, and phosphorus; and 3) less than 5% of athletes consumed adequate amounts of calcium, fiber, and water (de Sousa et al. 2008).

- Male and female adult Canadian athletes: 1) consumed well below the caloric recommendations for physically active persons, and 2) did not meet carbohydrate recommendations (Lun et al. 2009).
- In Brazilian adolescent tennis players: 1) caloric intake was 10% lower than daily energy expenditure in one-third of the athletes; 2) carbohydrate intake was below recommendations for physically active persons; and 3) fiber, calcium, potassium, magnesium, and folate values were below recommendations for 80%–100% of the athletes (Juzwiak et al. 2008).

These data make it evident that a future obstacle for sports nutritionists will be to ensure that athletes who attend training tables make wise decisions in regards to consuming foods that will optimize their hard work expended during practices and workout sessions. Deficiencies at the training table result in deficiencies in performance. More importantly, a bigger obstacle for scientists, practitioners, and athletes alike is to ensure that the majority of nonprofessional or noncollegiate athletes who do not have access to formal training tables possess adequate knowledge to make these same decisions.

1.3 CONCLUDING REMARKS

According to a recent scientific publication on the issue of sports nutrition education, athletes are interested in seeking accurate and practical nutritional advice (Chapman et al. 1997). These same authors also state, however, that there is "a lack of research focused on developing the most effective ways to educate athletes about sports nutrition" (p. 437). Fortunately, this book will present extensive research demonstrating that athletes benefit from a performance standpoint when they consume a well-balanced diet on a daily basis. While structuring a diet containing appropriate amounts of macronutrients (i.e., protein, carbohydrates, and fat) and micronutrients (i.e., vitamins and minerals) seems like a daunting task to some, this text will adequately address how athletes can do so in an effective and practical fashion. More specifically, this book will focus on the following aspects of sports nutrition:

- Provide a comprehensive description of the key macronutrients that fuel our daily metabolism and exercise training
- Discuss basic caloric needs and macronutrient-specific needs for various types of athletes and explain how those might differ from nonathletes
- Provide a comprehensive description of the key micronutrients, as well as fluid recommendations, that fuel daily metabolism and exercise training
- Provide a detailed explanation and rationale for the need for specific meal planning for athletes
- Address all these key issues from a training-table approach, including a discussion of various populations and current trends in the sports nutrition field

This text is an appropriate reference text for sport nutrition professionals, the informed layman, weekend and professional athletes, trainers and coaches, and/or anyone that works in the field of athletic performance and sports nutrition. In many instances, a proper reference is needed when examining the area of the training table because of the variables that exist when making recommendations to athletes depending on specific goals, type of athlete, or phase of training.

REFERENCES

Arnold, K. 2010. "Training table is here." http://irish.nbcsports.com/2010/01/19/training-table-is-here/

Chapman, P., R. B. Toma, R. V. Tuveson, and M. Jacob. 1997. Nutrition knowledge among adolescent high school female athletes. *Adolescence* 32: 437–446.

de Sousa, E. F., T. H. Da Costa, J. A. Nogueira, and L. J. Vivaldi. 2008. Assessment of nutrient and water intake among adolescents from sports federations in the Federal District, Brazil. *Br J Nutr* 99: 1275–1283.

Duellman, M. C., J. M. Lukaszuk, A. D. Prawitz, and J. P. Brandenburg. 2008. Protein supplement users among high school athletes have misconceptions about effectiveness. *J Strength Cond Res* 22: 1124–1129.

Grivetti, L. E., and E. A. Applegate. 1997. From Olympia to Atlanta: A cultural-historical perspective on diet and athletic training. *J Nutr* 127(5 Suppl): 860S–868S.

Heck, A. L., C. S. Barroso, M. E. Callie, and M. S. Bray. 2004. Gene-nutrition interaction in human performance and exercise response. *Nutrition* 20: 598–602.

Hulmi, J. J., V. Kovanen, H. Selanne, W. J. Kraemer, K. Hakkinen, and A. A. Mero. 2009. Acute and long-term effects of resistance exercise with or without protein ingestion on muscle hypertrophy and gene expression. *Amino Acids* 37: 297–308.

Juzwiak, C. R., O. M. Amancio, M. S. Vitalle, M. M. Pinheiro, and V. L. Szejnfeld. 2008. Body composition and nutritional profile of male adolescent tennis players. *J Sports Sci* 26: 1209–1217.

Lun, V., K. A. Erdman, and R. A. Reimer. 2009. Evaluation of nutritional intake in Canadian high-performance athletes. *Clin J Sport Med* 19: 405–411.

Pelly, F., H. O'Connor, G. Denyer, and I. Caterson. 2009. Catering for the athletes village at the Sydney 2000 Olympic Games: The role of sports dietitians. *Int J Sport Nutr Exerc Metab* 19: 340–354.

Section I

Caloric Demands of Sport

2 Energy Demands
Sedentary versus Active Individuals

Julie Kresta

CONTENTS

2.1 INTRODUCTION

Caloric intake and physical activity are popular topics today for many individuals because of the increased focus on living a healthy lifestyle. There are several health organizations that have developed recommendations on daily caloric intake for overall health and performance, with specifics for each of the macronutrients. Activity level is also directly linked to calorie demands. The greater the physical activity level of an individual, the greater the caloric intake needs. The reverse is true for sedentary individuals. In order to maintain weight and overall health, an excess of calories can be detrimental. The balance of energy intake and output is important to maintain health and fitness goals. For example, when intake exceeds output, this may lead to health problems such as obesity. Also, when intake is too low for the given output, this could lead to malnutrition and the inability to maintain physical performance.

These concepts are important for the general population as well as professionals in the health and fitness fields. They can use these concepts along with individual characteristics to develop exercise and diet prescriptions, because there is no one plan or recommendation that is appropriate for everyone. This chapter will discuss the general principles and physiology of caloric intake for all major macronutrients and how it pertains to both active and sedentary individuals. Subsequent chapters will then detail how these needs change based on the specific type of athlete as well as the goals of various athletes.

2.2 ENERGY

In order to sustain life, the consumption of macronutrients is crucial to provide energy. The energy requirement may differ depending on various individual factors such as the activity being performed or body composition; however, the average daily caloric requirement is approximately 2000 kcal for adult women and 3000 kcal for adult males (McArdle et al. 2001). Athletes, however, may require a much greater amount of calories per day to sustain their activity level. For example, weight lifters and body builders may consume an average of 3000 kcal/day, triathletes consume an average of 4800 kcal/day, and elite cyclists may consume close to 6000 kcal/day (McArdle et al. 2001). Several researchers suggest a caloric intake of 30 kcal/kg of fat-free mass per day as a lower threshold for active females (American College of Sports Medicine, American Dietetic Association, Dietitians of Canada 2009; Deuster et al. 1986; Kopp-Woodroffe et al. 1999; Loucks et al. 1998; Otten et al. 2006). The main energy-supplying dietary nutrients include carbohydrates, fats (lipids), and proteins. The metabolism of these macronutrients provides the body with the components needed to produce energy to fuel the demands of the body.

Taking a step back, we will now examine how foods are able to provide energy for the body. Food energy is measured using calories. By definition, a calorie is the amount of heat needed to increase the temperature of 1 kg or 1 L of water exactly 1°C. A kilocalorie (kcal) is equivalent to a kilogram calorie and is a more accurate unit of measure. For example, the average banana contains approximately 100 kcal. Therefore, the amount of energy in a banana is sufficient to raise the temperature of 100 L of water by 1°C. Food energy is also expressed as joules (J) or kilojoules (kJ). The conversion from kcal to kJ is to multiply the kcal by 4.184 (McArdle et al. 2001). To keep things uniform and simplified, the descriptions of energy needs, demands, and contents throughout the book will use the term calories (abbreviated as kcal).

Bomb calorimeters are used to measure the total energy value of foods using the principle of direct calorimetry. These calorimeters measure the heat of combustion, which is the heat released from complete oxidation of the food. The heat of combustion for carbohydrates varies slightly based on the specific variation of the atoms. For example, glucose equals 3.74 kcal/g and glycogen equals 4.19 kcal/g. The average value of 4.2 or 4 kcal is typically used to represent 1 g of carbohydrate. Lipids are able to produce more energy at an average of 9.4 or 9 kcal/g. This is primarily due to lipids having more hydrogen molecules available for subsequent oxidation compared with carbohydrates and proteins. As with carbohydrates, this value also varies

TABLE 2.1

Atwater General Factors for Major Macronutrients

	Atwater General Factors
Dietary carbohydrate	4 kcal/g
Dietary lipid	9 kcal/g
Dietary protein	4 kcal/g

depending on the structure of the fatty acids within the lipid. The energy in protein depends on the type of protein as well as the nitrogen content. The average heat of combustion for protein, however, is approximately 5.65 kcal/g. However, the net energy is only 4.6 kcal/g. This difference comes from the body's inability to oxidize the nitrogen component of the protein molecule. For simplicity and more practical uses, the Atwater general factors of 4, 9, and 4 kcal/g are typically used for carbohydrates, lipids, and protein, respectively (Table 2.1) (McArdle et al. 2001).

Once the calories are consumed and assimilated through the process of digestion and absorption, this energy needs to be converted appropriately in order to produce biological work. As the first law of thermodynamics states, energy is neither produced, consumed, or used up but is transformed from one form to another. Therefore, the potential energy from the macronutrients must be transformed because the human body cannot use heat energy directly. Energy from the macronutrients consumed in our diet is passed through adenosine triphosphate (ATP), an energy-dense nucleotide or high-energy phosphate. As ATP is broken down, energy is released and directly transferred to the surrounding energy-requiring molecules to drive various processes in the body both at rest and during exercise.

The body is only able to store about 80–100 g of ATP at any given time; therefore, there are several metabolic pathways in the body that allow for a continual supply of ATP during rest and activity. Pathways for the anaerobic breakdown of phosphocreatine, glucose, glycerol, and carbon skeletons from deaminated amino acids are found in the cytosol. Specifically, the anaerobic pathways are comprised of the ATP-phosphocreatine system (ATP-PC system, also known as the phosphagen system) and glycolysis, which is the body's means of breaking down carbohydrates. The mitochondria contains aerobic pathways including the citric acid cycle, beta-oxidation, and the electron transport chain (McArdle et al. 2001). The relative contribution of each of these metabolic pathways is dependent on the activity being performed and the nutritional status of an individual, as well as the training status of an individual.

2.2.1 Determining Individual Caloric Needs

Prior to determining the caloric needs for an individual, it is important to measure energy expenditure. Total energy expenditure (TEE) is made up of basal or resting metabolic rate (BMR or RMR), thermal effect of food, and physical activity. RMR has been shown to represent about 60%–75% of TEE, whereas the thermal effect of food and physical activity have lesser roles of 10 and 15%–30%, respectively. Of these, physical activity is the variable with the greatest effect on TEE based on the amount and type of exercise chosen by the individual, as well as the volume of exercise that is performed on a regular basis.

The thermal effect of food is also able to be altered to influence TEE. There are two components involved with this variable: obligatory and facultative thermogenesis. Obligatory thermogenesis pertains to the energy needed to digest and absorb the nutrients in foods. Facultative thermogenesis is concerned with the stimulating effect of the sympathetic nervous system as a response to feeding. Thus, metabolic rates can increase after feeding during the digestion of foods and will decrease in states of fasting or starvation.

BMR reflects the amount of energy needed or heat produced by the body to be awake on a daily basis. Because BMR is difficult to measure in a laboratory setting, RMR is typically used to determine an individual's metabolic rate. This is usually just slightly greater than the BMR level. RMR is a method used to determine the energy required to sustain life in the resting state. It is typically represented as kcal/day and can vary based on individual characteristics such as gender, age, body composition, and activity level. It is tested in a fasting state and without having performed a recent bout of physical activity. This is also referred to as resting energy expenditure (REE) (McArdle et al. 2001).

There are direct and indirect methods of determining REE. The direct methods include using doubly labeled water or direct calorimetry. Because these methods are expensive and require specialized equipment, there have been indirect methods developed to estimate the caloric needs of an individual. One common example is by using indirect calorimetry, which measures oxygen consumption and carbon dioxide production during rest for a given amount of time (typically 20–30 minutes) to estimate energy expenditure in units of kcal/day (Nieman 2003).

Other methods include prediction equations developed using data collected from large subject pools. Frankenfield et al. (2005) compared four common prediction equations for REE in healthy nonobese and obese individuals in a systematic review. They included the Harris-Benedict (Harris and Benedict 1919), Mifflin-St. Jeor (Mifflin et al. 1990), Owen (Owen et al. 1986, 1987), and Food and Agriculture Organization/World Health Organization/United Nations University (FAO/WHO/UNU, 1985) equations. Frankenfield and colleagues determined that the Mifflin-St. Jeor equation was actually the most accurate of the four in predicting REE within 10% of the value measured. The four equations are shown in Table 2.2.

2.2.2 Energy Balance

It is important to balance the amount of energy intake (EI) and TEE in order to maintain body composition and overall health. EI includes all energy from dietary sources, fluids, and supplements, whereas TEE, as explained earlier, includes REE, thermal effect of food, and physical activity (American College of Sports Medicine, American Dietetic Association, Dietitians of Canada 2009). The most variable part of TEE is that of physical activity (Genton et al. 2010). The energy balance (EB) is specifically defined with the equation EB = EI − TEE (Uauy and Diaz 2005). A positive EB corresponds to an excess of energy stored in the body, which can lead to complications such as obesity. A negative EB would result in more calories

TABLE 2.2

Prediction Equations for RMR

Mifflin-St. Jeor (Mifflin et al. 1990)

Men	RMR = 9.99 × weight + 6.25 × height − 4.92 × age + 5
Women	RMR = 9.99 × weight + 6.25 × height − 4.92 × age − 161

Harris-Benedict (Harris and Benedict 1919)

Men	RMR = 66.47 + 13.75 × weight + 5.0 × height − 6.75 × age
Women	RMR = 665.09 + 9.56 × weight + 1.84 × height − 4.67 × age

FAO/WHO/UNU (Food and Agricultural Organization/World Health Organization/United Nations University, 1985)

Men 18–30 years	RMR = 15.3 × weight + 679	RMR = 15.4 × weight − 27 × height + 717
Men 31–60 years	RMR = 11.6 × weight + 879	RMR = 11.3 × weight + 16 × height + 901
Men >60 years	RMR = 13.5 × weight + 487	RMR = 8.8 × weight + 1128 × height − 1071
Women 18–30 years	RMR = 14.7 × weight + 496	RMR = 13.3 × weight + 334 × height + 35
Women 31–60 years	RMR = 8.7 × weight + 829	RMR = 8.7 × weight − 25 × height + 865
Women >60 years	RMR = 10.5 × weight + 596	RMR = 9.2 × weight + 637 × height − 302

All equations use weight in kilograms, height in centimeters (except for FAO/WHO/UNU, which uses meters), and age in years.

being expended and will result in the body using fat and lean tissue to fuel the body (American College of Sports Medicine, American Dietetic Association, Dietitians of Canada 2009). The nature of energy balance in an individual is always changing based on the current food intake and exercise habits of the individual and thus must be monitored on a regular basis to maintain ideal body weight.

2.3   HEALTHY ACTIVE INDIVIDUALS

Physical activity is defined as movement produced by skeletal muscles that results in an increase in energy expenditure (Bouchard et al. 1994; Caspersen et al. 1985; Nieman 2003; United States Department of Health and Human Services 1996). The American College of Sports Medicine (ACSM) and American Heart Association recently updated the regulations and definition of physically active. They recommend that adults between the ages of 18 and 65 years should partake in moderate intensity aerobic physical activity for at least 30 minutes a day for 5 days a week or 20 minutes of vigorous intensity activity for 3 days a week (Haskell et al. 2007). The United States Department of Health and Human Services and Department of Agriculture based their levels and definitions of physical activity from the recommendations of the Institute of Medicine, which are described in Table 2.3 (United States Department of Health and Human Services and United States Department of Agriculture 2005).

There is a distinction, however, between recreationally active individuals and athletes. Physical activity levels used in various calculations to estimate energy expenditure do not include standards for athletes. They use categories of sedentary, low active, active, and very active. An athlete would still most likely be above the very

TABLE 2.3

Description of Levels of Physical Activity

Physical Activity Level	Description
Sedentary	Lifestyle that includes only light physical activity associated with daily life
Moderately active	Lifestyle that includes physical activity equal to walking 1.5–3 miles per day at 3–4 mph, in addition to activity of daily life
Active	Lifestyle that includes physical activity equal to walking more than 3 miles per day at 3–4 mph, in additional to activities of daily life

active category depending on the sport and training program (American College of Sports Medicine, American Dietetic Association, Dietitians of Canada 2009; Zello 2006). Athletes can be further broken down into different subcategories based on the characteristics of their sport. The more recognized types include strength or power athletes and endurance athletes. These individuals utilize different energy systems during their training and competition and also have some differing nutritional concerns regarding fueling the body to perform.

With regular physical activity, the REE has been shown to increase with an increase in lean muscle mass (Gilliatt-Wimberly et al. 2001). Gilliat-Wimberly and colleagues examined the effects of physical activity on REE and body composition in adult females. They found significantly greater REE and lower body fat levels in active women compared with levels in their sedentary counterparts. Gilliatt-Wimberly et al. suggested that this was due to physical activity increasing the daily caloric expenditure, as well as the fact that fat-free mass helps to maintain an elevated REE (Gilliatt-Wimberly et al. 2001).

2.3.1 Caloric Needs

The daily caloric requirement for a healthy individual is dependent on the need to consume enough calories to meet energy expenditure and maintain body weight. The more active a person is, the greater number of calories they must consume in order to maintain weight. Essential calories reflect the amount needed to meet recommended nutrient intake from foods. Discretionary calories represent the difference between total energy requirements and essential calories. Table 2.4 shows an estimate of caloric needs for different age groups, genders, and levels of physical activity according to the United States Department of Health and Human Services and United States Department of Agriculture. Caloric intake is typically recommended to be greater for active individuals, as seen in the Table 2.4. The major macronutrients of carbohydrates, fats, and protein make up the majority of caloric intake in most individuals. The distribution of these macronutrients may depend on the type, duration, and intensity of physical activity.

2.3.1.1 Carbohydrate Needs for Healthy Active Individuals

Carbohydrates (CHO) are a major fuel source required not only for the body to sustain activity, but also for the brain to function adequately. There are three main

TABLE 2.4
Estimated Caloric Requirements for Healthy Individuals (kcal/day)

Gender	Age (years)	Physical Activity		
		Sedentary	Moderately Active	Active
Child	2–3	1000	1000–1400	1000–1400
Female	4–8	1200	1400–1600	1000–1800
	9–13	1600	1600–2000	1800–2200
	14–18	1800	2000	2400
	19–30	2000	2000–2200	2400
	31–50	1800	2000	2200
	>50	1600	1800	2000–2200
Male	4–8	1400	1400–1600	1600–2000
	9–13	1800	1800–2000	2000–2600
	14–18	2200	2400–2800	2800–3200
	19–30	2400	2600–2800	3000
	31–50	2200	2400–2600	2800–3000
	>50	2000	2200–2400	2400–2800

classifications of CHO including: monosaccharides (i.e., glucose and fructose), disaccharides (i.e., sucrose and lactose), and polysaccharides (i.e., glycogen and starch). Upon consumption of any CHO, the body will digest it into glucose for the most part, which is then taken up by the cells and used to produce ATP (Houston 2006). A detailed look at carbohydrates will be addressed later in Chapter 7.

The glucose molecule cannot freely enter through the cell membrane but requires a protein transporter to carry it across in most cases. In larger tissues, such as skeletal muscle and fat, glucose transporters (GLUT) are necessary. There are fourteen main isoforms, GLUT-1–14, which are thrown into three subclasses based on their primary sequences. The main isoforms related to glucose homeostasis include GLUT-1, -2, and -4 (Augustin 2010). GLUT-1 helps transport glucose across the blood-brain barrier (Brockmann 2009). GLUT-2 acts as a sensor for beta-cells in the pancreas, thus important in glucose-induced insulin secretion (Thorens 2001). Finally, GLUT-4 is of particular importance in skeletal muscle and is regulated by insulin levels. It acts as the rate-limiting step in insulin-regulated glucose uptake in skeletal and heart muscle, as well as adipose tissue (Huang and Czech 2007). Aside from insulin, skeletal muscle is also able to increase glucose uptake with exercise, which can also stimulate GLUT-4 receptors (Houston 2006).

Upon entering the cell, the fate of glucose is to be metabolized into ATP for energy. There are a number of detailed metabolic processes involved in the conversion of glucose to ATP via glycolysis, but an explanation of these processes is beyond the scope of this chapter. However, to provide an overview: glycolysis converts glucose to pyruvate, which is then converted to acetyl coenzyme A, which travels on to the citric acid cycle to ultimately produce ATP (Houston 2006). During exercise, a portion of this glucose can also be converted into lactate, especially if the intensity of the activity is increased.

As previously mentioned, exercise can play a role in glucose uptake that is independent of insulin. This is achieved primarily in two ways: first, exercise can increase GLUT-4 transporters in the sarcolemma, and second, exercise activates adenosine monophosphate-activated protein kinase (AMP-K). These mechanisms are not only active during the activity but may also continue for up to several hours afterwards. It is beneficial to have insulin-independent mechanisms for glucose uptake because exercise leads to a lower blood insulin concentration; therefore other methods are required to maintain uptake for activity.

Recently, the Institute of Medicine established acceptable macronutrient distribution ranges (AMDRs), which allow for some flexibility compared with the previous recommended dietary allowance (RDA) values developed in the 1990s. The ADMR for carbohydrate is 45%–65% of the total daily energy (Institute of Medicine 2005) for healthy individuals. Carbohydrates are especially important for active individuals because stored muscle glycogen provides a great amount of energy during anaerobic and aerobic exercise. Therefore, the majority of the daily calories, 55%–60%, should come from carbohydrate sources such as starches, grains, fruits, and vegetables (McArdle et al. 2001). Studies have shown that stored glycogen levels deplete during training, especially in endurance athletes, even when they are consuming 40%–60% carbohydrates in their diet. Therefore, it has been concluded that because glycogen synthesis rates depend on carbohydrate intake, athletes or individuals involved in intense training should consume closer to 10 g/kg/day to maintain muscle mass and glycogen stores (Brouns et al. 1989; Costill and Miller 1980; McArdle et al. 2001).

2.3.1.2 Fat Needs for Healthy Active Individuals

Fats (i.e., lipids) are a crucial fuel source during all activity, especially at lower intensities and longer durations. Lipids are stored in the body as triglycerides (i.e., triacylglycerols) in fat cells or adipose tissue. There are four major classifications of lipids with different roles in the body and chemical structures. These include: fatty acids, triacylglycerols (TAG), phospholipids, and sterols. In terms of fuel for activity, the main lipids involved are fatty acids and TAG (Houston 2006).

The average healthy adult is capable of storing between 2000 and 3000 calories of energy as glycogen in the liver and in skeletal muscles. Compare this number with the over 75,000 calories of energy that is stored as TAG molecules in adipose tissue. For example, an 80-kg male with a body fat percentage of 15% has approximately 92,400 calories of energy stored as fat. Upon consumption of fats in a meal, the lipids are digested into individual fatty acids, and if they are not required for immediate use as energy, they are stored as TAG molecules through a series of steps (Houston 2006).

When energy is required of fats, the process of lipolysis is initiated to break down a TAG molecule into a glycerol and three fatty-acid molecules. In order for energy to be pulled from fatty acids, they must first enter the cell from the blood and ultimately get transported into the matrix of the mitochondrion. Once there, the fatty acids are broken down through a process called beta-oxidation. For long-chain fatty acids, this mainly occurs in the skeletal muscle, and each cycle of beta-oxidation shortens the fatty acid by two carbons and produces one acetyl coenzyme A molecule that proceeds to the citric acid cycle to ultimately convert into ATP (Houston 2006). Again, the details of this process are beyond the scope of this chapter and will be discussed in a subsequent chapter.

The standard for fat intake is not as established as the other macronutrients. Instead, the recommendation is that lipid consumption should be no greater than 30% of the daily caloric intake, of which 70% should come from unsaturated fat sources (McArdle et al. 2001). Unsaturated fats include both polyunsaturated and monounsaturated fats. These are mainly found in plant sources such as nuts, vegetable oils, and olive oil (http://www.AHA.org), and some are associated with health-promoting benefits. Saturated fats should be minimal in the diet because they do not provide as sound a nutritional impact and have negative effects on overall health in the body. Saturated fats are mainly found in animal products and can lead to an increase in low-density lipoprotein cholesterol, which can increase an individual's risk of heart disease. Examples of these food sources include beef fat and dairy products made from whole or 2% milk. The AMDR for total fat is 20%–35% of the total daily energy intake (Institute of Medicine 2005).

It is important for active individuals to meet recommendations for the essential fatty acids, which are those that must be ingested through the diet and are necessary for optimal health and biological function. The two identified essential fatty acids are α-linolenic acid and linoleic acid. The RDAs for linoleic acid for males and females are 17 and 12 g/day, respectively. For α-linolenic acid, the RDA values are 1.6 and 1.1 g/day for males and females, respectively (Cialdella-Kam 2009).

2.3.1.3 Protein Needs for Healthy Active Individuals

Protein consumed in the diet is initially broken down into amino acids that are subsequently absorbed into the bloodstream. These amino acids make up the amino acid pool that is used to create cell proteins based on the various needs of the body, which is a constant process affected by multiple factors. Metabolism of amino acids mainly occurs in the liver and kidney. The liver (and to a smaller extent, the kidney) is also responsible for the synthesis of the nonessential amino acids. The bulk of amino acids found in the body are found in skeletal muscle; however, not much is metabolized there (Houston 2006).

The body is not capable of synthesizing all necessary amino acids; therefore, some must be obtained from the diet (i.e., essential amino acids). Approximately 2%–5% of the daily energy expenditure is from amino acids. Because the body is not able to store amino acids like CHO or fats, any amino acids not used for protein synthesis or other products are used for fuel. This can be done with the conversion into glucose or lipids to be used directly or stored in adipose tissue. The detailed metabolism of amino acids will be discussed in a later chapter. In brief, however, the amino group must first be removed, which will result in just a carbon skeleton that can be oxidized or used to produce glucose or fats, as previously mentioned. Most of the nitrogen from the amino group is excreted from the body (Houston 2006), and the level of excretion typically matches the protein intake of an individual.

The RDA for protein intake in adults is currently set at 0.8 g/kg of body weight/day (Institute of Medicine 2005; Phillips 2006). This level was determined as the amount needed to cover the basal loss of nitrogen for an individual and is appropriate for approximately 97.5% of the population (Institute of Medicine 2005). There is no tolerable upper limit established for protein intake, thus implying that there is no maximum amount of protein intake for healthy individuals. However, for those with some pre-existing health disorders, namely renal conditions, high protein intake is not recommended (Zello 2006). The AMDR for protein is 10%–35% of the total daily energy intake (Institute of Medicine 2005).

Protein requirements are greater for individuals who are physically active, especially strength- and endurance-trained athletes. Because protein is not used for energy during normal conditions, the need for increased protein intake is mainly due to the greater need for protein synthesis to build new muscle as well as repair muscle damage associated with exercise (Lamont et al. 1999, 2001; McKenzie et al. 2000; Phillips et al. 1993). Although the RDA is sufficient for most sedentary and active individuals, athletes average a daily protein intake of between 1.2 and 1.8 g/kg (McArdle et al. 2001). The International Society of Sports Nutrition position on protein intake indicates that a range of 1.4 and 2.0 g/kg/day is safe and effective for healthy active individuals to improve training adaptations. They also stress the importance of the timing of protein intake for active individuals to enhance variables such as recovery, immune function, and muscle growth and maintenance (Campbell et al. 2001). Protein can be found in several forms in the diet in sources from animal products to soy.

A study by Tarnopolsky et al. (1992) showed that whole-body protein synthesis was reduced in strength athletes consuming a low-protein diet (0.86 g/kg/day) compared with medium-protein (1.4 g/kg/day) and high-protein (2.4 g/kg/day) diets. The low-protein diet corresponds to the current recommendations for a healthy adult; however, in the strength-athlete population, it was not sufficient to allow for adequate rates of protein synthesis. Tarnopolsky et al. concluded that individuals involved in strength training require more protein than inactive counterparts. These requirements are also greater than the recommended daily protein intake for healthy males in the United States (Tarnopolsky et al. 1992).

2.4 HEALTHY SEDENTARY INDIVIDUALS

The standards for defining sedentary are somewhat vague and rely on the definition and interpretation of what is considered physically active. There are several organizations that provide information and definitions of physical activity, one of which being the ACSM. According to the ACSM, an individual is considered sedentary if they do not meet the requirements for physical activity. Thus, if an individual does not exercise at a moderate intensity for at least 150 minutes a week, they are considered sedentary (American College of Sports Medicine, American Dietetic Association, Dietitians of Canada 2009). A sedentary lifestyle is also a modifiable risk factor for cardiovascular disease.

2.4.1 CALORIC NEEDS

The caloric needs for sedentary individuals are primarily for weight maintenance or loss, depending on the personalized goals. The calories consumed on a daily basis are used for proper function of the body and organs because a sedentary individual is not in need of calories or energy for any physical activity. As seen in Table 2.4, a sedentary healthy adult should consume between 2000 and 2400 calories daily depending on the gender, with males being on the higher end of the range. When excess calories are consumed, they result in weight gain, which can lead to possible health complications. The macronutrient distribution for these calories may not differ much from their active counterparts.

2.4.1.1 Carbohydrate Needs for Healthy Sedentary Individuals

The CHO range is similar in sedentary individuals; however, the overall caloric intake should be lower. Most sedentary individuals should stay on the lower end of the range (45%–65% daily caloric intake) because they do not require as much energy for activity, and excess CHO (especially glucose) can lead to health complications over time and is the basis for the development of type 2 diabetes.

For sedentary individuals, the role of CHO is slightly different. CHO primarily serves as an energy source; however, when glycogen stores are maximized (as seen in sedentary individuals not needing energy for activity), excess CHO is converted to fat and stored in adipose tissue. Glucose is also the primary fuel source for nerve tissue and the brain, but these needs are easily met through a diet that is approximately 45% carbohydrates. Thus, even though CHO is not needed for any exercise, sedentary individuals still need to maintain adequate CHO levels in the diet to maintain central nervous system function (McArdle et al. 2001).

2.4.1.2 Fat Needs for Healthy Sedentary Individuals

Fat recommendations for active individuals are not much different than for inactive counterparts. As seen in Table 2.5, there is no established RDA; however, the AMDR suggests a fat intake of between 20% and 35% of the total daily caloric intake. Of this, only about 10% of these calories from fat should come from saturated fat sources (McArdle et al. 2001). Most health organizations suggest a fat intake below 30% (American Heart Association, http://www.americanheart.org) or even below 20% (American Cancer Society, http://www.cancer.org). There are also limitations set on cholesterol intake. The American Heart Association recommends less than 300 mg/day, with lower intakes being more optimal (Williams et al. 1980).

2.4.1.3 Protein Needs for Healthy Sedentary Individuals

A healthy sedentary individual should still maintain a protein intake in accordance with the RDA, which as mentioned previously is set at 0.8 g/kg of body weight/day. The RDA for protein is adjusted slightly depending on age. It is recommended that infants and growing children get as much as 2–4 g/kg of body weight/day of protein.

TABLE 2.5
Generalized Macronutrient Recommendations for Healthy Adults

		Carbohydrate	Fat	Protein
Inactive adults	RDA	130 g/day	No RDA	0.8 g/kg/day
	AMDR	45%–65%	20%–35%	10%–35%
Active adults	Current recommendations	55%–60%	20%–35%	1.2–1.4 g/kg/day

Pregnant and nursing women should also have slightly increased protein intakes but not to the extent of young children. In general, the protein requirement decreases as individuals age, although daily intake should not (McArdle et al. 2001).

The main need for this protein in a healthy sedentary individual is to maintain muscle mass and cell function because protein is used to repair and maintain cell integrity and function. This need of dietary protein for normal growth and repair is essential, even when an individual chooses a sedentary lifestyle. Aside from skeletal muscle, amino acids are also used to produce products for healthy cell function such as: hormones (i.e., serotonin, adrenaline, and noradrenaline), nucleotides, glutathione, creatine, and heme groups (Houston 2006).

2.5 BASIC DIFFERENCES ACROSS AGE GROUPS

Dietary recommendations change with age because of different issues that arise for various age groups. Some issues related to aging include: a greater prevalence of disease, decreased physical activity, and altered body composition in the direction of an increase in body fat, decrease in muscle or lean mass, and decrease in bone density (especially in women). The increase in fat mass associated with age is different than general obesity in that this increase is usually in the form of intra-abdominal fat. This fat type is more greatly linked to metabolic changes (i.e., insulin resistance and type 2 diabetes) and cardiovascular disease and thus is a general health concern for these individuals.

Fat-free mass decreases associated with age are primarily due to the progressive loss of muscle mass that occurs as we age, also referred to as sarcopenia. This can result in decreased muscle strength and performance. Muscle strength actually decreases by about 50% between the ages of 50 and 80 years, whereas muscle mass decreases by about 30% (Tseng et al. 1995). It should be noted that participating in resistance training and maintaining a diet that has adequate dietary protein are established means of slowing this loss of muscle mass as we age.

REE decreases with age by approximately 2%–4% a decade beginning at 30 years of age. This rate accelerates at 40 years in men and at 50 years in women. This decrease is mainly due to the decrease in fat-free mass, because there is no concrete evidence of age-related effects on thermogenesis. In addition to a decrease in REE, older individuals are less active, thus decreasing their total energy expenditure (Ritz 2001). The combination of these two factors directly leads to a change in body composition for the negative by increasing the amount of fat mass and decreasing the amount of metabolically active muscle mass.

The protein recommendations are similar for young and elderly healthy adults. There is an added concern of kidney function decline in elderly individuals with greater protein intake, but there is no established upper limit for this population or health outcome. There are also no definite recommendations for fat and CHO intake for older people that are different than those for their younger counterparts. However, it has been shown that elderly individuals oxidize less fat during rest (Arciero et al. 1995; Calles-Escandon and Driscoll 1994; Horber et al. 1996; Melanson et al. 1997; Sial et al. 1996) and rely more heavily on glucose for energy during exercise than fat (Sial et al. 1996). In physically active older individuals, energy-intake goals should be set to avoid weight loss in healthy individuals, especially those involved in resistance training. This can help to offset the sarcopenia effects seen with aging (Ritz 2001).

2.6 CONCLUSIONS

In order to sustain life, the body needs sufficient energy to function as well as to produce biological work. The calories consumed through the major macronutrients in the diet supply the body with this necessary energy and both a deficit and surplus of this energy supplied through the diet can have detrimental effects on both health and performance. The amount of calories needed depends on individual characteristics such as age, gender, body composition, and physical activity. There are several methods to estimate an individual's caloric needs by measuring or calculating energy expenditure and RMR, and this value can be used to assist in proper meal planning to match energy needs through the diet with the current level of energy expenditure.

There are some differences in energy demands between active and sedentary individuals. The primary dietary recommendations in terms of the percentage of total calories for each macronutrient are similar between activity levels with slight differences depending on the intensity of the activity. However, an active individual may need to consume a greater number of both calories and dietary protein to accommodate for their greater energy expenditure to fuel the activities that are not required by their sedentary counterparts. Table 2.5 summarizes the general macronutrient recommendations for healthy inactive and active individuals. This chapter introduced an overview of some of the macronutrient concerns for sedentary and active individuals, not necessarily athletes. Thus, from a training-table perspective, these individuals do not require the same nutritional demands as athletes. The following chapters will detail the three macronutrients plus energy demands for various types of athletes in a more specific fashion.

REFERENCES

American College of Sports Medicine, American Dietetic Association, Dietitians of Canada. 2009. Joint position statement: Nutrition and athletic performance. *Med Sci Sports Exerc* 32: 2130–2145.

Arciero, P. J., A. W. Gardner, J. Calles-Escandon, N. L. Benowitz, and E. T. Poehlman. 1995. Effects of caffeine ingestion on NE kinetics, fat oxidation, and energy expenditure in younger and older men. *Am J Physiol* 268: E1192–E1198.

Augustin, R. 2010. The protein family of glucose transport facilitators: It's not only about glucose after all. *Life* 62: 315–333.

Bouchard, C., R. J. Shephard, and T. Stephens. 1994. *Physical Activity, Fitness and Health: International Proceedings and Consensus Statement.* Champaign, IL: Human Kinetics.

Brockmann, K. 2009. The expanding phenotype of GLUT1-deficiency syndrome. *Brain Dev* 31: 545–552.

Brouns, F., W. H. Saris, J. Stroecken, E. Beckers, R. Thijssen, N. J. Rehrer, and F. tenHoor. 1989. Eating, drinking, and cycling: A controlled Tour de France simulation study, part I. *Int J Sports Med* 10: S32–S40.

Brouns, F., W. H. Saris, J. Stroecken, E. Beckers, R. Thijssen, N. J. Rehrer, and F. tenHoor. 1989. Eating, drinking, and cycling: A controlled Tour de France simulation study, part II. Effect of diet manipulation. *Int J Sports Med* 10: S41–S48.

Calles-Escandon, J., and P. Driscoll. 1994. Free fatty acid metabolism in aerobically fit individuals. *J Appl Physiol* 77: 2374–2379.

Campbell, B., R. Kreider, T. Ziegenfuss, P. La Bounty, M. Roberts, D. Burke, J. Landis, H. Lopez, and J. Antonio. 2001. International Society of Sports Nutrition position stand: Protein and exercise. *J Int Soc Sports Nutr* 4: 8.

Caspersen, C. J., K. E. Powell, and G. M. Christenson. 1985. Physical activity, exercise and physical fitness: Definitions and distinctions for health-related research. *Public Health Rep* 100: 120–131.

Cialdella-Kam, L. 2009. Macronutrient needs of active individuals. *Nutr Today* 44: 104–111.

Costill, D. L., and J. Miller. 1980. Nutrition for endurance sports: Carbohydrate and fluid balance. *Int J Sports Med* 1: 2–14.

Deuster, P. A., S. B. Kyle, P. B. Moser, R. A. Vigersky, A. Singh, and E. B. Schoomaker. 1986. Nutritional intakes and status of highly trained amenorrheic and eumenorrheic women runners. *Fertil Steril* 46: 636–643.

Food and Agricultural Organization/World Health Organization/United Nations University. 1985. Energy and protein requirements. In *Report of a Joint FAO/WHO/UNU Expert Consultation World Health Organization Technical Report Series 724*. Geneva, Switzerland: WHO.

Frankenfield, D., L. Roth-Yousey, and C. Compher. 2005. Comparison of predictive equations for resting metabolic rate in healthy non-obese and obese adults: A systematic review. *J Am Diet Assoc* 105: 775–789.

Genton, L., K. Melzer, and C. Pichard. 2010. Energy and macronutrient requirements for physical fitness in exercising subjects. *Clin Nutr*, 29: 413–423.

Gilliatt-Wimberly, M., M. M. Moore, K. Woolf, P. D. Swan, and S. S. Carroll. 2001. Effects of habitual physical activity on the resting metabolic rates and body compositions of women aged 35 to 50 years. *J Am Diet Assoc* 101: 1181–1188.

Harris, J. A., and F. G. Benedict. 1919. A biometric study of basal metabolism in man. In *Publication no. 279*. Washington DC: Carnegie Institute of Washington.

Haskell, W. L., I. M. Lee, R. R. Pate, K. E. Powell, S. N. Blair, B. A. Franklin, C. A. Macera, G. W. Heath, P. D. Thompson, and A. Bauman. 2007. Physical activity and public health: Updated recommendation for adults from the American College of Sports Medicine and the American Heart Association. *Med Sci Sports Exerc* 39: 1423–1434.

Horber, F. F., S. A. Kohler, K. Lippuner, and P. Jaeger. 1996. Effect of regular physical training on age-associated alteration of body composition in men. *Eur J Clin Invest* 26: 279–285.

Houston, M. E. 2006. *Biochemistry Primer for Exercise Science*. 3rd ed. Champaign, IL: Human Kinetics.

Huang, S., and M. P. Czech. 2007. The GLUT4 glucose transporter. *Cell Metabol* 5: 237–252.

Institute of Medicine. 2005. *Dietary Reference Intakes for energy, carbohydrate, fiber, fat, fatty acids, cholesterol, protein and amino acids*. Washington, DC: National Academies Press.

Kopp-Woodroffe, S. A., M. M. Manore, C. A. Dueck, J. S. Skinner, and K. S. Matt. 1999. Energy and nutrient status of amenorrheic athletes participating in a diet and exercise training intervention program. *Int J Sports Nutr* 9: 70–88.

Lamont, L. S., A. J. McCullough, and S. C. Kalhan. 1999. Comparison of leucine kinetics in endurance-trained and sedentary humans. *J Appl Physiol* 86: 320–325.

Lamont, L.S., A.J. McCullough, and S.C. Kalhan. 2001. Relationship between leucine oxidation and oxygen consumption during steady-state exercise. *Med Sci Sports Exerc* 33: 237–241.

Loucks, A. B., M. Verdun, and E. M. Heath. 1998. Low energy availability, not stress of exercise, alters LH pulsatility in exercising women. *J Appl Physiol* 84: 37–46.

McArdle, W. D., F. I. Katch, and V. L. Katch. 2001. *Exercise Physiology: Energy, Nutrition and Human Performance*, edited by P. Darcy. 5th ed. Baltimore, MD: Lippincott Williams & Wilkins.

McKenzie, S., S. M. Phillips, S. L. Carter, S. Lowther, M. J. Gibala, and M. A. Tarnopolsky. 2000. Endurance exercise training attenuates leucine oxidation and BCOAD activation during exercise in humans. *Am J Physiol Endocrinol Metab* 278: E580–E587.

Melanson, K. J., E. Saltzman, R. R. Russell, and S. B. Roberts. 1997. Fat oxidation in response to four graded energy challenged in younger and older women. *Am J Clin Nutr* 66: 860–866.

Mifflin, M. D., S. T. St. Jeor, L. A. Hill, B. J. Scott, S. A. Daugherty, and Y. O. Koh. 1990. A new predictive equation for resting energy expenditure in healthy individuals. *Am J Clin Nutr* 51: 241–247.

Nieman, D. C. 2003. Physical fitness defined. In *Exercise Testing and Prescription: A Health-Related Approach*. New York, NY: McGraw-Hill.

Otten, J., J. Hellwig, and L. Meyers. 2006. *Dietary Reference Intakes: The Essential Guide to Nutrient Requirements*. Washington DC: The National Academies Press.

Owen, O. E., J. L. Holup, D. A. Dalessio, E. S. Craig, M. Polansky, J. K. Smalley, E. C. Kavle, M. C. Bushman, L. R. Owen, M. A. Mozzoli, Z. Kendrick, and G. H. Boden. 1987. A reappraisal of the caloric requirements of men. *Am J Clin Nutr* 46: 875–885.

Owen, O. E., E. Kavle, R. S. Owen, M. Polansky, S. Caprio, M. A. Mozzoli, Z. V. Kendrick, M. C. Bushman, and G. Boden. 1986. A reappraisal of caloric requirements in healthy women. *Am J Clin Nutr* 44: 1–19.

Phillips, S. M. 2006. Dietary protein for athletes: From requirements to metabolic advantage. *Appl Physiol Nutr Metab* 31: 647–654.

Phillips, S. M., S. A. Atkinson, M. A. Tarnopolsky, and J. D. MacDougall. 1993. Gender differences in leucine kinetics and nitrogen balance in endurance athletes. *J Appl Physiol* 75: 2134–2141.

Ritz, P. 2001. Factors affecting energy and macronutrient requirements in elderly people. *Public Health Nutr* 4: 561–568.

Sial, S., A. R. Coggan, R. Carroll, J. Goodwin, and S. Klein. 1996. Fat and carbohydrate metabolism during exercise in elderly and young subjects. *Am J Physiol* 271: E983–E989.

Tarnopolsky, M. A., S. A. Atkinson, J. D. MacDougall, A. Chesley, S. Phillips, and H. P. Schwarcz. 1992. Evaluation of protein requirements for trained strength athletes. *J Appl Physiol* 73: 1986–1995.

Thorens, B. 2001. GLUT2 in pancreatic and extra-pancreatic gluco-detection (review). *Mol Membr Biol* 18: 265–273.

Tseng, B. S., D. R. Marsh, M. T. Hamilton, and F. W. Booth. 1995. Strength and aerobic training attenuate muscle wasting and improve resistance to the development of disability with aging. *J Gerontol (A Biol Sci Med Sci)* 50: 113–119.

Uauy, R., and E. Diaz. 2005. Consequences of food energy excess and positive energy balance. *Public Health Nutr* 8: 1077–1099.

United States Department of Health and Human Services. 1996. *Physical Activity and Health: A Report of the Surgeon General*. Atlanta, GA: United States Department of Health and Human Services, Centers for Disease Control and Prevention, National Center for Chronic Disease and Prevention and Health Promotion.

United States Department of Health and Human Services and United States Department of Agriculture. 2005. *Dietary Guidelines for Americans*. Washington, DC: United States Department of Health and Human Services.

Williams, O. D., R. L. Mowery, and G. T. Waldman. 1980. Common methods, different populations: The Lipid Research Clinics program prevalence study. *Circulation* 62 (Suppl 4): 18–23.

Zello, G. A. 2006. Dietary reference intakes for the macronutrients and energy: Considerations for physical activity. *Appl Physiol Nutr Metab* 31: 74–79.

3 Energy Demands for Endurance Athletes

Ronald W. Mendel

CONTENTS

3.1 INTRODUCTION

When it comes to sport and athletes, some of the most debatable and lively discussions revolve around questions such as "what makes an activity or event a sport?" or "how do you define an athlete?" Probably the most intriguing part about these discussions is that there is really no one correct answer, but we know it when we see it. Just as difficult to define for most is exercise. Many people have their own sense of what exercise is, just walk into any local gym or recreation facility and observe for a bit. You will undoubtedly see all kinds of people doing all kinds of exercise, but are they really exercising? Some are but some are most definitely not. Exercise is primarily distinguished from physical activity by its overall purpose. Exercise is a planned or structured activity that has the sole purpose of maintaining or increasing physical fitness. Exercise can then be more specifically categorized as primarily aerobic or anaerobic in nature and include areas such as cardiovascular endurance, muscular strength/endurance, or even agility.

The point here is to demonstrate the actual complexity of exercise and to stress the importance of operationally defining or at least being able to correctly identify the type of exercise and/or athlete so that appropriate training methods and nutritional interventions can be employed to enhance performance. This particular discussion does not include the "average Joe" who jogs four or five times per week for health reasons or to stay in shape. Although the metabolic pathways necessary for energy creation and overall macronutrient intake will also be required to fuel the exercise, this chapter will focus on the elite competitors in endurance sports.

3.2   ENDURANCE ATHLETES

A quick search attempting to define the endurance athlete will provide any number of definitions that include a phrase something like an endurance athlete has "a high level of aerobic fitness." Of course, what is meant by "a high level of aerobic fitness" is the ability of the cardiovascular and pulmonary systems to deliver sufficient blood to the working muscles that have the capacity to sustain intense activity for any prolonged period of time. Most often, the term aerobic capacity is used and is commonly described as the body's ability to consume and utilized oxygen. Obviously, the pulmonary, cardiovascular, and muscular systems are all involved. It is also often said that one's aerobic capacity is only as good as the weakest of those three systems.

Elite endurance athletes have been described as those that train or compete between 8 and 40 hours per week (Tarnopolsky et al. 2005). Endurance athletes can be further classified by their particular event or activity. Endurance events are classified as short distance (i.e., 10 km to a marathon), long distance (i.e., triathlon), and ultradistance (i.e., 161-km ultramarathon) events. The critical component to the classification of these events is the time spent in the activity. In other words, it takes less time to run a marathon than it does to complete a triathlon or an ultramarathon. The particular mode of exercise (cycling, swimming, running) will not be considered to any great degree, instead this chapter will focus on the nutritional requirements for these athletes and how they vary depending on the duration/distance involved in a specific event.

As briefly mentioned, these endurance events are generally classified by how long it takes to complete the event. Short-distance endurance events typically last on the order of 1–4 hours and include events such as marathons and sprint triathlons. The first modern marathon was run during the first Olympic Games in Athens in 1896 (Maron and Horvath 1978). Since 1897, the Boston Marathon has probably been the most famous and most attended marathon, certainly in the United States. Sprint triathlons have quickly become very popular and are a reduced version of a full triathlon. Triathlons began sometime in the 1920s in France, and the first modern swim/bike/run event to be called a triathlon was held at Mission Bay, San Diego, California on September 25, 1974. The Mission Bay Triathlon consisted of a 5-mile run, a 5-mile bike ride, and 600-yard swim. The sprint triathlons consist of a 750-m (0.47 mile) swim, 20-km (12.4 mile) bike ride, and 5-km (3.1 mile) run. Many versions exist between the sprint triathlon and the full (Ironman) triathlon including the Olympic triathlon, which is double the distance of "sprint" event. The Ironman triathlon is considered a long-distance endurance event and consists of a 3.86-km (2.4 mile) swim, 180-km (112 mile) bike ride, and 42.2-km (26.2 mile) run taking 8–10 hours to complete for elite level athletes. Finally, the ultimate endurance events include ultramarathons (~100 miles) or adventure races (i.e., Marathon of the Sands). The Marathon of the Sands is a race run in the Moroccan desert spanning 6 days and totaling 156 miles.

Maybe now you have a better sense of what a true endurance athlete might do. If the times and distances do not have your attention yet, what about the caloric intakes of these athletes? It should be obvious that the different events (short, long, and/or ultradistance events) will require unique amounts of caloric intake, and of course caloric expenditure will vary between events. Marathoners typically expend 2500–4000 kcal during the event, whereas Ironman triathletes expend some 8,000–11,000 kcal. In order to complete these physically demanding sports, the athletes should consume at least 35%–55% of the calories that are expended. For example, if a triathlete expends 9000 kcal, they should aim to consume 3150–4950 kcal during the race.

Many consume the calories primarily during the bike ride because it is more easily done in the saddle. Besides fluid intake, carbohydrates and protein make up the bulk of calories and are consumed in a variety of ways depending on the personal preference of an athlete. These are obviously special people who spend a great deal of time training. In fact, sometimes they spend more time training than they do in their event, especially the shorter distance events. In any case, these are the people we have designated endurance athletes, and these are the events that we are considering to be endurance events.

3.3 ENERGY SYSTEMS

It has often been said that when we train, we train energy systems. The type of training performed will directly impact which energy system will be most affected and therefore dictate what adaptations will occur and how much better performance will become. Adenosine triphosphate (ATP) is the energy currency of the cell and, when broken down, yields energy for muscular work. Three basic energy systems exist to provide ATP for skeletal muscle: the phosphagen system (immediate), glycolysis (short term), and the oxidative system (long term). The energy systems are generally referred to as either aerobic or anaerobic with the aerobic energy systems requiring the presence of oxygen to function, whereas the anaerobic systems do not require the presence of oxygen. Obviously, endurance events require the presence of oxygen, so the oxidative system will be of primary importance.

3.3.1 IMMEDIATE ENERGY SYSTEM

The phosphagen system (ATP-PC system) and first part of glycolysis (fast glycolysis) do not require oxygen and occur in the sarcoplasm of the skeletal muscle cell. Carbohydrates (CHO) are the only macronutrients to be metabolized without directly involving the presence of oxygen and are therefore essential and critical to anaerobic metabolism. It is important to understand that all three energy systems are in flux or active at all times. It is more a matter of which is primary or has a greater magnitude of contribution and is principally determined by the intensity and duration of the activity. The phosphagen system provides ATP for any immediate energy needs of the body along with high intensity activities lasting seconds (i.e., 8–12 seconds). The primary role of the phosphagen system is to rapidly replenish ATP to maintain the body's limited ATP stores during the onset of exercise.

Remember, both aerobic and anaerobic processes are going on at the same time, all the time. Anaerobic energy production is more rapidly available than aerobic energy. Athletes, even endurance athletes, rely heavily on anaerobic processes at the beginning of any bout of exercise (Figure 3.1) and during higher-intensity segments such as the final kick of a race (Figure 3.2). The phosphagen system is the primary anaerobic component at the beginning of any training bout or race. Ultimately, the reliance on the phosphagen system is dependent upon how well trained the aerobic system actually is. A more well-trained aerobic system will rely less on the immediate energy supplied by the phosphagen system. The phosphagen system's capacity is very short, so only a few to several seconds of this anaerobic energy production will

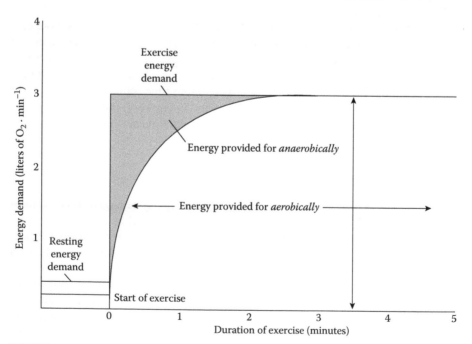

FIGURE 3.1   Onset of exercise. (Adapted from Foran, B., ed. 2001. *High-performance sports conditioning*. Champaign, IL: Human Kinetics.)

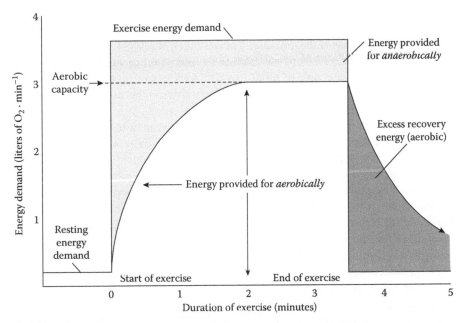

FIGURE 3.2 Anaerobic energy above aerobic capacity for the "final kick." (Adapted from Foran, B., ed. 2001. *High-performance sports conditioning.* Champaign, IL: Human Kinetics.).

come from the phosphagen system, with the remainder being supplied by the fast glycolytic energy system as the endurance athlete transitions to their more trained aerobic pathways.

3.3.2 Glycolytic Energy System

Glycolysis is simply the breakdown of carbohydrates (i.e., glucose) to generate ATP. The carbohydrate can either come from glycogen (stored CHO in muscle) or be taken from blood glucose to supply substrates for glycolysis. The end product of glycolysis is pyruvate, and this is the point whereby glycolysis becomes differentiated into fast or slow glycolysis and can be considered anaerobic or aerobic, respectively. Pyruvate can either be reduced to lactate (fast glycolysis—anaerobic) or shuttled into the mitochondria (slow glycolysis—aerobic) for further oxidation in the Krebs cycle after it is converted to acetyl coenzyme A (CoA). Higher-intensity exercise will require a faster rate of ATP resynthesis, so pyruvate will predominantly be reduced to lactate. Although this results in faster ATP resynthesis, it has limited duration because of the accumulation of H^+ ions that are produced during the production of lactate. The mechanisms of fatigue are beyond the scope of this chapter, but the accumulation of these products in the cell can have detrimental effects on overall functioning as levels increase during high-intensity exercise.

The point at which lactate clearance cannot keep pace with lactate production is known as the "lactate threshold." The intensity of activity, running speed for example, is the primary determinant of the lactate threshold and can be moved to a higher intensity (speed) with proper training. Marathoners typically run the majority of the race just below threshold intensity, which can be measured by lactate levels. In fact, if a marathoner were to have lactate measured during a race, it would probably be just slightly higher than if the measurement was taken at rest (~1 mmol/L). However, if the same lactate measurement was taken at the end of a race where the marathoner had "sprinted" the last couple of miles in a final kick to overtake an opponent, very high levels of lactate would be present in the bloodstream because of the increased utilization of carbohydrate in anaerobic glycolysis.

Slow glycolysis occurs when pyruvate is shuttled to the mitochondria and enters the Krebs cycle for ATP resynthesis. A quick review of basic metabolism reminds us that a majority of the ATP actually occurs from the reducing equivalents, nicotinamide adenine dinucleotide (NADH) and flavin adenine dinucleotide ($FADH_2$). These reducing equivalents are produced in glycolysis (when pyruvate is the product) and the Krebs cycle, with the majority produced in the Krebs. These reducing agents then enter the electron transport chain, which strips them of their electrons as they move down the chain. Oxygen accepts the final electron for the production of ATP through oxidative mechanisms. $NADH^+H$ produces approximately three ATPs and $FADH_2$ produces approximately two ATPs during oxidative phosphorylation.

This in actuality is how the majority of ATP is synthesized, not through direct synthesis of ATP via substrate-level phosphorylation. This occurs at a much slower rate but is maintained for a longer duration provided the intensity is low enough. Ultimately, the rate of metabolism is determined by the energy needs of the body, and glycolysis is no exception. If the energy (ATP) needs are high and oxygen consumption is unable to keep pace, pyruvate undergoes fast glycolysis; if the energy needs are lower and oxygen is able to be used for ATP generation, pyruvate proceeds through slow glycolysis. From this standpoint alone, proper carbohydrate intake is extremely important for optimal performance.

3.3.3 OXIDATIVE ENERGY SYSTEM

The oxidative system (long term) is the aerobic energy system that is responsible for ATP resynthesis at rest and during low- to moderate-intensity activities. Fats and carbohydrates are the primary macronutrients that supply this system, with a greater percentage provided by fat during periods of rest and throughout the day to fuel normal daily activities. As intensity of activity or exercise increases, the contribution from fat decreases while the reliance on carbohydrates increases. At maximal intensity, there is almost 100% reliance on carbohydrates as the fuel, thus favoring an anaerobic production of ATP. Through aerobic training and subsequent adaptations, the oxidative system becomes more efficient (increased ability to resynthesize ATP) in metabolizing fats at higher intensities, thereby decreasing the reliance on carbohydrate utilization and prolonging one's ability to exercise.

Fats (triglycerides) are broken down in adipose tissue into free fatty acids and transported to the working skeletal muscle cells. Additionally, free fatty acids can also be derived from intramuscular triglycerides during exercise. Regardless of the origin, free fatty acids then must go through beta-oxidation, which is a series of reactions that reduces the fatty-acid chain to smaller two-carbon fragments, resulting in the formation of acetyl-CoA. Acetyl-CoA enters the Krebs cycle, and ATP is resynthesized in the same fashion as it was from pyruvate that originated from carbohydrate. Remember, the contribution of ATP production is never derived from one energy system at any given time but relies on a constant demand of all three macronutrients, although fats and carbohydrates are the primary sources.

All three energy systems are on a continuum providing energy as directed by the energy demands of the body. The contribution of each energy system is driven by the intensity and duration of the activity to meet those needs. Immediate energy needs along with higher-intensity/shorter-duration activities are fueled by the phosphagen and fast glycolytic systems. As the intensity of activity decreases and the duration increases, oxygen is readily available to allow the oxidative system to supply the majority of the ATP needed to fuel exercise. The presence of oxygen is absolutely critical to the oxidation of fats, both during rest and exercise. The capacity of the oxidative system should be obvious as it predominates at rest but is also controlled by the intensity of activity. Only through proper training can we increase its ability to supply ATP at faster rates (higher intensity exercise). This increase in the oxidative capacity ultimately leads to the more efficient utilization and reliance on fat to fuel the exercise and reduce the reliance on carbohydrates. It has been well established that this carbohydrate (i.e., glycogen) sparing effect leads to improved performance in endurance events such as marathons, triathlons, and ultraendurance events.

Endurance and ultraendurance events ultimately rely on the oxidative relationship between carbohydrate utilization and fat metabolism. The previous section gave a brief overview of the individual energy systems and how they function, the time frame of when they predominate, and the capacity of each system to provide energy in the form of ATP. The following section will review the oxidative relationship of carbohydrates and fat and focus on their interaction because rarely, if ever, does the oxidation of these fuels occur in isolation, especially during endurance exercise.

3.4   ENERGY FOR ENDURANCE EXERCISE

Athletes are probably one of a few groups that actually understand the importance of eating, or at least one hopes they do. For the most part, people eat because they are hungry, bored, have a meeting, or "it's that time of the day." In actuality, eating is nothing more than an indirect way for humans to obtain macro- and micronutrients for bodily processes that provide for our survival and provide energy for physical work (i.e., skeletal muscle contraction). The approach presented here will not try to manipulate an athlete's diet for better performance, per se, but rather will provide information on and a rationale for eating to support training and competition.

The mindset of an endurance athlete should not focus on what to eat the morning before a race but should be set from a training-table approach that addresses the daily meals, snacks, and recovery formulations to fuel training to ensure that an athlete is adapting at an optimal rate. It might be a matter of semantics, but athletes should give this some thought and see whether it makes sense. Proper energy intake will allow for consistent and effective training while also helping in the process of recovering quickly, thus leading to optimal adaptations over the course of time. Appropriate and healthy eating, combined with proper training, will also help avoid losing days to injury and illness (Table 3.1).

TABLE 3.1

Caloric Expenditure during Exercise

Mode of Exercise	kcal/minute/kg of body weight
Swim	0.13–0.16
Bike	0.15–0.17
Run	0.10–0.20

Example: A 154-pound (70 kg) athlete that participates in a hard swim for 45 minutes would expend 504 calories: 0.16 (kcal) × 70 (kg) × 45 (minutes) = 504.

It is known that both carbohydrates and fat are used during rest and exercise in a reciprocal type fashion, and many factors (specifically exercise duration and intensity) influence the relative proportions of fat and carbohydrate use during exercise. At the initial onset of exercise, there is a transient drop in plasma-free fatty acid concentration because of the increased uptake by skeletal muscle. The plasma-free fatty acid concentration eventually increases as triacylglycerol breakdown (lipolysis) increases from the adipocytes and intramuscular triglyceride stores. As exercise intensity (as a greater percentage of aerobic capacity) increases from light to moderate, free fatty acid (fat) oxidation is the major energy source. With moderate-intensity exercise, there is an approximately equal contribution of ATP production from fat and carbohydrate fuel sources. As intensity of exercise continues to increase, a point is eventually reached whereby carbohydrate oxidation exceeds that of fat oxidation. This is known as the crossover effect. Once this threshold is crossed, the activity or exercise becomes progressively anaerobic in nature, and exercise capacity becomes reduced if the intensity continues to increase because of the limited carbohydrate stores and eventual depletion of these stores. This depletion of carbohydrate stores can be addressed with proper dietary intake before, during, and after exercise and will be discussed in greater detail later in the chapter. Even when exercise intensity is moderate in nature, but the duration exceeds an hour, a greater supply of energy is provided by fat metabolism through depletion of stored carbohydrates. This situation obviously sets up the need for consumption of carbohydrates during training or competition that exceeds 60 minutes in duration.

Many positive and critical adaptations occur from aerobic exercise training, but perhaps none is as important as the enhanced capacity for fat oxidation during endurance exercise. This enhanced capacity for fat oxidation provides for a reduced reliance on carbohydrate stores during prolonged submaximal exercise at a higher intensity. This, in effect, spares carbohydrate stores, thereby delaying fatigue or the subsequent reduction in intensity that accompanies carbohydrate depletion and potentially ketosis. The maximal rate of energy production via fat oxidation increases with aerobic training, which translates into higher endurance capacity at a given exercise intensity.

Other adaptations that occur in and around skeletal muscle from aerobic training include improved blood supply to the muscle cells via increased capillary density and hemoglobin concentration. This is important for increased blood supply to working muscle and allows for increased oxygen and nutrient delivery along with increased removal of carbon dioxide and other waste products. There is also an increase in the number and size of mitochondria, as well as an increased number of oxidative enzymes that regulate these metabolic pathways. The mitochondrial adaptation is of significance because all oxidative pathways occur in the mitochondria of a cell, and additionally a final step of fat metabolism (i.e. beta-oxidation) occurs in the matrix of the mitochondria. Finally, aerobic adaptations include an increase in lactate threshold so that lactate accumulation does not exceed lactate production until later in exercise. This scenario contributes to fatigue and inhibits the body's ability to burn fat, which increases the rate at which glycogen is broken down. In the end, all of these adaptations help the athlete become more efficient in using fat as the primary fuel source during exercise, thereby delaying depletion of muscle glycogen and the accompanying fatigue or reduction in performance and increasing the endurance capacity of an athlete.

3.5 GENERAL MACRONUTRIENT RECOMMENDATIONS

Dietary reference intakes (DRIs) represent a new and more comprehensive approach for nutritional recommendations for people. The DRI has become an umbrella term that encompasses specific recommendations including the recommended dietary allowance (RDA), estimated average requirement, adequate intakes, and upper tolerable intake levels. Most are familiar with the RDAs, which represent the average daily food intake that sufficiently meets all the nutrient requirements of approximately 97%–98% of all healthy individuals in a group. The RDA represents the goal each individual should strive to attain in their daily diets and includes the six classes of nutrients (carbohydrates, fats, protein, vitamins, minerals, and water), but our focus will primarily examine the macronutrient needs of endurance athletes.

3.5.1 CARBOHYDRATES

The general recommendation for carbohydrate intake for normal people is approximately 40%–55% of total caloric intake, which equates to approximately 300 g for a total of 1200 kcal of energy. Most sports nutritionists recommend a higher-carbohydrate diet for those that are engaged in heavy training and want to optimize performance, and this is particularly true for athletes that participate in marathons, triathlons, and ultraendurance types of races. Recommendations for those individuals suggest carbohydrate intakes up to 65%–70% of total calories consumed. Remember, ingestion of 3150–4950 kcal and potentially more can be expected during an ultraendurance event. This means that carbohydrate consumption will range from 788 to 1238 g. In fact, there is some evidence that ultraendurance athletes will expend ~17,000 kcal during the course of a 24-hour race, of which 9000 kcal come from carbohydrate metabolism. Assuming maximal glycogen storage (2000–2500 kcal), this athlete will consume 7000–7500 kcal of carbohydrates throughout the race (1750–1875 g) (Mendel, unpublished data). It is quite obvious that reduced carbohydrate intake during training or scheduled rest periods is not advisable or recommended for these athletes. Diets that severely restrict carbohydrate intake such as the Atkins diet should be avoided at all costs for athletes engaging in endurance events.

3.5.2 FATS

Recommendations for average people suggest that no more than 30% of total calories be consumed from fats. This further breaks down into <10% from saturated fats, 10% from monounsaturated, and 10% from polyunsaturated sources on a day-to-day basis. In addition, recommendations also focus on weekly servings of fish high in omega-3 fatty acids. Generally speaking, endurance athletes do not have significant difference in fat intake compared with normal people. Data on fat loading for ergogenic effects has been equivocal at best. Horvath (2000) examined male and female runners consuming diets of 16% and 31% fat for 4 weeks. The results showed a decreased endurance run in the lower fat group compared to the higher fat. Brown and Cox (2000) showed no ergogenic effect in endurance-trained cyclists over a period of 12 weeks when subjects consumed a high-fat (47% of total calories) compared to a high-carbohydrate diet (69% of total energy). Although no conclusive data exist for fat consumption in endurance athletes, at worst, no ergogenic effect exists. There is no evidence to suggest a decrease in performance with a higher fat intake. The key recommendation is to make sure to ingest fats normally (no less than 20%) with the focus of keeping saturated fats to a minimum.

3.5.3 PROTEIN

The RDA for dietary protein intake for normal people is 0.8 g/kg of body weight. There is much debate over this topic of recommended and optimal levels of protein consumption. Factors such as age, gender, and protein type convolute this topic even further. However, our examination of protein will focus on the needs of those athletes participating in endurance and ultraendurance exercise. Van Erp-Baart et al. (1989) reported that endurance cyclists consumed approximately 3.0 g/kg of body weight/day of protein. This is definitely on the upper end of protein ingestion with a recommended intake of 1.8 g/kg of body weight. This recommendation varies depending on the source; thus a general range for endurance athletes would most likely land between 1.2 and 1.8 g/kg of body weight/day. It seems that endurance training has a protein-sparing effect, i.e., the better trained a person is, the lower the protein breakdown and oxidation during exercise. As training and competition time increase, so does food intake. With increasing food intake, the amount of protein automatically increases because many of the food products consumed by these athletes contain protein (gels, bars, and sports drinks) and provide an exogenous source of amino acids during exercise that can plug into metabolism in several places in the exercising body.

3.6 ENDURANCE EXERCISE

Endurance athletes require different amounts of food and fluid than do recreational athletes and for the most part require more than power or team-sport athletes. Four factors generally make up one's ability for success: genetics, training, nutrition, and recovery. As you can see, three are within one's control, training, nutrition, and recovery, whereas one has no control over genetic makeup. As for the three factors that are within your control, much of your training and even recovery will be dependent upon your daily nutrition (training table), which makes knowing what to eat and when to eat absolutely vital to adaptations to training and subsequent competition performance. In fact, what you eat on a daily basis and how you train are intimately linked to performance. The importance of nutrient intakes and timing is magnified when it involves a high-level to elite athlete, because simple nutritional deficiencies can be the difference in competition. The nutrients (both macro- and micronutrients) and fluids consumed daily provide the fuel necessary for performing. Proper diet can also reduce or inhibit the incidence of a compromised immune system, which leads to illness and even the occurrence or reoccurrence of injuries that impact training and performance. Therefore, whether you are a competitive athlete or one who likes a good challenge, your ability to properly fuel your body for what it needs is a critical component to training, competition, performance, and of course overall health.

3.6.1 Short Range (Sprint)

Shorter-range endurance events are those that last for more than one hour up but only up to three or four hours depending on the athletes' abilities. It is important to distinguish these short-range endurance events from those of longer or ultraendurance status because the nutritional requirements for athletes competing in the different events are quite different. Short range events are performed at a higher intensity than the others and therefore rely more heavily on both the anaerobic and aerobic energy systems. Total energy expenditure during a marathon is approximately 3000 kcal. Typically then, athletes should consume 1000–1500 kcal during the race. Previous discussion of the energy systems reminds us that carbohydrates are critical for higher-intensity exercise and can be used in both the aerobic and anaerobic pathways. The other important consideration is that the training time for these shorter range events is far greater than the actual time spent in competition. Because of this, proper nutrition during training may be slightly different than the nutritional game plan for competition. It may also be that the recreational aspect of the event is more important than the competition or performance, so the training may not be optimal. In that case, one might make the argument that race-day nutrition becomes even more important to get you through the event as well as possible.

3.6.1.1 Pre-event Nutrition

It is imperative to fully maximize carbohydrate stores prior to exercise, especially in shorter sprint-type events. The good news is that an athlete is in complete control of this issue and can maximize their carbohydrate stores through fairly simplistic nutritional guidelines. Approximately 500 g of total carbohydrates are stored as glycogen, of which 400 g are found in skeletal muscle and the remaining 100 g are in the liver in the average well-fed athlete consuming the normal intake of carbohydrates. As mentioned previously, extended fasting (even overnight) or reduced-carbohydrate diets will have a significant impact on glycogen storage. In fact, carbohydrate loading is useful in expanding the amount of carbohydrate that can be stored as glycogen.

A classic method of carbohydrate loading is to increase carbohydrate intake and reduce exercise training volume (i.e., tapering training) 1 week prior to competition. Carbohydrate intake should increase to approximately 75% of total calories while training volume is decreased. The 2 days prior to competition, carbohydrate intake should be about 600–700 g/day. Assuming adequate glycogen storage, events lasting less than 1 hour are not impacted by glycogen depletion; thus a normal well-fed athlete should just focus on approximately 6–8 g/kg of body weight/day. However, higher-intensity events that last longer than 1 hour are definitely impacted by glycogen depletion; thus, 1–2 days prior to the event is an important time for "topping off" the tank in terms of glycogen storage.

No one single precompetition meal exists, and so athletes should experiment with a variety of foods during training. The night or morning before a race is not the right time to try something different, because every individual is different and it is unknown how different athlete's bodies will respond to different food choices and practices. It is natural to tend to ingest a higher amount of carbohydrate-rich foods the day or two before competition, but it is important to understand that you should not overdue it. Remember, this should be a "topping off," not "filling up" time. As for the morning of the event, the simple rule is to eat something and make the majority of those calories from carbohydrates. Your meal should be 2.5–4 hours before your competition, and you should consume 13–14 kcal/kg of body weight, with 70%–80% coming from carbohydrates. It is also important to be self-aware. Athletes vary widely in what they can tolerate and how their bodies respond to different types of food. For example, you do not want to be in the bathroom when the gun sounds because you did not time your meal correctly. Well-tolerated fluids should also be a staple of your pre-event nutrition plan. Water, sports drinks, and even milk, as long as tolerated by the athlete, should be consumed up to 2 hours before the event. This time frame will allow any excess fluid to be excreted as well as to allow adequate digestion and absorption of the prerace meal.

When an athlete is training and competing in events that last more than 60 minutes, a sports drink is certainly your best option for multiple reasons. Not only do sports drinks replace fluids and electrolytes lost via sweating and metabolism, they also provide the body with an ideal concentration and formulation of carbohydrates for fuel. This exogenous carbohydrate will either be used in place of the depleted glycogen stores or be used before tapping into additional glycogen stores, thereby delaying fatigue and providing the opportunity for a race-finishing kick.

Consumption of sports drinks during endurance events should be accompanied by the consumption of gels, energy bars, or even real food to help maintain steady blood-sugar levels throughout an event and provide the body with adequate fuel as the duration of an event increases. For example, a Powerbar gel contains a total of 110 kcal (CHO = 27 g; sodium = 200 mg; potassium = 20 mg; caffeine = 50 mg), and a Gatorade endurance-formula drink contains 100 kcal (CHO = 28 g; sodium = 400 mg; potassium = 180 mg), both of which are optimally formulated for consumption during these types of events.

Again, the most difficult aspect of any type of sports nutrition is making specific recommendations for each individual athlete. Everyone is so different to begin with, but other factors such as age and fitness level are significant as well. In general though, 25–60 g of carbohydrate/hour of activity after the first hour should be consumed. It appears that approximately 60–70 g/hour is the maximal rate that muscle can use, so that is the upper limit to carbohydrate consumption. Obviously, the higher the intensity and the longer the duration, the greater the amount of carbohydrate that should be consumed. Regardless of how much an individual athlete chooses to consume during exercise or a competition, the main goal still should be that the food choices are tolerable to the athlete. Otherwise, no benefit will be received, and performance could actually be compromised.

3.6.1.2   Recovery from Short Range Events

The "window of opportunity" to replenish carbohydrate stores after exercise is relatively small and should begin immediately. Again, consumption of 1 g/kg of body weight within 30 minutes should be the goal. Some people cannot eat solid food during this post-exercise period; thus those athletes should get their carbohydrates and calories for recovery via fluids (i.e., sports drinks). Beyond replenishing your carbohydrate stores, muscle-repair processes need fuel and building blocks (i.e., amino acids) as well; thus the addition of fast-absorbing protein (whey protein) should be consumed as well during the recovery period. Many sports drinks now contain protein if food is not an option. Whatever your choice, consumption of CHO and protein within 30 minutes of exercise cessation is critical to proper recovery and preparation for the next training or event. Further discussion involving post-exercise nutrition is discussed in Chapter 13.

3.6.2   Long Distance (Traditional)

Long-distance endurance events or the more traditional endurance (Ironman) events are those that last 6–12 hours. Obviously proper training is required to make events like this not only possible but maybe even enjoyable. Proper training is only possible with the necessary nutrition for the body to sustain the enormous energy expenditure that accompanies these events. Total energy expenditure during a triathlon can reach 10,000 kcal. Interestingly, recreational runners primarily rely on carbohydrates for the first hour and then fat gradually increases in importance. Elite runners maintain a relatively constant pace at a higher intensity (80%–85% of aerobic capacity).

A good guide is to consume 300–400 kcal/hour of the race with items such as bananas, Powerbars, Gatorade, etc. An interesting component of these events, along with the ultraendurance events, is the need to fuel the body when it does not feel like it needs it. On the other hand, when stomach distress is wreaking havoc, you still need to provide adequate energy and fluid to the system. It should be noted again that not all individuals are the same, and so there is no one single nutritional intervention that will serve everyone the same. There are only guidelines and recommendations that should be experimented with during training in hopes of finding the right formula for you.

As with the shorter events, being well hydrated and well fueled (topped off glycogen stores) is paramount to success in events of longer duration. Pre-event nutritional plans should focus on making sure that total glycogen stores are optimized (approximately 400 g in skeletal muscle and 100 g in the liver) by carbohydrate loading about 1 week prior to competition (see Chapter 13 for a detailed look at carbohydrate loading). Along with carbohydrate loading, increasing fluid intake is also necessary to help with glycogen storage. Because of the length of the event and increased likelihood of prolonged sweating, proper fluid intake prior to the event is warranted, but the consumption of plain water only should be monitored. Hyponatremia is a very common occurrence in long range endurance events and will negatively impact performance. Hyponatremia is a condition of low sodium concentration in the blood. This can occur by ingesting too much plain water thereby diluting the concentration in the blood or by heavy sweating of sodium. Regardless of the mechanism by which hyponatremia occurs, hyponatremia is detrimental to performance and health with extreme cases being life threatening. Thus an increase in salt intake in the days leading up to an event should also be part of the nutritional plan for longer distance endurance athletes to help with delaying and/or hopefully preventing hyponatremia.

Carbohydrate, salt, and fluid should be the major concerns for the pre-event nutritional plan. A high-carbohydrate breakfast should be consumed the morning of the event with the meal occurring 2.5–4 hours before the start time of the event. This window of time will allow your body enough time to digest, absorb, and assimilate the nutrients necessary for the work ahead. Much the same as with the shorter events, a meal before an endurance event should consist of 13–14 kcal/kg of body weight, with 70%–80% coming from carbohydrates. Consume protein at one-quarter of the amount of carbohydrate. In other words, if you consume 100 g of CHO, you should consume approximately 25 g of lean dietary protein. The remainder of the calories should come from fat sources that are naturally present in an athlete's food choices. Hydration is critical and should be ongoing up to 90 minutes prior to the start. Again, this will provide enough time to rid the body of excess fluid. If plain water is the beverage of choice (500 mL) or the only choice, salt tablets might be used to help alleviate the potential for hyponatremia caused by dilution of sodium in the blood. However, an athlete might want to consult with their doctor or maybe more importantly their sport nutritionist to see what approach would be ideal for both performance and health purposes.

Much more extensive research has been conducted on nutritional strategies during longer-distance endurance events and is divided into three components: fluid, fuel, and electrolytes. Fuel and electrolytes generally become used up or lost through the excessive time and effort spent in exercise. As already mentioned, stored carbohydrate accounts for only 2000 calories (500 g), and electrolytes such as sodium and potassium are lost in sweat at high rates during these types of events, especially if environmental conditions are extreme. Fluid consumption becomes critical by helping maintain hydration levels for proper sweat production to keep the body's core temperature in a safe and optimal range while simultaneously providing energy (i.e., carbohydrate) and electrolytes (i.e., sodium, potassium, chloride, etc.) through sports drinks.

Drinking early and often is important in the process. The thirst mechanism is activated by an increase in plasma osmolality caused by a decrease in plasma fluid. Once the thirst mechanism has been activated, dehydration has already occurred, and the athlete will be behind on his recommended fluid intake. Therefore, the recommendation is to ingest 2–8 ounces (60–250 mL) of an electrolyte-carbohydrate solution (sports drink) every 15–20 minutes during prolonged exercise. A variety of factors can alter this need for individual people, so it is critical to be self-aware and monitor such things as body-weight losses during training. Body weight is a simple measure of how much fluid was lost with sweating. One should look to match fluid loss to avoid performance-decremental dehydration. Knowing body-weight losses during prolonged exercise will also help gauge intake needs during exercise (see Chapter 10 for a detailed discussion on fluid-replacement strategies).

Carbohydrate intake recommendations are similar to shorter distance events and call for consumption of 25–60 g/hour after the first hour. Twenty-five g/hour is probably too little, so the aim should be 50–60 g/hour. Trial and error is an important step in determining your specific needs and should only be determined or practiced in training, not competition. An athlete should strive to consume as much carbohydrates as is personally tolerable during their event, and the importance of this grows the longer the event becomes. Electrolyte ingestion should focus on sodium intake. Very rarely will you find a sport drink, gel, or bar formulated for endurance athletes without an appreciable level of sodium. Through proper consumption of these types of nutritional aids during competition, an athlete will typically consume enough sodium unless they are an abnormally heavy sweater. The nutritional plan during a longer-distance event should provide fluid to maintain hydration, provide energy in the form of carbohydrate, and also provide electrolytes (sodium) to prevent hyponatremia.

3.6.3 Ultraendurance

Ultraendurance events are very much all-inclusive activities that take hours and sometimes days to complete (i.e., 50-mile, 100K, 100-mile, and 24-hour runs). Cycling, adventure racing, and hiking and winter-sport adventures should not be left out of the conversation. The major difference between long-distance and ultraendurance events is that ultraendurance events are run at a slower pace with a lot more food consumption (Eberle 2007). Think about it this way: you eat and drink during a normal 24-hour period when the energy demands are relatively low. Imagine not eating or drinking when you are exercising for 15+ hours straight. Ultraendurance events are as much about nutritional awareness and strategy as they are about training. Pre-event nutrition recommendations mimic the shorter and longer distance events and will not be repeated here except for saying that maximal glycogen storage and optimal hydration status is key. Starting in a depleted state in terms of glycogen storage or fluid balance would be magnified early on in these types of events, would definitely limit performance, and would in some cases prevent an athlete from completing such an extreme task.

Nutrition during the ultraendurance event has somewhat of a two-fold approach. It is certainly warranted that the appropriate fuel, electrolyte, and fluid balance be met, but it is also necessary to realize some of the other challenges that are present in extreme events such as these. To begin though, the energy demands of an ultraendurance event are very similar to a longer-distance event, except for the much greater duration that is required in these events. Because of the increased time, intensity is reduced significantly. The general guideline of 50–60 g of CHO/hour remains the goal for an ultraendurance athlete. Because of the extreme duration, the CHO consumption needs to begin immediately and continue until the ultraendurance distance is complete. Athletes can easily expend 400–500 calories per hour during ultra races, and so the ability to replenish the energy is required to maintain a race intensity even though the overall negative energy balance is normal (Eberle 2007).

Carbohydrates are the primary macronutrient for the energy requirements of the ultraendurance athlete. As we know, the limited glycogen stores provide fuel for higher-intensity exercise and can be depleted rather quickly and are nowhere close to the energy requirements that it takes to complete these types of events. However, the sheer amount of time spent running or cycling is absolutely detrimental to the glycogen stores and is more relevant to these ultraendurance events than intensity alone. Therefore, it is essential to regularly provide exogenous carbohydrates to inhibit or delay glycogen depletion as much as possible.

Post-race nutrition is always critical and even more so after ultraendurance events. Not only do you need to refuel the body after the extreme energy expenditure, but repair of the muscular system is important. Protein intake of 1.5–2.0 g/kg of body weight/day is recommended for ultraendurance athletes to help reduce the subsequent muscle damage after a race (Burke and Read 1987; Khoo et al. 1987). Also, micronutrient considerations (zinc, iron, vitamin B_6, and riboflavin) must be addressed and usually are met through the consumption of a balanced diet. The extreme nature of ultraendurance events often affects the digestive system in such a way that "real" food is not always an option (Applegate 1989); thus each athlete should aim to take the nutritional approach that is the most tolerable for that athlete.

3.7   RECOVERY

Recovery is absolutely critical to an endurance athlete's success in both training and competition. It can take a few different forms including fuel replenishment (glycogen resynthesis), work capacity, muscle function, and immune function. Immediate recovery focuses on the "window of opportunity" whereby the rate of glycogen synthesis is optimized if 1.5 g/kg of body weight of carbohydrates are consumed immediately after exercise and at 2-hour intervals thereafter (Ivy et al. 1988). Doyle and Sherman (1991) also found a high rate of glycogen resynthesis by feeding subjects 0.4 g of CHO/kg of body weight every 15 minutes during the 4 hours immediately after exercise. Although some debate exists as to the most optimal amount of carbohydrates consumed immediately post-exercise, there is no debate regarding the 2-hour window of opportunity that follows glycogen-depleting exercise for the greatest rate of glycogen replenishment. As for type of carbohydrates ingested immediately post-exercise, Blom et al. (1987) found glucose to increase the rate of glycogen resynthesis nearly twofold over fructose. Other work has shown that the rate of glycogen resynthesis seems to be independent of the form (i.e., solid versus liquid) of carbohydrates ingested immediately post-exercise (Reed et al. 1989) (see Chapter 13 for a detailed discussion of post-exercise nutrition). Thus eating early and often following all types of endurance exercise is recommended to maximize recovery, regardless of whether it is a 3-hour training session or a competitive event.

We know that muscle glycogen levels are depleted following a marathon, but this is also accompanied by a decrease in muscular strength and work capacity by almost

50% (Sherman et al. 1984). This lowered muscular strength has been shown to still be present up to one week following the event, whereas glycogen levels and work capacity were back to normal. Likewise, Keizer et al. (1987) found that even when muscle glycogen levels returned to normal 24 hours after glycogen-depleting exercise, work capacity was still reduced. Therefore, muscle glycogen recovery is an extremely important consideration in recovery but does not guarantee fully recovered muscle function. The extent of muscle damage that occurs during these types of endurance events must also be considered when replenishing muscle glycogen levels. Furthermore, it has been reported that damage to skeletal muscle can inhibit the uptake of glycogen in the muscle, thus contributing to this hampered ability of the muscle to recover (Costill et al. 1990; Doyle and Sherman 1991; O'Reilly et al. 1987). Thus a combination of tissue damage and reduced glycogen levels are most likely to contribute to the reduced muscle function seen following endurance events and heavy training. This effect highlights not only the importance of proper nutrition from a training-table standpoint but also how a properly structured training regimen allows for ample time for recovery so that long-term training adaptations are not compromised.

Although immediate recovery of glycogen, the ability to work maximally, and optimal muscle function are significant issues in proper recovery from endurance events, immune function cannot be overlooked in endurance athletes because of the nature of long-duration endurance exercise. The incidence of depressed immune function during times of high volume of training has been shown to increase the risk of illness, especially upper respiratory illness (URI) (Gleeson et al. 1995; Peters et al. 1996). The "J" curve (Figure 3.3) models the risk of illness as it relates to exercise volume and intensity (Nieman 1994).

As can be seen, excessive volume of strenuous endurance exercise can suppress immune function leading to an increased risk of illness. This is of significance because this chapter addresses athletes who specifically engage in events that are excessive in volume and strenuous in nature. This "open window" theory suggests that suppression of some of the immune variables make the body more susceptible, which may increase the risk of URI (Pedersen and Bruunsgaard 1995). Up until recently, many exercise immunology studies only examined pre-exercise resting levels and immediately post-exercise levels of various immune variables (Chinda et al. 2003; Gannon et al. 1997; Nieman et al. 2007a), whereas some measured up to 2 hours post-exercise (Henson et al. 2000; Ibfelt et al. 2002; Nieman et al. 2007b) and 24 hours post-exercise (Scharhag et al. 2005). More recently, Kakanis et al. (2010) increased sampling points to include pre-exercise, immediately post-exercise, and 2, 4, 6, 8, and 24 hours post-exercise. Of significance in this study, validation of the open window theory was found by confirming the presence of lower immune cell numbers. In particular, natural killer cell (NK) numbers were found to be depressed significantly at 4, 6, and 8 hours post-exercise compared with pre-exercise levels. NK cells are part of the immune systems' first line of defense. The reduction of NK cells so late following strenuous endurance exercise may have serious implications for multiple training bouts in a day or for ultraendurance competitions whereby the immune system may face chronic suppression of NK cell count and therefore make the athlete more susceptible to illness and potential injury (Topic Box 3.1).

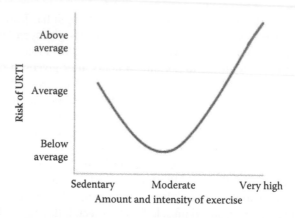

FIGURE 3.3 "J" curve. Relationship between exercise volume and intensity with risk of upper respiratory tract infections. (Adapted from Nieman, D. C. 1994. *Med Sci Sports Exerc* 26: 128–139.)

TOPIC BOX 3.1   NUTRITIONAL SUPPLEMENTS TO ATTENUATE EXERCISE-INDUCED IMMUNOSUPPRESSION

Because endurance athletes are more susceptible to upper respiratory tract infections because of their heavy and constant training, they need to find alternative methods to reducing the incidence of these conditions because reducing training is not an option. Some specific nutritional supplements (vitamin C, glutamine, and carbohydrates) have been tested on the immune response to intense and prolonged exercise.

- **Vitamin C:** 600 mg/day for 3 weeks has been shown to reduce upper respiratory tract infection (Peters, 1996).
- **Glutamine:** Although not a definitive solution, decreased glutamine levels have a direct effect in the reduced proliferation rates of lymphocytes which may impair immunity (Castell, 1997; Rohde, 1996).
- **Carbohydrates:** Probably the most well-established link to immunosuppression, CHO supplementation before, during, and after exhaustive exercise has been associated with higher plasma glucose, reduced cortisol response, and less fluctuation in blood immune cell counts. All of this suggests that reduced physiological stress occurs with CHO ingestion (Nieman, 1998).

3.8   EVERYDAY NUTRITIONAL GUIDE

Whether it is during training or competition, providing adequate fuel to the body for endurance athletes is not just about before, during, and after exercise. Instead, it is about a concerted daily effort to provide the body with the appropriate nutrients in proper amounts. This approach is the basis for the concept of the training table, which achieves to help athletes structure their approach to nutrition on a day-to-day basis (see Chapter 5 for detailed discussion of meal planning). Certainly the DRI is a legitimate jumping-off point, but endurance athletes have special needs, especially the total number of daily calories needed to match, but not exceed, their daily caloric expenditure based on their current training volume.

Elite endurance cyclists, runners, swimmers, and triathletes have reported energy intakes between 22 and 93 calories/kg of body weight/day (Klaas and Saris 1991). On average, these endurance athletes consumed 55 calories/kg of body weight daily, which equates to a 70-kg athlete consuming approximately 3800 calories a day. Most endurance athletes tend to graze, eating multiple small meals and snacks throughout the day rather than eating on the traditional three-meal plan. In general, six food types are essential to provide the energy and nutrients to sustain optimal training and competition for endurance athletes. These food types include fruits, vegetables, grains-legumes, lean meats, low-fat milk products, and fats/sweets (Houtkooper 1992). Of course, what is not included in this list is water. These categories of food types can be found in the food guide provided by the United States Department of Agriculture at www.MyPyramid.gov.

3.8.1 CARBOHYDRATES

All endurance athletes should be consuming quality carbohydrates on a daily basis to supply approximately 60% of total calories daily depending on the current needs of the athlete. If your training consists of 1 hour/day, you should be consuming ~6 g of carbohydrates/kg of body weight. When training 2 hours per day, your carbohydrates intake should equal ~8 g/kg of body weight. Those endurance athletes that train for 3 or more hours daily should consume roughly 10 g of carbohydrates/kg of body weight/day. For example, a 26-year-old 115-pound female triathlete will need to consume 2100 kcal of carbohydrates, whereas a 30-year-old 160-pound male will consume approximately 3000 kcal of energy from carbohydrates to fuel training.

Foundational carbohydrate nutrition begins with whole grains, and endurance athletes should focus on consuming whole-wheat breads, tortillas, bagels, cereals, and even waffles. Whole-wheat pastas along with brown rice and whole-grain crackers are ideal food choices as well. Legumes, fruits, and vegetables are also high-carbohydrate foods that should be a staple of an endurance athlete's diet. Legumes include dried beans and dried peas. Fiber is also important and can be found in apples, bananas, dates, figs, and berries. In general, the athlete should always strive to select fruits and vegetables that are fresh and have not been processed.

3.8.2 PROTEIN

An endurance athlete's protein needs range from 1.0 to 1.7 g/kg of body weight daily (Houtkooper 1992). Sherman and Maglischo (1991) have also indicated that some endurance athletes require even more protein on a daily basis (2.0 g/kg of body weight). Although these recommendations are slightly higher than more current recommendations (1.2–1.4 g/kg of body weight), they are certainly comparable (Kreider et al. 2010; Rodriguez et al. 2009). Higher-protein foods include lean cuts of meat (i.e., beef, chicken, eggs, fish, lamb, and turkey) and low-fat milk products of skim or 1% milk and yogurt. Most energy bars, shakes, and meal-replacement products that are focused on sports nutrition will also contain ample amounts of dietary protein as well. Thus there are a multitude of factors that go into proper food selection to provide the body with the optimal array of protein on a day-to-day basis and establish the basis of a sound training table.

3.8.3 FATS

Fat seems to be consumed on the ends of the quantity spectrum. Athletes either consume too much or too little. Endurance athletes should consume approximately 1 g/kg of body weight daily. Mono- and polyunsaturated fats should be the focus and can be found primarily in fish, nuts, seeds, certain oils, and milk products. Most of an endurance athlete's energy comes from fat oxidation, so too little fat consumption is unwarranted and in some cases has been shown to limit or hamper performance when chronic consumption of dietary fat is less than 20% of total caloric intakes. Also, fat plays an integral role in hormone production, especially testosterone and other androgen hormones. Fat is definitely an important component of an endurance athlete's daily food intake, but overall the focus should be on optimal consumption of these fats without exceeding recommended intakes.

3.9 CONCLUSIONS

Endurance events are generally classified by how long the event takes to complete and can range from short (1–4 hours), long (6–12 hours), to ultra (24+ hours). It is quite obvious that providing enough energy to the body for these events is of primary importance. With that being said, the day of the actual "event" plays only a part small; the role of daily nutrition in regards to the training table is of utmost importance to ensure that the fuel needs for chronic training are optimal, otherwise the actual endurance event suffers in regards to performance. The major metabolic pathway for endurance sports is the oxidative system, which is a very sustainable energy system that can theoretically last forever if the proper fuel sources are continuously supplied at the optimal rate. The major fuel sources that endurance athletes rely on include muscle and liver glycogen, blood glucose, and stored fat (intramuscular and adipose tissue). In order to train and compete successfully, a full understanding of the appropriate nutrients serving as the fuel source is essential for both the athlete and/or the professional that is working with an athlete attempting to optimize performance.

Carbohydrates are the most critical energy source for endurance exercise for several reasons. Because of the body's limited ability to stockpile carbohydrate stores, depletion of stored carbohydrates (muscle and liver glycogen) is the primary cause of fatigue. In other words, approximately 2000 kcal of energy can be stored as carbohydrates, and these stores can be depleted quite easily during long-duration events. It is the depletion of these carbohydrate stores that is one of the primary factors that defines fatigue as inability to maintain exercise intensity. In contrast, athletes will effectively never deplete their fat stores during training or competition because of the gross amount stored even in the leanest of individuals. It is recommended that endurance athletes consume anywhere from 55% to 75% of their total calories as carbohydrates depending on multiple factors, including the training volume of an athlete and whether or not an athlete is in a precompetition phase and is looking to glycogen "load." This corresponds to anywhere from 6 to 10 g of carbohydrates/kg of body weight.

Not only is daily consumption of carbohydrates important, but the consuming of carbohydrates during the event is essential as well, otherwise performance will most definitely suffer. Consumption during the event should be 35%–55% of the energy expended during the event. Pre-event nutrition should focus on "topping off" the glycogen stores, whereas nutrition during the event helps maintain glycogen stores and supply a steady stream of exogenous carbohydrates into the bloodstream to be utilized by the working muscle and other glucose-requiring processes in the body. Post-exercise consumption of carbohydrates is crucial for faster glycogen resynthesis and for overall recovery to prepare the athlete for the next training bout or competition session.

Fats and protein are also an important fuel for endurance athletes on a daily basis. Equivocal data exist in regards to fat loading, but endurance athletes should definitely not reduce their fat intake below 20% of total calories. Protein is also important during exercise; however the contribution as an "energy" source does not compare to that of carbohydrates and fat. When the body is depleted of its carbohydrate stores, intensity of exercise must decrease or a new source of carbohydrates must become available. Protein is quite often the source of new carbohydrate that forms in a process known as gluconeogenesis as the duration of a bout of endurance exercise increases. Most recommendations of protein intake for endurance athletes are 1.2–1.8 g/kg of body weight/day. Some have demonstrated consumptions of 3.0 g/kg of body weight (Van Erp-Baart et al. 1989). Protein consumption immediately following endurance exercise is valuable in decreasing muscle soreness and decreasing further protein breakdown from skeletal muscle.

Proper carbohydrate ingestion should be the primary consideration for endurance athletes while also being mindful of protein and fat intake on a daily basis. Carbohydrates can be used in either aerobic or anaerobic metabolic pathways and are central to an athlete's ability to maintain exercise intensity. It should also be recognized by endurance athletes that proper timing of carbohydrate ingestion can also impact exercise performance, not only before and after exercise but during as well. Athletes have always known the importance of training and recovery to performance, but even the most well-designed training and recovery regimens will fall short if energy supply is inadequate.

REFERENCES

Applegate, E. 1989. Nutritional concerns of the ultraendurance triathlete. *Med Sci Sports Exerc* 21: S205–S208.

Blom, P. C. S., A. T. Hostmark, O. Vaage, K. R. Kardel, and S. Maehlum. 1987. Effect of different post-exercise sugar diets on the rate of muscle glycogen synthesis. *Med Sci Sports Exerc* 19: 491–496.

Brown, R., and C. Cox. 2000. High-fat vs. high-carbohydrate diets: Effect on exercise capacity and performance of endurance trained cyclists. *New Zealand J Sports Med* 28: 55–59.

Burke, L. M., and R. D. Read. 1987. Diet patterns of elite Australian male triathletes. *Physician Sportsmed* 15: 140–155.

Castell, L.M., J.R. Poortmans, R. Leclercq, M. Brasseur, J. Duchateau, and E.A. Newsholme. 1997. Some aspects of the acute phase response after a marathon race, and the effects of glutamine supplementation. *Eur J Appl Physiol* 75: 47–53.

Chinda, D., S. Nakaji, T. Umeda, T. Shimoyama, S. Kurakake, N. Okamura, T. Kumac, and K. Sugawara. 2003. A competitive marathon race decreases neutrophil functions in athletes. *Luminescence* 18: 324–329.

Costill, D. L., D. D. Pascoe, W. J. Fink, R. A. Robergs, and S. I. Barr. 1990. Impaired muscle glycogen resynthesis after eccentric exercise. *J Appl Physiol* 69: 46–50.

Doyle, A. J., and W. Sherman. 1991. Eccentric exercise and glycogen synthesis. *Med Sci Sports Exerc* 23: S98.

Eberle, S. 2007. *Endurance Sports Nutrition.* Champaign, IL: Human Kinetics.

Foran, B., ed. 2001. *High-performance sports conditioning.* Champaign, IL: Human Kinetics.

Gannon, G., S. Rhind, M. Suzui, P. Shek, and R. Shepard. 1997. Exercise-enhanced natural killer cell cytotoxic capacity of peripheral blood is not affected by the opioid antagonist naltrexone. *Med Sci Sports Exerc* 29: 297.

Gleeson, M., W. McDonald, A. Cripps, D. Pyne, R. Clancy, and P. Fricker. 1995. The effect on immunity of long-term intensive training in elite swimmers. *Clin Exper Immunol* 102: 210–216.

Henson, D. A., D. C. Nieman, S. L. Nehlsen-Cannarella, O. R. Fagoaga, M. Shannon, M. R. Bolton, J. M. Davis, C. T. Gaffney, W. J. Kellin, M. D. Austin, M. E. Hjertman, and B. K. Schilling. 2000. Influence of carbohydrate on cytokine and phagocytic responses to 2 h of rowing. *Med Sci Sports Exerc* 32: 1384–1389.

Horvath, P. 2000. The effect of varying dietary fat on performance and metabolism in trained male and female runners. *J Amer Coll Nutr* 19: 52–60.

Houtkooper, L. 1992. Food selection for endurance sports. *Med Sci Sports Exerc* 24: S349–S359.

Ibfelt, T., E. Peterson, H. Bruunsgaard, M. Sandmand, and B. Pedersen. 2002. Exercise-induced change in type 1 cytokin D8+ T cells is related to a decrease in memory T cells. *J Appl Physiol* 93: 645–648.

Ivy, J. L., M. C. Lee, J. T. Broznick, and M. J. Reed. 1988. Muscle glycogen storage after different amounts of carbohydrate ingestion. *J Appl Physiol* 65: 2018–2023.

Kakanis, M. W., J. Peake, E. W. Brenu, M. Simmonds, B. Gray, S. L. Hooper, and S. M. Marshall-Gradisnik. 2010. The open window of susceptibility to infection after acute exercise in healthy young male elite athletes. *Exerc Immunol Rev* 16: 119–137.

Keizer, H. A., H. Kuipers, G. van Kranenburg, and P. Geurten. 1987. Influence of liquid and solid meals on muscle glycogen resynthesis, plasma fuel hormone response, and maximal physiological working capacity. *Int J Sports Med* 8: 99–104.

Khoo, C. S., N. E. Rawson, M. L. Robinson, and R. J. Stevenson. 1987. Nutrient intake and eating habits of triathletes. *Ann Sports Med* 3: 144–150.

Klaas, R. and W. M. H. M. Saris. 1991. Limits of energy turnover in relation to physical performance, achievement of energy balance on a daily basis. *J Sports Sci* 9: 1–15.

Kreider, R. B., C. D. Wilborn, L. Taylor, B. Campbell, A. L. Almada, R. Collins, M. Cooke, C. P. Earnest, M. Greenwood, D. S. Kalman, C. M. Kerksick, S. M. Kleiner, B. Leutholtz, H. Lopez, L. M. Lowery, R. Mendel, A. Smith, M. Spano, R. Wildman, D. S. Willoughby, T. N. Ziegenfuss, and J. Antonio. 2010. ISSN exercise & sport nutrition review: Research and recommendations. *J Inter Society Sports Nutr* 7: 1–43.

Maron, M. B., and S. M. Horvath. 1978. The marathon: A history and review of the literature. *Med Sci Sports Exerc* 10: 137–150.

Nieman, D. C. 1994. Exercise, upper respiratory tract infection and the immune system. *Med Sci Sports Exerc* 26: 128–139.

Nieman, D.C. 1998. Influence of carbohydrate on the immune response to intensive, prolonged exercise. *Exerc Immunol Rev* 4: 64–76.

Nieman, D. C., D. A. Henson, S. J. Gross, D. P. Jenkins, J. M. Davis, E. A. Murphy, M. D. Carmichael, C. L. Dumke, A. C. Utter, S. R. McAnulty, L. S. McAnulty, and E. P. Mayer. 2007a. Quercetin reduces illness but not immune perturbations after intensive exercise. *Med Sci Sports Exerc* 39: 1561–1569.

Nieman, D., D. Henson, G. Gojanovich, J. M. Davis, C. Dumke, A. Utter, A. Murphy, S. Pearce, S. McAnulty, and L. McAnulty. 2007b. Immune changes: 2 h of continuous vs. intermittent cycling. *Inter J Sports Med* 28: 625–630.

O'Reilly, K. P., M. J. Warhol, R. A. Fielding, W. R. Frontera, C. N. Meredity, and W. J. Evans. 1987. Eccentric exercise-induced muscle damage impairs muscle glycogen repletion. *J Appl Physiol* 63: 252–256.

Pedersen, B., and H. Bruunsgaard. 1995. How physical exercise influences the establishment of infection. *Sports Med* 19: 393–400.

Peters, E., J. Goetzsche, L. Joseph, and T. Noakes. 1996. Vitamin C as effective as combinations of anti-oxidant nutrients in reducing symptoms of upper respiratory tract infections in ultramarathon runners. *South African J Sports Med* 11: 23–27.

Reed, M. J., J. T. Broznick, N. C. Lee, and J. L. Ivy. 1989. Muscle glycogen storage postexercise: Effect of mode of carbohydrate administration. *J Appl Physiol* 66: 720–726.

Rohde, T., D.A. MacLean, A. Hartkopp, B.K. Pedersen. 1996. The immune system and serum glutamine during a triathlon. *Eur J Appl Physiol* 74: 428–434.

Rodriguez, N. R., N. M. DiMarco, and S. Langley. 2009. A critical examination of dietary protein requirements, benefits and excesses in athletes. *J Sports Nutr Exerc Metabol* 17. S58–S76.

Scharhag, J., T. Meyer, H. Gabriel, B. Schlick, O. Faude, and W. Kindermann. 2005. Does prolonged cycling of moderate intensity affect immune cell function? *Brit J Sports Med* 39: 171–177.

Sherman, W. M., and F. W. Maglischo. 1991. Minimizing chronic athletic fatigue among swimmers: Special emphasis on nutrition. *Sports Science Exchange* 4(35).

Sherman, W. M., L. E. Armstrong, T. M. Murray, F. C. Hagerman, D. L. Costill, R. C. Staron, and J. L. Ivy. 1984. Effect of a 42.2-km footrace and subsequent rest or exercise on muscular strength and work capacity. *J Appl Physiol* 57: 1668–1673.

Tarnopolsky, M., M. Gibala, A. Jeukendrup, and S. M. Phillips. 2005. Nutritional needs of elite endurance athletes. Part I: Carbohydrate and fluid requirements. *Euro J Sport Sci* 5: 3–14.

Van Erp-Baart, A. M., W. H. Saris, R. A. Binkhorst, J. A. Vos, J. A., and J. W. A. Elvers. 1989. Nationwide survey on nutritional habits in elite athletes. *Inter J Sports Med* 10 (Suppl 1): S3–S10.

4 Energy Demands for Strength–Power Athletes

Chris N. Poole and Colin D. Wilborn

CONTENTS

4.1 INTRODUCTION

The activities and sports that strength–power athletes engage in stress the body's tissues and metabolic systems in a unique manner. Thus, it is vital to understand how these activities stress the body so one has the knowledge to develop and implement nutritional strategies and practices for athletes that will promote optimal performance on a daily basis. This chapter will explain the energy demands of strength–power athletes by discussing: 1) what is unique about strength–power athletes, 2) the energy systems utilized during strength–power activities, 3) macronutrient recommendations and caloric requirements for strength–power athletes, 4) nutrient timing for strength–power athletes, and 5) recovery considerations following exercise. After reading this chapter, the general practitioner should have the competency to provide strength–power athletes with scientifically based nutritional strategies designed for success from a training-table prospective.

4.2   WHAT IS UNIQUE ABOUT STRENGTH–POWER ATHLETES?

The movements executed during strength–power activities vastly differ from those associated with aerobic or endurance-related exercise. To help the reader understand this concept, we will begin by defining what exactly strength and power are and how they relate to this subset of athletes. Strength in the athletic domain refers to the ability to exert force through skeletal muscle on external objects. Examples of exhibiting strength through sport-related movements are performing a bench-press exercise, an offensive lineman blocking a defender, or two basketball players fighting over a loose ball. Most often, strength is thought of as belonging strictly in a weight room; however, all sports, especially strength–power sports, rely heavily upon strength as an aspect of performance.

There are several classifications, or levels, of strength that can be performed by an athlete. Maximal strength is the maximal amount of force that can be exerted on an object through a single effort or attempt. A one-repetition maximal squat or bench-press lift is an ideal example of this type of strength. Endurance strength, or muscular endurance, is the ability to exert a certain amount of force on an object over an extended period of time. Performing the bench-press exercise at the NFL combine (225 lbs as many times as possible in one set before failing) exemplifies this rather well. There are some sports, such as power lifting, that rely primarily on maximal strength. Most strength–power sports and activities are dependent on various combinations of maximal and endurance strength; therefore most strength and conditioning programs focus on improving both of these aspects before in-season competition begins. A football offensive lineman may only have to block for two seconds on one particular play, but the quarterback may require seven seconds of good blocking on the subsequent down to locate an open receiver. Dynamic strength is often referred to as the ability to possess or utilize strength during specific competition movements. Coaches often refer to certain players that are not necessarily "weight-room strong" but are among the strongest out on the field or on the court. In most circumstances, dynamic strength takes precedence over weight-room strength, because in the end, what separates winning and losing is a player's performance on game day, not his off-season maximal lift on the bench-press exercise.

Strength and power are often coupled with one another, even though they contain different properties. Power is defined as the rate at which work is performed and can be calculated by $P = W/T$, where P = power, W = work, and T = time to completion. Thus, power movements are usually described as very quick, explosive bouts, whereas strength-related movements are performed in a much slower fashion. A power lifter will never perform a bench-press lift at the same rate as a basketball player jumps for a rebound. Muscular strength necessitates precision and control, where power compromises strength to gain quickness and explosiveness, which decreases the time needed to perform a given task. It is now clear that an inverse relationship exists between strength and power and that strength–power athletes must find an appropriate balance of both strength and power through extensive training to meet the demands of their respective sporting activities.

4.3 ENERGY SYSTEMS UTILIZED DURING STRENGTH–POWER ACTIVITIES

Before discussing the energy demands of strength–power athletes, it is imperative to understand the functioning of involved energy systems specifically related to these forms of activities. As described in the previous section, strength–power athletes perform single to very brief, intermittent bouts of exercise that are primarily reliant upon muscular strength and power. Consequently, anaerobic energy systems, or energy systems that operate without oxygen being present, will supply the majority of energy in the form of adenosine triphosphate (ATP) to the working muscles during strength–power activities. The phosphocreatine and glycolytic energy systems are able to generate ATP at a rapid rate but for a short duration, resulting in an increase in lactate production and a subsequent decrease in exercise intensity (Karlsson and Saltin 1970) if the exercise bout continues for a prolonged period of time. These energy systems are preferentially used in type II muscle fibers (i.e., type IIa and type IIx fibers), which are characterized by their anaerobic properties (Table 4.1). Type II muscle fibers are neurally activated and recruited during high intensity or anaerobic exercise. As a result of the physiological nature of strength–power activities and their utilized energy systems and muscle-fiber types, it is now easy to comprehend why these athletes must intermittently rest and recover in order to maintain 100% effort during a competition. However, it should be noted that the phosphocreatine and glycolytic energy systems can become more efficient through proper training techniques and nutritional strategies (Greenhaff et al. 1993; Hill et al. 2007), which enables an athlete to sustain a high exercise intensity for a longer period of time.

4.3.1 PHOSPHOCREATINE SYSTEM

The phosphocreatine (PCr) energy system is the initial provider of ATP at the onset of exercise. When an athlete transitions from a standstill to an all-out sprint, PCr generates the necessary ATP at a rapid pace to restore the ATP that is currently being

TABLE 4.1
Muscle Fiber Types and Their Characteristics

Characteristic	Type I	Type IIa	Type IIx
Force production	Low	High	Very high
Power output	Low	High	Very high
Fatigue resistance	High	Moderate	Low
Endurance	High	Moderate	Low
Contraction speed	Slow	Fast	Fast
Fiber diameter	Small	Intermediate	Large

hydrolyzed and degraded to adenosine diphosphate (ADP) and adenosine monophosphate. The PCr reaction is as follows:

$$ADP + CP \leftrightarrow ATP + Creatine$$

ADP accepts an additional phosphate group from a creatine phosphate (CP or PCr) molecule to form ATP and creatine. This is a reversible reaction catabolized by the enzyme creatine kinase. The PCr energy system can generate ATP at a very rapid rate; however, because PCr is stored in low amounts within muscle, it cannot act as the main supplier of ATP for longer duration or continuous activities (Cerretelli et al. 1980). Specifically, the amount of PCr stored within muscle is enough to fuel the body for only a matter of seconds during all-out, high-intensity exercise conditions. When PCr stores within the muscle deplete after this short period of time, exercise intensity will decrease significantly, and an alternate means to acquire more ATP becomes necessary if exercise is to continue anaerobically.

The body stores a limited quantity of ATP at all times (i.e., enough to last 2–4 seconds without ATP resynthesis), thus necessitating the body's energy systems to synthesize ATP when it begins to deplete during physical activity. The phosphocreatine system does exactly this by using the creatine kinase reaction to rapidly synthesize and return ATP concentrations to pre-exercise levels. Furthermore, type II muscle fibers (fast-twitch fibers) house more PCr than type I fibers (slow-twitch fibers) (Karatzaferi et al. 2001). Therefore, athletes with higher percentages of type II muscle fibers, which will oftentimes be strength–power athletes, have the potential to regenerate ATP faster through the PCr energy system during anaerobic bouts of exercise.

4.3.2 GLYCOLYSIS

During the high-intensity exercise that strength–power athletes regularly engage in, an alternate source of ATP becomes necessary when PCr stores are exhausted. Therefore, glycolysis predominates the ATP production process during anaerobic exercise after approximately 10 seconds, and this energy system can produce ATP without oxygen at a high enough rate for 2–3 minutes before exercise intensity is sacrificed to regain a homeostatic state within the body. Glycolysis is the breakdown of a glucose molecule, either from intramuscular glycogen stores (glycogen is the storage form of glucose in humans) or free-form glucose traveling through the blood to working muscles. Free-form glucose originates from glycogen breakdown in the liver or from digested carbohydrates that have been catabolized to the simple sugar, glucose, which can be absorbed and transported to skeletal muscle for storage or instant ATP production.

Glycolysis consists of a series of catalytic reactions that result in the resynthesis of ATP at a somewhat slower rate than what transpires during the PCr system. Although this feature can be detrimental at times, especially during high-intensity exercise, glycolysis can in fact produce more ATP than the PCr system, because it has a much greater supply of glycogen and glucose compared with PCr stores, respectively. One common trait that glycolysis and PCr share is that their processes/reactions occur in the sarcoplasm of muscle fibers.

The end product of glycolysis is pyruvate, which has one of two fates depending on the physiological conditions within the cell: 1) pyruvate can be converted into lactate if oxygen is not present (anaerobic conditions), and 2) pyruvate can be transported into the mitochondria if oxygen is present (aerobic conditions). If energy or ATP is needed at a very high rate as during a bout of resistance exercise, pyruvate will preferentially convert to lactate, because this reaction will result in a faster rate of ATP resynthesis. However, the duration of ATP regeneration from lactate production is limited; thus exercise intensity will be compromised after a matter of minutes or even seconds during high-intensity exercise. On the other hand, if exercise intensity is lower, resulting in lower energy demands within the cell, oxygen will be present, and pyruvate can enter the mitochondria for further oxidation. This process is a more efficient means of producing ATP compared with that of lactate production, because ATP can continue to be resynthesized as long as oxygen is present and exercise intensity remains low enough. Oftentimes, strength–power athletes will not undergo this method of ATP production during exercise, because the intensity and metabolic demands associated with their sporting activities are too high.

The formation of lactate is made possible by the enzyme lactate dehydrogenase. A common misconception is that lactic acid is the end result of this biochemical reaction. The actual products are lactate (the anion molecule of lactic acid) and a hydrogen proton (H^+). Lactate is generally thought of as the cause of muscle fatigue, the burning sensation we feel inside our muscles. Conversely, the H^+ accumulation that accompanies lactate production is what most scientists believe to cause muscle fatigue by reducing intracellular pH, inhibiting glycolytic reactions, and possibly interfering with processes directly involved with muscle contraction (Nakamaru and Schwartz 1972). Although an increase in H^+ accumulation decreases exercise intensity, it serves as a protective mechanism against muscular injury by limiting exercise when the body is overly stressed and fatigued. Furthermore, lactate can be diminished via oxidation within the muscle fiber where it originated or be transported through the blood to other muscle fibers to undergo oxidation (Mazzeo et al. 1986). Another method of lactate clearance is through the Cori cycle, in which lactate is transported to the liver and converted to glucose for later energy production via glycolysis, which results in a constant source of glucose production during exercise.

4.3.3 Aerobic Metabolism

At any given time, whether it be during a resting state or during exercise, all energy systems contribute to ATP production to some degree. Strength–power athletes, as mentioned earlier, primarily utilize anaerobic energy systems to generate ATP. Thus, aerobic means of generating ATP will likely be used more so during the recovery period following a high-intensity exercise bout. During recovery when oxygen is readily available to bind to pyruvate, the end product of glycolysis, pyruvate enters the mitochondria to initiate the Krebs cycle. This energy system continues ATP production that began during glycolysis by producing two ATP molecules via guanine triphosphate, six nicotinamide adenine dinucleotide (NADH) molecules, and two flavin adenine dinucleotide ($FADH_2$) molecules. The NADH and $FADH_2$ molecules are transported to the electron transport chain, where the hydrogen atoms are used to create ATP and water.

Fat is also used as a substrate for ATP production during aerobic metabolism. Triglyceride molecules can be broken down to free fatty acids and glycerol. Through a process called beta-oxidation, fatty acids can be used to form acetyl-CoA, the beginning substrate for the Krebs cycle. ATP production via fatty acids serves as the body's most efficient method of creating energy for biological work. For strength–power athletes, however, this energy system is primarily utilized to return the body to a homeostatic condition following exercise, because it can only be relied upon when exercise intensity is minimal. Thus, aerobic athletes that exercise at lower intensities compared with strength–power athletes take advantage of aerobic metabolism to sustain exercise duration.

4.4 MACRONUTRIENT AND GENERAL INTAKE RECOMMENDATIONS

The energy demands of strength–power athletes surpass the general macronutrient recommendations of sedentary individuals and even those that meet the recommended requirement of daily physical activity. Therefore, strength–power athletes must eat accordingly by consuming far more calories than the typical individual to enhance performance, allow for adequate recovery between exercise bouts, and alleviate any chances for injury. The following paragraphs outline general intake recommendations for strength–power athletes.

4.4.1 Carbohydrates

The amount of carbohydrate stores within the liver and skeletal muscle highly influence exercise performance of strength–power athletes, and as discussed earlier, glycogen is a primary substrate for ATP regeneration during high-intensity exercise. It has been shown that a 45-minute lower-body resistance exercise routine can deplete muscle glycogen stores by 23%, 40%, and 44% in type I, type IIa, and type IIx muscle fibers, respectively (Koopman et al. 2006). In many cases, strength–power athletes engage in sporting activities or high intensity training lasting more than an hour. Such an exercise bout can significantly deplete intramuscular and liver glycogen stores to the extent where exercise intensity (i.e., strength and power), and therefore performance, will be impaired. Consequently, the amount of carbohydrates consumed on a daily basis becomes a critical factor in the performance of strength–power athletes.

The amount of glycogen stored in the body at any given time is the result of the amount of carbohydrates consumed through the diet and the amount used during exercise and everyday activity. It is recommended that strength–power athletes consume 55%–60% of total energy intake in the form of carbohydrates (Lambert et al. 2004), which would equate to 5–6 g/kg/day. However, it is appropriate to individualize the amount of carbohydrates needed for athletes, because different strength–power sporting activities may require athletes to consume more or less carbohydrates on a daily basis to meet specific energy demands. For instance, if carbohydrate intake is less than optimal during high-intensity or high-volume training sessions, the quality of the workout may be compromised, leading to subpar training adaptations over time. Strength–power athletes should consume the majority of carbohydrates in the form of complex, low-to-moderate glycemic indexed foods that contain high-quality nutrients such as whole grains, fruits, and vegetables. The exception to this recommendation is during the recovery period following an exercise bout or training session when an athlete is attempting to replenish glycogen stores at a quick rate. This will be highlighted in the recovery considerations section of the chapter.

4.4.2 PROTEIN

Protein requirements for athletes have been a hot topic for many years. Athletes, including those participating in strength and power sporting activities, utilize protein for optimizing training adaptations, exercise recovery, and the prevention and treatment of injuries. Proteins are made of amino acids that are linked together by peptide bonds. Two classifications of amino acids exist: 1) nonessential amino acids, which can be synthesized in the body and therefore do not need to be consumed through the diet, and 2) essential amino acids, which cannot be synthesized by the body and therefore must be consumed on a daily basis. Foods that are lacking one or more of the essential amino acids are said to be incomplete protein sources, whereas foods that contain all of the essential amino acids are said to be complete protein sources. Athletes should focus on consuming the majority of their daily requirements of protein from complete protein sources, because research has shown that nonessential amino acids are not necessary for stimulating muscle protein synthesis (Tipton et al. 1999b). The essential and nonessential amino acids and quality sources of complete proteins can be found in Table 4.2.

TABLE 4.2
Essential and Nonessential Amino Acids and Quality Sources of Complete Protein

Essential AA	Nonessential AA	Complete PRO Sources
Histidine	Alanine	Whey
Isoleucine	Arginine	Casein
Leucine	Asparagine	Whole eggs
Lysine	Aspartic acid	Milk and other dairy
Methionine	Cysteine	Beef
Phenylalanine	Glutamic acid	Poultry
Threonine	Glutamine	Fish
Tryptophan	Glycine	Soy
Valine	Proline	
	Serine	
	Tyrosine	

The recommended daily allowance of protein is currently 0.8 g/kg/day. Studies have indicated that this amount is insufficient for meeting the needs of athletes (Lemon et al. 1992; Tarnopolsky et al. 1992) attempting to increase muscle mass, because it may be necessary to approach 2 g/kg/day for some athletes engaged in strenuous strength training (Lemon 1998). Therefore, a recommendation of 1.5–2.0 g/kg/day is more appropriate for attaining the goals of strength–power athletes, which translates into 150–220 g of protein/day for a 220-pound (100 kg) strength–power athlete.

4.4.3 FATS

The dietary intake of fat for strength–power athletes can closely resemble the recommended intake of the average adult. Fat is an indispensible macronutrient that assists the digestion and absorption of fat-soluble nutrients found in fruits and vegetables. Because strength–power athletes continually try to maintain a positive energy balance, it may be necessary for these individuals to consume slightly more fat throughout the day than the average person (Venkatraman et al. 2000). Therefore, it is recommended that strength–power athletes consume 30% of their total daily caloric intake from fats, of which no more than 10% come in the form of saturated fats. The majority of this fat intake should come in the form of monounsaturated and polyunsaturated fatty acids. Mono- and polyunsaturated fatty acids help to improve cholesterol and triglyceride levels in the blood (Colussi et al. 2004), prevent cardiovascular and other related diseases (Sacks and Katan 2002), as well as improve insulin sensitivity (Minami et al. 2002) to reduce the risk for developing type II diabetes. Additionally, a beneficial role of increasing daily fat intake, specifically saturated fats, is that circulating testosterone levels seem to be better maintained compared with a low-fat diet (Hamalainen et al. 1983). Cholesterol is the starting point for testosterone synthesis. Therefore, obtaining more fats through dietary intake, specifically cholesterol, may result in more testosterone production and higher circulating levels of testosterone throughout the day. Recently, it was recognized that older individuals consuming a high-cholesterol diet were better able to increase strength and muscle mass over a 12-week resistance exercise program than those consuming a diet low in cholesterol (Riechman et al. 2007). It should be noted that these individuals did not experience any detrimental effects to blood-lipid profiles while increasing dietary cholesterol. No such research has been conducted with athletes, but the possibility exists for increased cholesterol intakes to increase testosterone profiles and training adaptations in younger populations.

Good food choices to obtain dietary fat are as follows: monounsaturated fatty acids are found in olive, peanut, and canola oil, along with peanuts and avocados. Polyunsaturated fatty acids are found in the same food stuffs as monounsaturated fatty acids, as well as corn, sesame, soy, and fish such as salmon and tuna. Saturated fatty acids are characterized as solid fats at room temperature and can be consumed through meat, dairy, and poultry products. Trans-fatty acids should be avoided, meaning that the strength–power athlete should stay away from processed and packaged foods such as cookies, pastries, and other baked goods, along with chips, fried fast food, and margarine because trans-fatty acids have no performance benefits but also have a detrimental effect on health.

4.5 CALORIC REQUIREMENTS OF STRENGTH–POWER ATHLETES

In regards to the diet of strength–power athletes, one must first consider the daily energy requirements that are necessary to maintain muscle mass and overall body weight, optimize performance, and prevent overtraining symptoms that are often associated with high intensity, strenuous exercise. To fulfill these scenarios, the athlete must first intake enough calories on a daily basis to account for the daily calories expended. The total daily energy expenditure (TDEE) of strength–power athletes can be accounted for by three factors: 1) the basal metabolic rate (BMR), 2) energy expended during physical activity, and 3) the thermic effect of food. The BMR is the minimum amount of calories needed to continue or maintain life and usually equates to 60%–70% of the total amount of calories expended each day. This includes the metabolic cost of the body's organs, tissues, and physiological processes (not including digestion), which is directly determined by one's gender, body composition, body size, and age. The daily physical activity level of an individual is the most inconsistent component of one's TDEE, because it accounts for approximately 10%–30%. Lastly, the thermic effect of food makes up the third and smallest component of TDEE, which is approximately 5%–10%. This is the cost of energy related to the digestion and absorption of nutrients. These three factors must be considered when attempting to achieve a desired energy balance for both weight-loss (fat) and weight-gain (skeletal muscle) strategies.

4.5.1 CALCULATING CALORIC REQUIREMENTS

Many methods are presently used to calculate the daily energy requirements of athletes. In particular, indirect calorimetry is a preferred method utilized in laboratory settings that requires a metabolic cart to measure the quantity of oxygen consumed by the body. Knowing the amount of oxygen consumption, energy expenditure can be precisely calculated. Such techniques are not easily accessible to the average athlete. Therefore, it becomes necessary for other readily available measures to be used. One of the most often used ways to calculate BMR or resting metabolic rate is through the use of the Harris-Benedict equations (Harris and Benedict 1919). Males and females have their own separate equations, because men generally have a higher metabolic rate than women. Variables that are factored into the equations include body weight (kg), body height (cm), and age. All three of these variables directly affect the metabolic rate of an individual and therefore need to be taken into consideration to obtain the most accurate BMR prediction possible. For men, the equation is as follows:

$$\text{BMR (calories/day)} = 66.5 + (13.75 \times \text{weight in kg}) + (5.003 \times \text{height in cm})$$
$$- (6.775 \times \text{age in years})$$

TABLE 4.3
Physical Activity Level Factors

Activity factor	Activity level
1.53	Sedentary or lightly active
1.76	Active or moderately active
2.25	Vigorously active

Use the appropriate physical activity level factor from the table to calculate daily energy expenditure. Multiply the BMR by the physical activity level factor that best describes the athlete. Most athletes will fall into the vigorously active category.

For women, the equation is as follows:

$$\text{BMR (calories/day)} = 655.1 + (9.5663 \times \text{weight in kg}) + (1.85 \times \text{height in cm}) - (4.676 \times \text{age in years})$$

After calculating the BMR for a male or female athlete, you must determine the activity factor (Table 4.3) that represents the athlete's daily physical activity level. Once this factor is determined, multiply the calculated BMR by the activity factor (BMR × activity factor) to calculate the overall daily energy expenditure. This information can then be a useful tool in determining the amount of calories an athlete needs daily to meet his desired body-weight goal.

4.5.2 BODY-WEIGHT GOALS

If an athlete desires to maintain his current weight, the BMR determined by the Harris-Benedict equation multiplied by the activity factor must be equal to the total caloric intake of the athlete on a daily basis. If the athlete desires to gain or lose weight, alterations need to be made to the dietary plan in an effort to meet the desired outcomes.

To gain weight, the athlete must consume more calories than his or her energy expenditure. One pound of muscle is approximately 2500 kcal, meaning that an athlete should consume an extra 300–500 kcal beyond normal energy requirements to promote muscle hypertrophy without promoting excess gains in fat mass. This equates to 2100–3500 extra kcal per week, which can oftentimes be a difficult task for some athletes. Fortunately, one is not limited by eating only whole foods, as various nutritional supplement products such as protein and meal replacement powders can be supplemented into the diet to meet both additional calorie and/or protein needs.

If an athlete desires to lose weight, the amount of calories he or she consumes daily must fall short of the athlete's energy expenditure. One pound of fat is approximately 3500 kcal. Therefore, it is recommended that the athlete consume 500 fewer kcal per day in order to reach a 3500 kcal deficit, or one pound of fat loss, over a week long period. Furthermore, this method provides a safe and effective way of losing fat without having to compromise muscle mass.

No matter the body-weight goals of an athlete, certain nutritional practices should be adopted by all athletes. Specifically, a daily meal plan (see Chapter 5) consisting of 4–6 meals, with smaller snacks disbursed between the meals, will promote a favorable anabolic environment within the body while maintaining a high metabolic rate and low-to-moderate elevations in circulating insulin levels. These conditions are advantageous for packing on lean muscle tissue and decreasing body fat, both of which are goals of any competitive strength–power athlete.

4.6 NUTRIENT TIMING AND RECOVERY CONSIDERATIONS FOR STRENGTH–POWER ATHLETES

Over the past 25 years, nutrient timing and exercise recovery have undoubtedly gained much attention in the eyes of researchers interested in performance nutrition. The following paragraphs will highlight the nutrient timing and recovery considerations that have proven to be effective practices for strength–power athletes striving to enhance performance. Numerous research studies have been performed on the effects of CHO and protein (PRO) supplementation prior to, during, and after exercise on endurance-performance parameters. Because our focus is on strength–power athletes, studies concentrating on strength or power activities in conjunction with nutritional intervention will be discussed.

4.6.1 BEFORE EXERCISE

In regards to the literature pertaining to nutrient timing before or after resistance exercise, far fewer studies have analyzed the impact of CHO or PRO ingestion during the pre-exercise time period on muscle protein synthesis following exercise or performance measures over a chronic training duration than postexercise supplementation. A study by Tipton et al. (2001) compared the response of 6 g of essential amino acids (EAA) and 35 g of CHO immediately before or after a bout of resistance exercise on muscle protein synthesis in six subjects. This group of researchers found that supplementation prior to resistance exercise proved more effective at stimulating muscle protein synthesis and overall protein balance than supplementing immediately following exercise. A follow-up study by the same research group compared whole proteins (whey), as opposed to amino acids and CHO, ingested either before or after resistance exercise on muscle protein synthesis. It was concluded that pre- and postexercise supplementation had similar effects on overall protein balance. Another investigation by Anderson et al. (2005) had participants resistance train for 14 weeks and ingest a CHO or PRO supplement before and after each workout. The PRO supplement was superior for increasing both type I and type II muscle fiber cross-sectional area, as well as improving squat-jump height. Collectively, these studies show that pre-exercise ingestion of amino acids and CHO or whole proteins can create an anabolic environment within the body to promote muscle growth; however, carbohydrate supplementation alone provided at pre- and postexercise is unable to initiate anabolism, which is a primary goal of the strength–power athlete.

Another factor that can affect strength–power performance during prolonged workouts is the amount of glycogen available for energy production. It is widely accepted that fatigue occurs when glycogen stores become depleted and that carbohydrate supplementation can delay fatigue during prolonged bouts of exercise (Coyle et al. 1983). It is therefore important for strength–power athletes to intake a carbohydrate bolus along with protein to maximize performance during the workout along with enhancing the recovery/remodeling processes after exercise.

4.6.2 During Exercise

Research focused on nutrient administration during strength–power activities has been conducted far less than that of pre- and postexercise. Nonetheless, it is worth noting a few studies that have unveiled important strategies that can potentially benefit strength–power athletes. Lambert et al. (1991) examined the effects of a glucose polymer solution or a placebo administered to resistance-trained subjects prior to and intermittently during fifteen sets of knee extensions at 80% of their predetermined ten-repetition maximum on performance. When given the glucose polymer solution, the subjects were able to complete more sets and repetitions compared with placebo ingestion. Bird et al. (2006) observed the effects of a 6% CHO solution, 6% CHO with 6 g of EAA solution, or placebo ingested during resistance exercise over a 12-week training program on markers of protein synthesis and muscle hypertrophy. CHO with EAA ingestion resulted in a 26% reduction in muscle protein breakdown and the greatest increase in type I and type II muscle cross-sectional area compared with the other groups. These studies demonstrate that carbohydrate ingestion during strength–power activities may maintain exercise intensity, whereas combined ingestion of carbohydrates and protein helps to minimize the catabolic response and maximize muscle hypertrophy over the course of a chronic training period. Some athletes may not have the luxury of utilizing nutrient-timing strategies during exercise, so these athletes should take advantage of the pre- and postexercise nutrition strategies described prior to and after this section of the chapter.

4.6.3 Postexercise

Numerous research studies have been carried out evaluating the effects of postexercise supplementation of carbohydrates and protein on performance and training adaptations, and this window should be highly emphasized by the strength–power athlete in order to maximize adaptations. The following is a general consensus of the published literature and its implications to strength–power athletes.

It has been shown that postexercise consumption of carbohydrates immediately or soon after resistance exercise improves overall protein balance primarily by decreasing protein breakdown (Borsheim et al. 2004; Roy et al. 1997). However, if the goal is to create a positive protein balance and substantially increase protein synthesis after exercise, other supplementation strategies must be implemented. It is well established that ingestion of EAA or protein after resistance exercise promotes a positive protein balance and muscle protein synthesis (Esmarck et al. 2001; Tipton et al. 1999a, 2004), which translates to muscle mass gains over the course of time. The timing of these nutrients, however, becomes important to stimulating the anabolic response after exercise. If protein or EAA are ingested immediately (Esmarck et al. 2001) or one hour (Tipton et al. 2004) following a resistance-exercise bout, protein synthesis, along with a net positive protein, balance occur. If the timing of postexercise protein is delayed until two hours after the exercise bout, a net positive protein balance is not reached (Esmarck et al. 2001). These studies demonstrate that it is crucial to supplement during the postexercise period as soon as possible to initiate an anabolic response in the body. Missing this window from a training-table prospective is one of the worst things that a strength–power athlete could do on a day-to-day basis.

Other studies have compared different types of protein ingested after resistance exercise on muscle protein synthesis and muscle hypertrophy. Whey and casein proteins increase muscle protein synthesis to a similar degree when ingested one hour after resistance exercise (Tipton et al. 2004), whereas milk proteins (whey and casein) may be superior for increasing muscle protein synthesis acutely after resistance exercise (Tang et al. 2009) and muscle mass over a chronic resistance training program (Hartman et al. 2007). In conclusion, the timing and type of protein ingested after exercise can affect acute and chronic variables related to muscle mass, strength, and performance.

4.6.4 OTHER CONSIDERATIONS

Nutritional supplementation for strength–power athletes is not limited to carbohydrate and protein ingestion. Other supplements have proven effective for increasing performance in strength–power activities. Table 4.4 displays these supplements and provides scientific references supporting each supplement's use for the interested reader.

TABLE 4.4
Other Supplements for Strength–Power Athletes

Supplement	Function/Benefits
Creatine[A]	-Increases strength and muscle mass
	-Increases anaerobic exercise performance
Beta-Alanine[B]	-Increases muscle carnosine levels
	-pH buffer
	-Improves exercise/training volume
β-Hydroxy β-methylbutyrate[C]	-Decreases muscle damage
	-May improve strength in untrained populations

[A] Buford et al. 2007; Preen et al. 2001; Vandenberghe et al. 1997; Volek et al. 1999.
[B] Hill et al. 2007; Hoffman et al. 2008.
[C] Knitter et al. 2000; Nissen et al. 1996.

4.7 CONCLUSION

Strength–power athletes utilize anaerobic energy systems to create ATP for high intensity, short bursts of exercise. Nutritional strategies must be implemented to ensure that these athletes are mentally and physically prepared to undergo stressful exercise conditions and to fully recover and promote training adaptations that will improve performance in the future.

REFERENCES

Andersen, L. L., G. Tufekovic, M. K. Zebis, R. M. Crameri, G. Verlaan, M. Kjaer, C. Suetta, P. Magnusson, and P. Aagaard. 2005. The effect of resistance training combined with timed ingestion of protein on muscle fiber size and muscle strength. *Metabolism* 54: 151–156.

Bird, S. P., K. M. Tarpenning, and F. E. Marino. 2006. Independent and combined effects of liquid carbohydrate/essential amino acid ingestion on hormonal and muscular adaptations following resistance training in untrained men. *Eur J Appl Physiol* 97: 225–238.

Borsheim, E., M. G. Cree, K. D. Tipton, T. A. Elliott, A. Aarsland, and R. R. Wolfe. 2004. Effect of carbohydrate intake on net muscle protein synthesis during recovery from resistance exercise. *J Appl Physiol* 96: 674–678.

Buford, T. W., R. B. Kreider, J. R. Stout, M. Greenwood, B. Campbell, M. Spano, T. Ziegenfuss, H. Lopez, J. Landis, and J. Antonio. 2007. International Society of Sports Nutrition position stand: Creatine supplementation and exercise. *J Int Soc Sports Nutr* 4: 6.

Cerretelli, P., D. Rennie, and D. Pendergast. 1980. Kinetics of metabolic transients during exercise. *Inter J of Sports Med* 55: 178–180.

Colussi, G. L., S. Baroselli, and L. Sechi. 2004. Omega-3 polyunsaturated fatty acids decrease plasma lipoprotein(a) levels in hypertensive subjects. *Clin Nutr* 23: 1246–1247.

Coyle, E. F., J. M. Hagberg, B. F. Hurley, W. H. Martin, A. A. Ehsani, and J. O. Holloszy. 1983. Carbohydrate feeding during prolonged strenuous exercise can delay fatigue. *J Appl Physiol* 55: 230–235.

Esmarck, B., J. L. Andersen, S. Olsen, E. A. Richter, M. Mizuno, and M. Kjaer. 2001. Timing of postexercise protein intake is important for muscle hypertrophy with resistance training in elderly humans. *J Physiol* 535: 301–311.

Greenhaff, P. L., A. Casey, A. H. Short, R. Harris, K. Soderlund, and E. Hultman. 1993. Influence of oral creatine supplementation of muscle torque during repeated bouts of maximal voluntary exercise in man. *Clin Sci* 84: 565–571.

Hamalainen, E. K., H. Adlercreutz, P. Puska, and P. Pietinen. 1983. Decrease of serum total and free testosterone during a low-fat high-fibre diet. *J Steroid Biochem* 18: 369–370.

Harris, J., and F. Benedict. 1919. *Biometric Study of Basal Metabolism in Man.* Washington, D.C.: Carnegie Institiute of Washington.

Hartman, J. W., J. E. Tang, S. B. Wilkinson, M. A. Tarnopolsky, R. L. Lawrence, A. V. Fullerton, and S. M. Phillips. 2007. Consumption of fat-free fluid milk after resistance exercise promotes greater lean mass accretion than does consumption of soy or carbohydrate in young, novice, male weightlifters. *Am J Clin Nutr* 86: 373–381.

Hill, C. A., R. C. Harris, H. J. Kim, B. D. Harris, C. Sale, L. H. Boobis, C. K. Kim, and J. A. Wise. 2007. Influence of beta-alanine supplementation on skeletal muscle carnosine concentrations and high intensity cycling capacity. *Amino Acids* 32: 225–233.

Hoffman, J. R., N. A. Ratamess, A. D. Faigenbaum, R. Ross, J. Kang, J. R. Stout, and J. A. Wise. 2008. Short-duration beta-alanine supplementation increases training volume and reduces subjective feelings of fatigue in college football players. *Nutr Res* 28: 31–35.

Karatzaferi, C., A. de Haan, R. A. Ferguson, W. van Mechelen, and A. J. Sargeant. 2001. Phosphocreatine and ATP content in human single muscle fibres before and after maximum dynamic exercise. *Pflugers Arch* 442: 467–474.

Karlsson, J., and B. Saltin. 1970. Lactate, ATP, and CP in working muscles during exhaustive exercise in man. *J Appl Physiol* 29: 596–602.

Knitter, A. E., L. Panton, J. A. Rathmacher, A. Petersen, and R. Sharp. 2000. Effects of beta-hydroxy-beta-methylbutyrate on muscle damage after a prolonged run. *J Appl Physiol* 89: 1340–1344.

Koopman, R., R. J. Manders, R. A. Jonkers, G. B. Hul, H. Kuipers, and L. J. van Loon. 2006. Intramyocellular lipid and glycogen content are reduced following resistance exercise in untrained healthy males. *Eur J Appl Physiol* 96: 525–534.

Lambert, C. P., M. G. Flynn, J. B. Boone, T. J. Michaud, and J. Rodriguez-Zayas. 1991. Effects of carbohydrate feeding on multiple-bout resistance exercise. *J Strength Cond Res* 5: 192–197.

Lambert, C. P., L. L. Frank, and W. J. Evans. 2004. Macronutrient considerations for the sport of bodybuilding. *Sports Med* 34: 317–327.

Lemon, P. W. 1998. Effects of exercise on dietary protein requirements. *Int J Sport Nutr* 8: 426–447.

Lemon, P. W., M. A. Tarnopolsky, J. D. MacDougall, and S. A. Atkinson. 1992. Protein requirements and muscle mass/strength changes during intensive training in novice bodybuilders. *J Appl Physiol* 73: 767–775.

Mazzeo, R. S., G. A. Brooks, D. A. Schoeller, and T. F. Budinger. 1986. Disposal of blood [1-^{13}C]lactate in humans during rest and exercise. *J Appl Physiol* 60: 232–241.

Minami, A., N. Ishimura, S. Sakamoto, E. Takishita, K. Mawatari, K. Okada, and Y. Nakaya. 2002. Effect of eicosapentaenoic acid ethyl ester v. oleic acid-rich safflower oil on insulin resistance in type 2 diabetic model rats with hypertriacylglycerolaemia. *Br J Nutr* 87: 157–162.

Nakamaru, Y., and A. Schwartz. 1972. The influence of hydrogen ion concentration on calcium binding and release by skeletal muscle sarcoplasmic reticulum. *J Gen Physiol* 59: 22–32.

Nissen, S., R. Sharp, M. Ray, J. A. Rathmacher, D. Rice, J. C. Fuller, Jr., A. S. Connelly, and N. Abumrad. 1996. Effect of leucine metabolite beta-hydroxy-beta-methylbutyrate on muscle metabolism during resistance-exercise training. *J Appl Physiol* 81: 2095–2104.

Preen, D., B. Dawson, C. Goodman, S. Lawrence, J. Beilby, and S. Ching. 2001. Effect of creatine loading on long-term sprint exercise performance and metabolism. *Med Sci Sports Exerc* 33: 814–821.

Riechman, S. E., R. D. Andrews, D. A. Maclean, and S. Sheather. 2007. Statins and dietary and serum cholesterol are associated with increased lean mass following resistance training. *J Gerontol A Biol Sci Med Sci* 62: 1164–1171.

Roy, B. D., M. A. Tarnopolsky, J. D. MacDougall, J. Fowles, and K. E. Yarasheski. 1997. Effect of glucose supplement timing on protein metabolism after resistance training. *J Appl Physiol* 82: 1882–1888.

Sacks, F. M., and M. Katan. 2002. Randomized clinical trials on the effects of dietary fat and carbohydrate on plasma lipoproteins and cardiovascular disease. *Am J Med* 113(Suppl 9B): 13S–24S.

Tang, J. E., D. R. Moore, G. W. Kujbida, M. A. Tarnopolsky, and S. M. Phillips. 2009. Ingestion of whey hydrolysate, casein, or soy protein isolate: Effects on mixed muscle protein synthesis at rest and following resistance exercise in young men. *J Appl Physiol* 107: 987–992.

Tarnopolsky, M. A., S. A. Atkinson, J. D. MacDougall, A. Chesley, S. Phillips, and H. P. Schwarcz. 1992. Evaluation of protein requirements for trained strength athletes. *J Appl Physiol* 73: 1986–1995.

Tipton, K. D., T. A. Elliott, M. G. Cree, S. E. Wolf, A. P. Sanford, and R. R. Wolfe. 2004. Ingestion of casein and whey proteins result in muscle anabolism after resistance exercise. *Med Sci Sports Exerc* 36: 2073–2081.

Tipton, K. D., A. A. Ferrando, S. M. Phillips, D. Doyle, Jr., and R. R. Wolfe. 1999a. Postexercise net protein synthesis in human muscle from orally administered amino acids. *Am J Physiol* 276: E628–E634.

Tipton, K. D., B. E. Gurkin, S. Matin, and R. R. Wolfe. 1999b. Nonessential amino acids are not necessary to stimulate net muscle protein synthesis in healthy volunteers. *J Nutr Biochem* 10: 89–95.

Tipton, K. D., B. B. Rasmussen, S. L. Miller, S. E. Wolf, S. K. Owens-Stovall, B. E. Petrini, and R. R. Wolfe. 2001. Timing of amino acid-carbohydrate ingestion alters anabolic response of muscle to resistance exercise. *Am J Physiol Endocrinol Metab* 281: E197–E206.

Vandenberghe, K., M. Goris, P. Van Hecke, M. Van Leemputte, L. Vangerven, and P. Hespel. 1997. Long-term creatine intake is beneficial to muscle performance during resistance training. *J Appl Physiol* 83: 2055–2063.

Venkatraman, J. T., J. Leddy, and D. Pendergast. 2000. Dietary fats and immune status in athletes: Clinical implications. *Med Sci Sports Exerc* 32(7 Suppl): S389–S395.

Volek, J. S., N. D. Duncan, S. A. Mazzetti, R. S. Staron, M. Putukian, A. L. Gomez, D. R. Pearson, W. J. Fink, and W. J. Kraemer. 1999. Performance and muscle fiber adaptations to creatine supplementation and heavy resistance training. *Med Sci Sports Exerc* 31: 1147–1156.

5 Meal Planning for Athletes

Amanda Carlson-Phillips

CONTENTS

5.1   INTRODUCTION

The science of sports nutrition has taught us how to utilize nutrients and their timing to help to elevate an athlete's ability to perform. Through the integration of exercise physiology, nutrition, and endocrinology, we have been able to come up with fairly specific nutrition recommendations to give to an athlete to enhance recovery, improve strength, mediate fatigue, and speed recovery. However, even with the granularity that the science has given us, this extensive body of scientific research becomes obsolete if the athletes themselves do not change their nutritional behaviors.

An athlete who utilizes and executes an ideal nutrition strategy is not guaranteed to become a better athlete, but fueling the body efficiently and effectively can make a good athlete great or a great athlete better.

As a society, we most often look at nutrition and food as a means to gain or lose weight. Many teams and strength coaches consult with nutrition professionals specifically to work with their "body composition" athletes. It is this particular mindset that is beginning to evolve yet still keeps many athletes from utilizing nutrition to assist in performance and recovery. Athletes are sometimes hesitant about going to a nutritionist or addressing their nutrition because they do not want to be on a *diet*.

5.2   MEAL- AND TRAINING-TABLE PLANNING FOR ATHLETES

Meal planning in a literal sense means figuring out the calories that the athlete needs to meet their demands, making sure that the macronutrient breakdowns makes sense for the athlete's needs, identifying a recovery solution for fueling times around training and games, and then printing out a few perfect planned days for the athlete to follow. Meal planning is simply one tool that is a part of a performance nutrition program. Creating a meal plan is actually the final step, the action phase of nutritional work with an athlete that if not reinforced with education, coaching, a positive nutrition environment, and continuous support, will more than likely not be successful, and the sample meal plan developed for the athlete will end up in the trash or put somewhere where it will begin to collect dust. Another form of meal planning specifically for the athlete is in the form of a training table. The training table for the athlete is oftentimes the real-food version of the meal plan because the athletes are eating the majority of their meals from the training table. Therefore, when thinking of creating great nutritional strategies for your athlete, there are both the individual recommendations and the training-table set-up and execution to consider.

The training table can take on many forms. It can be an elaborate set-up at a beautiful Division I athlete dining hall, a post-workout spread, or even something as simple as prepacked snack boxes prepared for an athlete's air travel. The training table is oftentimes the most powerful vehicle when it comes to the athlete executing on their nutritional recommendations, so the better you can make the food environment or the training table, the better the chance the athlete will fuel their body to their recommendations.

5.2.1   QUALIFICATIONS

The question of who should be giving out the nutrition knowledge to the athlete is often a touchy subject. There are many people and fitness professionals (certified personal trainers, conditioning coaches/professionals, athletic trainers, and strength coaches) who are very knowledgeable about an athlete's physiology, the demands of their sport and how nutrition plays a role in performance; however, they may not be qualified to deliver detailed nutrition information. In addition, there may be those who are "qualified" as registered dietitians to deliver information to athletes, but they themselves are not as knowledgeable as other fitness professionals in the field.

Many certifications granted through organizations like the American College of Sports Medicine, the National Strength and Conditioning Association, and the National Academy of Sports Medicine require that the fitness professional demonstrate a certain level of knowledge regarding basic nutrition prior to achieving certification status. The International Society of Sports Nutrition has taken their certification (Certified Sports Nutritionist or CISSN) one step further with minimum education requirements as well as a vigorous exam with a heavy focus on the raw science of sports nutrition. This knowledge should equip them with the skills necessary to help them provide general nutrition recommendations and suggestions to their athletes. However, referral to a nutrition professional is needed when an athlete presents a situation that requires medical nutrition therapy (disease state or eating disorder) or when the level of recommendations moves beyond that of general guidelines and into personalized recommendations.

This blurred scope of practice is due to the fact that sports nutrition is a unique, multidisciplinary field that requires many professionals to work together. Athletic trainers, strength and conditioning coaches, coaches, athletic directors, and even food-service providers all must come together in order to provide the most effective service, information, and guidance to the athlete (Santana et al. 2007).

5.2.1.1 The Registered Dietitian

There are laws that regulate dietitians and nutritionists through licensure, statutory certification, or registration. Dietetics practitioners are licensed by states to ensure that only qualified, trained professionals provide nutrition services or advice to individuals requiring or seeking nutrition care or information. The issue of licensure and scope of practice can be confusing because each state is slightly different in how they word who can do what when it comes down to providing nutrition information. In states where there is licensure, only licensed dietetics professionals can provide nutrition counseling. Nonlicensed practitioners may be subject to prosecution for practicing without a license. States with certification laws limit the use of particular titles (e.g., dietitian or nutritionist) to persons meeting predetermined requirements; however, persons not certified can still practice.

It is critical that you determine the laws within the state you are working in to determine the legality of scope of practice within the world of nutrition. There is loose regulation in some states as to who can give out nutritional advice, and in some instances, those that do not possess adequate knowledge may be providing nutritional guidance. If you are a professional and not a registered dietitian and find yourself needing to give out nutritional information and advice, it is important to find a professional that you trust to collaborate with. Just as you would not expect a registered dietitian who is not an expert in strength and conditioning to give out training programs, do not give out nutrition prescriptions if you yourself do not meet the qualifications. If you are an athlete looking for nutritional guidance, then you want to find someone who not only has the qualifications to really dig deep into your nutritional needs but also has the experience and working knowledge to be able to relate the science to your particular needs. For both allied professionals and athletes alike, working with a registered dietitian (RD) will help to provide better solutions and a more integrated team of experts for the athlete.

5.2.1.2 A Sports Dietitian

Sports dietitians are experienced registered dietitians who apply evidence-based nutrition knowledge in exercise and sports. They assess, educate, and counsel athletes and active individuals. They design, implement, and manage safe and effective nutrition strategies that enhance lifelong health, fitness, and optimal performance (American Dietetic Association 2008). The American Dietetic Association (ADA) has taken steps to help distinguish qualified dietitians most knowledgeable in the area of sports nutrition by creating a specialty certification, Board Certified Specialists in Sports Dietetics (CSSD). CSSD certification is offered by the Commission on Dietetic Registration for RDs who have specialized experience in sports dietetics.

5.2.1.2.1 What Are the Responsibilities of a Sports Dietitian?

A comprehensive sports nutrition program will provide both individuals and teams nutrition counseling and education to enhance performance. The sports nutritionist plays many roles and has many responsibilities. The ADA has put together a "job description" for the sports nutritionist (Steinmuller et al. 2009). Each one of these objectives is equally important. The role and responsibilities of the sports nutritionist go far beyond the assigning of calories and include:

- Counseling individuals and groups on daily nutrition for performance and health
- Translating the latest scientific evidence into practical sports nutrition recommendations
- Tracking and documenting outcomes of nutrition services
- Serving as a food and nutrition resource for coaches, trainers, and parents
- Providing sports nutrition education for health/wellness programs, athletic teams, and community groups
- Maintaining professional competency and skills required for professional practice

There are confidentiality requirements and considerations to be aware of when working with athletes. When working with an athlete, you are gathering, assessing, and analyzing personal health information. The Health Insurance Portability and Accountability Act was created to provide a national standard for the handling of medical information. The key to the privacy act is to ensure that a person's protected health information is not inappropriately distributed to others. The rule broadly defines protected health information as individually identifiable information maintained or transmitted by a covered entity in any form or medium (Michael and Pritchett 2002).

5.2.2 What Does This All Mean to the Trainer or the Nutritionist?

There will be times where the nutrition information you gather will be used in a collaborative effort with other members of the athlete's performance team. It is a good practice to let the athlete know what you plan to do with their health information up front. Disclose who you would like to communicate with about their health information and get the athlete's permission to do so. If there is ever any question as to what to do with an athlete's information, get their permission before communicating their health information to other individuals or practitioners in any way. It is always best to err on the side of caution with the athlete's private information by getting a signed document. Always disclose to the athlete what you are going to share and why and then get a signed document stating that the athlete acknowledges the disclosure of that information.

5.3 DEVELOPING THE ATHLETE'S NUTRITIONAL PLAN

The goal of any nutrition program is to provide the athlete with the knowledge and tools to make good nutrition feel normal and easy. When the statements morph from "Why do I have to eat this post-workout snack right after my workout?" to "I can't believe I forgot to plan my post-workout snack—I am swinging by the convenience store to pick up chocolate milk," you know that the athlete has created a lasting positive nutritional habit and that smart sports nutrition is their nutrition normal. From a training-table perspective, this is a primary goal because it is important to teach and reinforce the idea that an athlete's day-to-day meals and snacks are vital in regards to their long-term performance goals.

A good plan makes nutrition seem approachable, action oriented, applicable, and nonclinical. It spans from strategies for everyday eating to how to eat before, during, and after practices/games/matches. Nutrition becomes the training partner to the athlete and just as important as a warm-up or cool-down routine. There are many levels in which to reach an athlete and assist in meal planning. Nutritional education and meal planning needs to mirror the planning process implemented in sport and in training for sport. Just as there are progressions and various cycles to skill training, when training the body to be stronger and have more aerobic and anaerobic capacity, there has to be a logical nutrition progression to get the best chances for change and implementation.

A great football player did not get that way overnight. By the time he shows up on the field his freshman year of college, he has had over 10 years of experience with the game. A middle-distance runner has been training their technique and capacity for a good majority of their life. They simply did not wake up one day and say "I want to run 800 m, *fast*."

Although nutrition should be made simple for the athlete and presented in a way that makes changes seem easy to make, it should not be expected that the athlete will grasp and be able to make the changes that are needed as a result of a 1-hour nutrition talk at the beginning of the season. A football quarterback is not presented with a playbook through a 90-minute lecture and then expected to go out and successfully run the plays on the field. Therefore, in developing effective nutritional programming, it needs to be viewed as another training technique, another play, and an integrated part of the entire team's strategy. Strategies should be developed at each phase of the nutrition programming continuum. Understanding and competencies must be exhibited to move on to the next phase of the process. Focus on any of the phases will help the athlete to improve their performance nutrition, but a clear

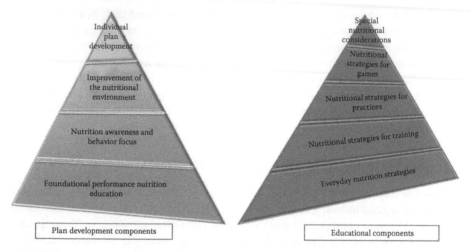

FIGURE 5.1   Athletes' Performance, Inc., nutritional programming pyramid.

progression through each of the levels will be the most effective (see Figure 5.1 for an illustration of this progression).

The development of the athlete's plan should include specific plans for both training days and game/race days. The athlete spends the bulk of his time training; therefore it is critical to incorporate plans for nutrition, hydration, and recovery that they can follow on a day-to-day basis. Recovery is one of the main limiting factors to performance; therefore it is important to design a protocol of before-, during-, and after-workout nutrition to ensure adequate protein and carbohydrates in a timely fashion to enhance recovery from the session at hand. The third phase of program development is a game- or race-day strategy, which will focus on what is needed to fuel, hydrate, and recover the body from the stress of competition.

As the athlete's nutritional plan development begins, be sure to take into consideration the athlete's desire to improve the fueling for their performance but also to look at them as the whole person. Great nutritional programs go beyond the grams of carbohydrate, protein, and fat. It is the relationship developed with the athlete and the coaching staff that sets the athlete up for successful nutrition improvement. It is important to realize that athletes are often just as busy as or even busier than the general population. Even with the help of a coach, nutritionist, trainer, and others, athletes find themselves facing the same pitfalls as the nonathlete: poor planning and poor implementation resulting in poor adaptation and performance during training and competition.

5.3.1   NUTRITION EDUCATION: CAN IT CHANGE BEHAVIORS AND HABITS?

The really tough part about nutrition is that it is a behavior and a habit. Athletes are held accountable by others for showing up at practices or training session. Their performance on their particular field of play is also tracked and reviewed. However, when it comes to nutrition, it is mostly the athlete alone who is holding himself accountable. Therefore, if a good knowledge base is not in place to ground the athlete's good nutritional decisions, then the motivation to make great nutritional choices may dwindle.

One of the key questions that researchers have been trying to evaluate is whether or not nutrition education enhances the athlete's overall nutritional knowledge and additionally whether that knowledge will actually lead to an improvement in nutritional choices. In 1996, Taramella and Kemler found that athletes who took a nutrition course were not significantly more knowledgeable than those who did not take a structured nutrition course. They also found that overall the athletes indicated a low degree of certainty for their answers. This study indicated the need for effective tools and interventions to help guide athletes to good nutritional decisions. There has been a lot of forward progress since 1996 as sports nutrition has evolved into a deeper science and practice, yet still, many coaches (Gibson et al. 2010) and athletes simply do not have the knowledge necessary to support appropriate sports nutrition behaviors. As an athlete, the majority of "advice" that they receive will typically come from their coaches; thus, the lack of knowledge here results in a potentially direct negative effect on the athlete if the nutritional and/or training advice is not accurate.

Many of the nutritional programs have been developed out of the need for the prevention or treatment of eating disorders, the consequences of the female athlete triad, and heat/hydration-related illness. These are all conditions or situations that can lead to serious health detriment for the athlete; however, the treatment approach to broad-based sports nutrition alienates those athletes who do not present a clinical issue yet are chronically over, under, or inadequately fueled to meet the demands of their sport and their body's recovery needs.

In 2001, the attitudes, beliefs, and knowledge of Division I freshman football players was evaluated. The groups were found to have normal eating patterns (eating 3.6 times/day) and were eating out quite frequently (4.8 times/week). When the athletes chose to eat out, fast-food restaurants were their destination of choice (55%). The group's educational level was weak, with an average score of 5.55 of 11 on a nutrition aptitude test on the most basic performance nutrition areas. Interestingly, the athletes expressed a great interest in learning about nutrition. The players were interested in a variety of topics at varying levels:

- 97% in nutrition for peak performance
- 81% in tips for weight gain
- 71% in eating out
- 52% in weight control
- 48% in cooking demonstration and meal preparation
- 39% in grocery store tools

This study clearly showed that these young players could benefit and were interested in performance nutrition education and programming (Jonnalagadda et al. 2001).

Another study in 2004 evaluated the dietary intake of football players. This study found that on average the players were under-fueled in comparison with standards set for their age and activity level. They were also deficient in both carbohydrate and protein. Although there are clear issues in both under-reporting and over-reporting with dietary recalls and analysis, the results still indicate an inadequate fueling strategy (Cole et al. 2005). Recent studies still indicate the same findings as previously mentioned. America's Cup sailors were found to be under-fueled for their energy demands, averaging macronutrient intake of 43% carbohydrate, 18% protein, and 39% fat (Bernardi et al. 2007), and a study of a group of 72 elite female Australian athletes also were not meeting minimal carbohydrate recommendations of >5 g/kg/day (Heaney et al. 2010). Although the populations represented in these studies may not be similar to the group with whom you work, the overarching principles are the same in that there tends to be a lack of nutrition education and strategy for many athletes.

Athletes receive their nutritional information from a variety of sources; however, it remains consistent that a good majority of the information is coming from strength and conditioning coaches or athletic trainers (Jacobson et al. 2001); therefore, it becomes increasingly important to ensure that the right information is being delivered or that priority is placed on developing a relationship with a dietitian to share the programming work with the rest of the athletic team to insure the information that athletes receive coincides with their goals both individually and as a team.

In developing nutritional programs, it is important to think of a more holistic approach of mindset, habits, behaviors, beliefs, and hard-science recommendations. Nutritional science often forgets about the fact that there are so many reasons why we choose to eat what we eat:

- Traditions
- Family/business eating
- Time constraints
- Stress
- Physiologic hunger

All of these need to be taken into consideration in working with groups and individuals. When preparing the group educational strategy, think about the priorities for the season and what will be available for the athlete to actually execute. Do not make recovery education a priority if the time and resources are not going to be allotted to actually assist the athlete in following through with a team recovery solution. Do not make foundational nutrition a focus if post-game meals are only going to consist of burgers, pizza, or what is left over from the restaurants at the stadium. There needs to be consistency from the educational message to the environment where the nutritional strategy is actually implemented or more simply put—where the athletes are going to eat.

5.3.1.1 Group Education

Group education is a powerful tool. It creates a sense of community and also a common thread of nutritional concepts and expectations. Large group sessions can be great at setting expectations for the team, but large group sessions should then be broken into small group sessions. Ideas for breakouts would be: rookies, veterans, position specific, injured athletes, weight gain, weight loss/body composition, or evaluated knowledge level. Smaller and tailored groups allow for further customization of the recommendations. A baseball pitcher is going to have different needs than that of an outfielder. A wide receiver will have much different needs than that of an offensive lineman. Thus, the training table of each of these athletes is quite variable. Group education sessions should also, if possible, be done for the coaching staff, the training staff, and the medical staff. All that are involved with the team need to have some sort of brief on what the strategies, expectations, and key nutrition objectives are for the season so that they can become a part of the support structure.

Educational sessions should be general with specific recommendations. Athletes need a list of what they should be doing, grocery shopping for, or eating at McDonald's—a little theory and then more take-home action items (Topic Box 5.1).

TOPIC BOX 5.1 TAKING INTO CONSIDERATION THE ENVIRONMENT: EASY WAYS TO GET ATHLETES TO MAKE LASTING CHANGE

- **Recovery area:** Create a recovery area outside of practices or training rooms. This recovery area should house all the necessary things for creating perfect pre- and post-workout nutrition. This area should be easily accessible and be a pass through point between leaving the training field or floor and the locker room. Placement of this area will ensure a reminder to get timely pre- and post-workout nutrition.
- **Hydration station:** Don't just have water jugs, have a hydration station. Individualized hydration solutions should be determined for your athletes based on their body composition goals, sweat rate, electrolyte loss, and overall fuel needs during practices, games, or training. Having a hydration station with water, powdered or pre-mixed sports drinks, and packaged electrolytes will allow athletes to prepare their hydration solution. Near this area should be a scale that has a chart for athletes to weigh in and weigh out of their sessions so that athletes can establish the success of their hydration during their session.
- **Training table:** There should be a strategy as to how the food room is set up or the buffet line flows. Placing all "healthy" items on the line may be setting the system up for disaster. Make sure to include 20%-30% of items that are not ideal for those who may not be ready to fully make all nutritional changes. An athlete with mediocre choices is better than an under fueled athlete. Another idea is to put descriptions on the foods. Full nutrition information can be overwhelming, so often a "stoplight" approach works well. Green dots for great choices, yellow dots for middle of the road choices and red dots for the choices that are not ideal. Athletes generally are low on the fruit and vegetable intake and may miss the mark on their high fiber

carbohydrates. Set up the line in a way that supports your educational initiatives. It should be in the following order:

1. Fruits and veggies: Add as much color to the plate as possible. Putting these at the front of the line (preferably cut up for increased consumption) will prevent athletes from filling their plate with other things first.
2. High octane carbs: Provide a mixture of ideal high fiber carbs and those more traditional carbs to ensure variety so that athletes eat.
3. Lean proteins.
4. Healthy fats.
5. Hydrators.

- **Integration of nutrition evaluation and consultation**: If possible, it is great to have the nutrition evaluation take place by an RD as a rotation during pre- and post-season medical evaluations. This integrates it into the entire process. Additional work with the RD should also, ideally, take place close to the training room or field of play. The health center or hospital just does not feel performance-based. The closer the nutrition is to the sport, the more integrated it will become and the more front of mind it will be for the athlete. Athletes may not make another appointment to see the RD in another building, but they will definitely stop by their office if it is right near the training floor.

5.4 MEAL PLAN DEVELOPMENT

The difference between offering an athlete nutritional advice and creating a true nutrition plan is the method in which you approach the athlete. A good nutrition plan will mimic traditional standards of care. A formalized set of processes and procedures to develop structured plans and systems is the most efficient way to develop plans for athletes (Clark 1999; Lacey and Pritchett 2003; Rosenbloom 2005, 2007). The more organized the gathering of information and the more detailed the delivery of the program, the more the athlete will get from the education and guidance they receive. From a nutritional standpoint, the ADA's Nutrition Care Process is a good model to follow when working with an individual or team. The ADA adopted the Nutrition Care Process and Model in 2003 in hopes of implementing a standardized process of providing high-quality care to patients. This same model can be utilized in the development of a nutrition plan for athletes. The phases of the Nutrition Care Process are: 1) nutrition assessment, 2) nutrition evaluation, 3) nutrition intervention/ education, and 4) nutrition monitoring and evaluation (Lacey and Pritchett 2003).

5.4.1 Steps in Developing an Athlete's Nutrition Game Plan

5.4.1.1 Step 1: Assess the Athlete

The assessment of the athlete is the first step to creating an effective plan. This is the time to get to know the athlete and to understand their situation and their objective data. You can sit down with the athlete one on one or you can develop a question-naire for the athlete to fill out by hand or electronically. The information to gather includes:

- Anthropometric data: Measured height, weight, and circumference data.
- Biochemical data: Lab values can provide more detailed data; however, it is important to note the physiologic state of the athlete when the blood is drawn at the time. Both dehydration and intense training can cause changes in blood volume that can skew the interpretation of blood work. In addition, food and beverage intake can alter certain blood tests (cholesterol, triglycerides, etc.).
- Sport, position, and point in season or phase of training: Prescribing correct nutrient and hydration recommendations will depend on their sport, posi-tion within that sport, and point in their season. Different positions within the same sport can have vast differences in nutrient needs. This concept of altering an athlete's food intake to correlate with where they are in their season is called nutrition periodization. Periodizing nutrition to the phase of training is very important. A football player in the beginning of his off season will have decreased caloric needs than when he starts to ramp up to two practices a day. It is critical to individualize the athlete's recommenda-tions beyond just their sport.
- Nutrition knowledge: It is important to be aware of what the athlete knows and what they do not know. Develop a system or a "quiz" to gauge the athlete's basic knowledge of the performance nutrition fundamentals (i.e., macronutri ent function, meal timing, recovery nutrition, hydration, game-day nutrition).
- Stage of change: The transtheoretical model (Prochaska et al. 1994) is extremely useful in counseling athletes. Sometimes we judge nutritional success as getting the grams of carbohydrate recommended, drinking the perfect hydration mix, and having the exact amount of carbohydrate and protein in the post-workout recovery shake. This can mean success for some athletes, whereas success for others may mean cutting down on their fast-food intake. The transtheoretical model developed by Prochaska and DiClemente is useful in determining a nutritional counseling strategy (Dandoval et al. 1994). The goal is to help the athlete go from stage to stage and to help them permanently adopt a new positive behavior or extinguish a behavior that does not enhance performance (Topic Box 5.2). Moving too quickly through the stages or developing plans for athletes who are not ready will lead to noncompliance and "failure."
- Current dietary habits and intake:
  - 24-hour or 3-day dietary recall.
  - Food habits, for example, How often do you grocery shop? How often do you eat out? How much water do you drink per day? How many meals do you eat per day? How many days per week do you eat break-fast? What dietary supplements do you use? How consistent are you with those dietary supplements?
- Allergies, dislikes, intolerances, and cultural or religious considerations.
- Medications: It is critical to check for drug-nutrition interactions.

- Injuries: Acute injuries can have an effect on their training and activity load, but overtraining injuries may be a sign of poor nutritional intake.
- Goals and timeline: Understanding the athlete's goals and timeline will help shape your strategy for education and coaching. The NFL draftee may be working on a tight timeline to prepare himself for the draft, whereas the elite speed skater may be looking for a plan to help her peak for a competition that is nine months away.

5.4.1.2   Step 2: Nutritional Evaluation

This step is the analysis of the assessment to determine the athlete's calorie needs. This can be done by measuring the athlete's resting metabolic rate or utilizing

---

TOPIC BOX 5.2   STAGES OF CHANGE

1. **Pre-contemplation** is the stage of resistance because the athlete believes either "I don't want to" or "I can't." They may not see the benefit of a change and be benignly ignorant. For example, a successful baseball player that eats a cheeseburger, fries, and a soda before each game does not see why he should change his behavior. The elite distance runner eats very little, if anything, prior to races, yet still does well; therefore, she does not see the need to add more fuel prior to and during her runs. Sports nutrition professionals need to help them see the pros of change that can overcome the cons.
2. **Contemplation** is the stage where ambivalence is present. It is important here to discuss why the athlete wants to change and then link those reasons to the behavior-change strategy. A plan should not yet be discussed in this stage.
3. **Preparation** is the stage where the athlete will most often reach out. They are gathering up all the information needed to make a change. "What should I eat before a game?" "What should I get at the grocery store?" At this stage it is important to start developing a plan and discussing what appropriate goals would be.
4. **Action** is when the athlete is actively working to make changes. He is working on the plan that you developed for him. At this stage, it is important to focus on helping him foresee obstacles, motivate him through setbacks and lapses, continue to provide him with evidence as to the positive outcomes of his behavior change, and always be there to support him through the process. He needs you to be a nutritional coach at this stage.
5. **Maintenance** is the final stage where you help the athlete identify times when he may revert into old behaviors and what to do when he starts to see himself falling off the wagon. At this stage you let your athlete go, knowing and assuring him that he is capable, but letting him know that you will always be there for support.

an energy expenditure equation and then accounting for activity. If the athlete is looking to gain or lose weight, add or subtract 500–1000 calories per day from the basal metabolic rate + activity total. This should produce a 1–2-pound weight loss or gain per week. The degree of weight loss or gain will depend on the athlete's genetic makeup, degree of positive energy balance, number of rest/recovery days per week, and the type of training phase they are in (American Dietetic Association 2009).

Next it is important to address the athlete's goals or issues (i.e. cramping, weight management, fatigue, soreness). When identifying something that you want to work on with the athlete, be sure to state the issue consistently with: 1) problem, 2) etiology, and 3) signs and symptoms (Rosenbloom 2005), for example: "Female soccer player has extreme fatigue and cramping toward the end of practices and toward halftime in games, which is hindering her performance. This is related to low daily energy intake that is not meeting her needs, inadequate fluid intake during matches, and the lack of a carbohydrate/electrolyte drink while playing." By setting up the issues in this way, it will give you a clear path into additional recommendations beyond general needs for the athlete.

Next you need to figure out the athlete's carbohydrate, protein, and fat needs dependent upon sport, position, and stage of training. It is important to create guidelines for: 1) everyday, 2) recovery, and 3) game or event day. There are two ways to express these values: g/kg of body weight or percent of total calories. Utilizing g/kg of body weight gives the athlete a more exact recommendation and is recommended, but critical thinking must be applied, and the percentage of total calories needs to be evaluated secondary to an athlete's total energy intake. For example, if a 60-kg female endurance athlete at the high end of her training would fall into the 7–10 g/kg range, this would put her at 420–600 g of carbohydrate; but if her total caloric intake is 2800 calories/day, this would be 60%–85% of her total calories. Sixty percent makes sense, but 85% does not. That is why it is important to check macronutrient guidelines when you translate research-based recommendations into reality.

5.4.1.2.1 Everyday

- Carbohydrate: 5–7 g/kg/day for general training needs and 7–10 g/kg/day for increased needs because of endurance training or for strength and power athletes enduring multiple training sessions per day (American Dietetic Association 2009; Burke et al. 2001).
- Protein: 1.2–1.7 g/kg/day depending upon sport and intensity of training (American Dietetic Association 2009; Phillips 2006).
- Fat: Remainder of needed calories. The amount of fat should be at least 1 g/kg/day and no less than 15% of total calories (American Dietetic Association 2009).
- Hydration: The Institute of Medicine's recommendations for fluid intake are 2.7 L/day for women and 3.7 L/day for men. Determine an exact amount of fluid for your athlete to consume. A range of 0.5–1 oz/pound/day depending

upon activity throughout the day will help to give greater direction for fluid intake.

- Multivitamin/fish oil/ergogenic aids: The necessary amounts must be determined from analysis of their dietary intake. These recommendations should be made under the supervision of a dietitian and/or doctor and need to be in accordance with the athlete's rules on banned substances.

5.4.1.2.2   Recovery Nutrition

Pretraining or practice: The optimal carbohydrate (CHO) and protein (PRO) content of a pre-exercise meal is dependent upon a number of factors including exercise duration and fitness level (Kreider et al. 2010).

- General guidelines recommend ingestion of 1–2 g CHO/kg and 0.15–0.25 g PRO/kg 3–4 hours before exertion (Kerksick et al. 2008).
- Pre-exercise ingestion of essential amino acids or PRO alone increases muscle protein synthesis. In addition, ingesting PRO + CHO pre-exercise has been shown to produce significantly greater levels of muscle protein synthesis (Kerksick et al. 2008).
- 17–20 oz fluid (water or sports drink) in the 2 hours prior to training and then an additional 10 oz of fluid 10–20 min prior to training (Casa et al. 2000).

During training or practice: Fluid intake is critical during training and practice.

- It is important to make sure the athlete understands that he needs to drink enough fluid to prevent no more than a 2% decrease in body weight during his training (Casa et al. 2000).
- If exercise duration increases beyond 60 minutes, a sports drink containing carbohydrates and electrolytes is beneficial. This CHO source should supply 30–60 g of CHO/hour and can typically be delivered by drinking 1–2 cups of a 6%–8% CHO solution (8–16 fluid ounces) every 10–15 minutes (Kerksick et al. 2008).
- Mixing different forms of CHO has been shown to increase muscle CHO oxidation from 1.0 g of CHO/minute to levels ranging from 1.2 to 1.75 g of CHO/minute, an effect that is associated with an improvement in time-trial performance; therefore, glucose, fructose, sucrose, and maltodextrin can be used in combination, but large amounts of fructose are not recommended because of the greater likelihood of gastrointestinal problems (Kerksick et al. 2008).
- The addition of protein to the during-workout beverage is debated in the literature, but it has been recommended that the addition of PRO to CHO at a ratio of 3–4:1 (CHO:PRO) has been shown to increase endurance performance during both acute exercise and subsequent bouts of endurance exercise (Kerksick et al. 2008).
- The research suggests that CHO, alone or in combination with PRO, during resistance exercise increases muscle glycogen stores, offsets muscle

damage, and facilitates greater training adaptations after acute and prolonged periods of resistance training (Kerksick et al. 2008).

- Keep the athlete well fueled and hydrated to support his needs. Do not forget about taste. If the beverage is not to the athlete's liking, he will not drink it, and then you will not help the athlete stay hydrated, which is the most important priority during training.
- After training or practice is a critical period for the athlete. So many athletes do not eat anything in the post-workout period where simply adding a meal, chocolate milk, or a whole-food snack will facilitate the recovery process. Making specific recommendations for the athlete will give them more exact guidelines to follow, therefore creating more of a customized solution. The post-workout nutrition beverage or food should consist of both carbohydrate and protein (Kerksick et al. 2008). Liquid is often better tolerated than solid food because some athletes experience appetite suppression with intense exercise.
- Use a repletion factor of 1.2–1.5g/kg of body weight dependent upon the amount of glycogen depletion and the intensity of exercise (American Dietetic Association 2009; Kerksick et al. 2008).
- Ratio should be 2:1 to 4:1 of carbohydrate to protein.
  - Protein: 0.3–0.4 g/kg
  - Carbohydrate: 0.8–1.2 g/kg
- Engineered supplements, like protein shakes and bars, can be utilized here especially because they are convenient. However, other less expensive alternatives like chocolate milk have been shown to be effective in helping with recovery (Karp et al. 2006).
- Get a combination of carbohydrate and protein within the first 30 minutes after the completion of training and then get the athlete to eat again about 1 hour later. Make recommendations on the exact number grams of protein and carbohydrates, but something is ultimately better than nothing (Kerksick et al. 2008).

5.4.1.2.3 Game/Event-Day Nutrition

If the athlete has been following the everyday and recovery recommendations, when they reach the day of their event or game, they should be well prepared. The focus of game/event-day nutrition is to get the body fueled and hydrated without upsetting the stomach. Game-day nutrition should be practiced, and nothing new should be done on the day of the event.

There are general recommendations for the training table and eating around competition. Typically when there is an evening or afternoon competition, the largest meal is 3–4 hours prior to the event. If there is a morning competition, then the goal is to eat about 2 hours prior to the event. There are documented guidelines for the consumption of macronutrients prior to the athletes' event to improve performance, but when it comes down to it, the athlete will decide the amount of food they feel best consuming. It is the role of the support staff (dietitian, ATC, strength coach) to educate them on the importance of fueling and get them to consume as close to the recommendations as possible.

Pre-game carbohydrate recommendations are as follows (Kerksick et al. 2008):

- 1 hour prior = 0.5 g of carbohydrates/kg of body weight
- 2 hours prior = 1 g of carbohydrates/kg of body weight
- 3 hours prior = 1.5 g of carbohydrates/kg of body weight
- 4 hours prior = 2 g of carbohydrates/kg of body weight

The dietary protein needs at this time should be consumed at 0.15–0.25 g of PRO/kg (Kerksick et al. 2008), and additionally this pre-game meal should include some healthy fat (omega-3 fats or monounsaturated or polyunsaturated oils), as well with the focus on limiting the quantity at this time. The National Athletic Trainers Association's position paper recommends 17–20 fluid ounces of water or sports drink 2–3 hours before exercise and an additional 10 fluid ounces 10–20 minutes prior to exercise (Casa et al. 2000), but discussion of fluid requirements will be addressed in more detail in a subsequent chapter (Chapter 10). If athletes have problems tolerating food prior to events, sports drinks and gels offer a great option. With that being said, the keys to success in the pre-game scenario are

1. Plan ahead.
2. Do not experiment the day of the event.
3. Know the restaurants in the area.
4. Pack a cooler full of snacks and fluid.

5.4.1.3   Step 3: Nutritional Intervention/Education

One may assume that an athlete, especially a highly trained athlete, has a vast knowledge of their own physiology and the nutrient demands of their sport and that their coaches or others who work with them on a daily basis would also have that knowledge; however, this is often not the case. When working with an athlete and in the development of their plan, start with the basics and general education and then build into personalization and customization. Just as an athlete must develop foundational basics of their particular sport first, it is very difficult to fine-tune when the foundation knowledge is not there. Starting with the basics is critical. With some athletes they may be covered quickly, but these basic concepts must still be covered. A sports nutritionist creates and implements a strategy to improve the problems identified during the assessment.

During the assessment process, the nutritionist will start to gain a sense as to what the athlete understands and what they would like to learn about. It is important to mix in what the athlete finds interesting with the basics that they need to have a deeper understanding of. Education should build awareness and understanding so that it increases the likelihood of the athlete improving their nutritional habits. The education should touch on the foundational and performance topics that were previously outlined in this chapter. The nutritionist must then help the athlete to set realistic and performance-based goals. Again, it is up to the nutritionist to blend the athlete's expectations and a true goal that will have a healthy progress rate and an end result of increased performance.

After the education is complete and the foundation of knowledge has been built or improved upon, it is time to set up the athlete's plan for all phases of their training and competition cycle. The plan should match the current phase the athlete is in but also give an element of foreshadowing how the plan will and should evolve with the athlete's phases of training through the season. So many times, the athlete sees the nutritionist and thinks it is a one-time occasion. Just as an athlete develops skills and strength and there is a consistent progression through the season or training cycle, the athlete must start to see nutrition as their training partner that ebbs and flows with the season and the training.

The recommendations could come in the form of simple strategies or in full-blown meal plans. For many athletes, the meal plan is too overwhelming, and simple behaviors can prove to be better ways to improve performance. Simple strategies like "eat minimally processed carbohydrate" or "have a recovery meal after every training session" may be as extensive as the plan needs to be. However, there will be those that really want the next level of planning and desire exact recommendations. When determining the needs of the athlete, remember to have a system of checks and balances by working with both g/kg of body weight and percentages of total calories to find a realistic recommendation for the athlete (Burke et al. 2001; Kreider et al. 2010).

In this day in age, there are very few nutrition consultations or talks that do not address the topic of supplements. It is the sports nutritionist's responsibility and duty to make sure they discuss supplement safety with the athlete. Many athletes are unaware of the fact that supplements may contain ingredients that are not on the label or that there may be an issue with the accuracy in labeling. It is important to check the athlete's respective governing body (NCAA, NFL, MLB, World Anti-Doping Agency, etc.) to find their banned substance lists. It is then important to find third-party testing organizations that the organizations support. Finally, it is critical to remind the athlete that the responsibility falls upon them and if they take a dietary supplement of any kind that contains a banned substance that they will be held responsible and be reprimanded according to their governing body's specific rules. The following websites provide information for these athletes: http://www.nsf.org, http://www.informed-choice.org, and http://www.informed-sport.com.

There are a few other key items to remember in the nutrition plan set-up and coaching. Make sure to set up realistic systems for the athlete to attain success. Whether it be exact prescriptions for before-, during-, and after-workout nutrition, specific products that would work well for the athlete, simple meals for before and after competition, coordination with food service, or even potentially a meal delivery service, it is critical to help the athlete set up a system of planning and implementation. All plans also need to take into consideration any food intolerances, allergies, religious beliefs, cultural influences, strong likes and dislikes, ability to cook, access to food, restaurants commonly visited, and socioeconomic status when developing the plan. Converting knowing to doing is a huge part of the battle and a critical issue for the long-term success of the athlete. Next, help the athlete to see their nutritional path in a sequence of small steps while still keeping the end goal in sight. Showing how all of these small steps lead to the big payoff in the end will help to keep the athlete motivated and on course. Finally, the athlete is rarely alone in their endeavors and may have deep networks of support systems. Educate those who have personal relationships with the athlete (i.e., wife, family members, others working with the athlete).

The last thing to remember when coming up with the athlete's plan and coaching him through it is that it should address the needs of the athlete and help to alleviate an issue that you found in the assessment. Also, ensure that it is something that the athlete wants to work on. The nutritionist is a guide in the process, helping to give direction and support as the athlete navigates through this new way of thinking about food as fuel for their performance.

5.4.1.4   Step 4: Nutrition Monitoring and Follow-Up

An athlete who comes to see the nutritionist one time to get a plan and then never returns will not have the same success as someone who is being monitored. There are many ways to monitor the athlete:

- Weight monitoring: Daily or weekly weights should be tracked depending upon the needs and mindset of the athlete. Some athletes respond well to daily weights, whereas others become fixated on the number on the scale. This is up to the discretion of those working with the athlete (Dionne and Yeudall 2005).
- Body fat monitoring: Monthly body-fat measures are a good way to track changes in lean body mass versus fat mass beyond what the scale tells the athlete.
- Hydration monitoring: This consists of weighing athletes in before and after sessions to assess hydration practices.
- Habit monitoring.
- Energy monitoring.
- Intake monitoring.
- Personal contact and relationship building: It is important to set up how you are going to communicate with the athlete. Staying in touch with the athlete is critical for their success. Formal appointments or checkups can be effective, but time consuming. Utilizing technology can be extremely helpful. E-mail checkups are quick and easy. A simple text message can be a great reminder and keep the athlete on track. If you have the ability to attend the athlete's practice, games, training sessions, or strength and conditioning sessions, do so as much as you can.

The more the sports nutritionist is integrated into all parts of the athlete's life and sport, the more impact he will have. Set realistic timelines to achieve the goals the athlete is looking for. If weight loss or weight gain is the goal, it is the nutritionist's job to set realistic goals. A healthy weight gain or weight loss is going to be no more than two pounds/week. Using simple tools to allow the athlete to check in with their habits can be extremely helpful.

Be sure to discuss the progress with the different members of the athlete's training team. It is crucial to share the information that you and the athlete have decided to share in order to show progress and gain reinforcement or support from the other coaching staff on the athlete's progress or need to continue to focus in on the behavior-change process.

5.5 MEAL PLANS

A meal plan is a tool. One tool does not work well for all athletes. A tool that gives options and flexibility works as a good common denominator, but still some athletes need very specific recommendations. Before creating the actual meal plan for the athlete, it is good to take a step back and really ask what the meal plan is for. It is also important to ask yourself what it means if the athlete is successful when it comes to the meal plan.

The goal is not to have the athlete follow everything exactly. The goal is for the athlete to become aware of what they are eating, improve upon the quality of their choices, start to understand the amounts that are right for them, and in one, three, or six months tell you that they either were more aware of what they were eating or that they were eating the right foods, at the right times, in the amounts that were perfect for them. Ultimately, we want the athlete to become an intuitive eater. We want eating frequently, cleanly, and consistently to be second nature. However, to get to that point we must give the athlete a guide or blueprint, a description and understanding of serving sizes, and examples to follow.

A modified exchange system seems to work well as a guide for the athlete (Figure 5.2). The meal plans in this chapter serve as starter guides. Work with an RD to help

Exchange	Example of 1 Serving		
Grains "Come back to earth" Look for >3g Fiber/Serving	1/3c Brown rice 1/2c High fiber cereal 1/2c Beans 1/2 Baked sweet potato	1 Slice whole grain bread 1/2c Oatmeal 1/2c Corn 1 Granola bar	6" Whole grain tortilla 1/2c Grits 1/2 Baked potato 5 Whole grain crackers
Proteins "Less legs the better" Look for lean proteins	3oz Fish / Shrimp 3oz Lean pork 1/2c Beans	3oz Chicken / Turkey 1c Low fat milk / Yogurt 1Tbs Peanut butter	3oz Lean beef 2 Eggs / 4 Egg whites 1/2oz Raw nuts
Dairy Look for low fat dairy "skim" or "1%"	1/2 Cottage cheese 1 Small string cheese	8oz Low fat milk 1/2 Low fat soy milk	6oz Low fat fruit-flavored yogurt
Fruits "Eat the rainbow" Choose whole fruit over juice	1 Small apple 1/4c Watermelon 1/2 Banana 14 Grapes 1 Small pear	12 Cherries 1c Melon 3/4c Pineapple 2Tbs Dried fruit 1/2c Fruit salad	1.25c Strawberries 1 Medium orange 1c Mixed berries 1 Small kiwi 6oz 100% Juice
Vegetables "Eat the rainbow" 1 Serving =	Lettuce / Spinach Green beans Tomato / Tomato sauce Bell peppers Summer squash	Broccoli Cauliflower Salsa Stir fry vegetables 6oz Vegetable juice	Asparagus Onions Carrots Zucchini
Fats "Eat fats that give back" look for unsaturated fats	1 Tbs Peanut butter 10 Black olives 2Tbs Seeds 1/4 Avocado	1Tbs Almond butter 2Tbs Flax seed 1.5tsp Olive oil 3Tbs Guacamole	11 Almonds 8 Pecans 7 Walnuts 3Tbs Low fat salad dressing

FIGURE 5.2 Athletes' Performance, Inc., modified exchange system.

determine the correct calories for your athlete. From there you can pick one of the starter nutrition blueprints. After you have picked the right nutrition blueprint range, then you can start to build sample meals.

5.5.1 MEAL BUILDER INSTRUCTIONS

1. First familiarize yourself with your calorie goal. This number is located in the upper left-hand corner of your meal builder.
2. The next section details a practical template to implement these recommendations. For instructional purposes, we will refer to this as the template.
3. "Fueling" times are represented by the six columns across the top of the template, whereas food groups and supplements are represented by the ten rows of the template. The numbers located within the body of the template are the recommended number of servings from each food/supplement group at each fueling time. Located at the bottom of the template is a detailed breakdown of the number of calories, grams of carbohydrate, grams of protein, and grams of fat provided at each fueling time.
4. Underneath the template are drop-down boxes detailing a list of "best bet" foods and supplements from each row of the template. The number to the left of each food item signifies one serving. For example, one slice of whole-wheat bread equals one grain serving. Each serving may be used interchangeably. Therefore, if you tire of whole-wheat toast at breakfast you can replace it with any of the foods listed in the grain column. You are only limited by your creativity.
5. You are now prepared to build customized meals that will provide sustainable fuel throughout the day as well as power you through your training session.

Helpful hints:

- Plan your meals around protein.
- Include a variety of colors within each meal/snack. Strive for at least three at every meal.
- Try adding fats like nuts and seeds to grains or vegetables to add some crunch.
- If you have a favorite dish, break down the ingredients and see which food group they fall into.
- Write out your meal plan for an entire week, transfer this plan to a grocery list, and then implement the plan!

5.5.2 EXCHANGE LIST

Each of the items listed in Tables 5.1 through 5.6 equates to one serving from each of the groups. Look at your meal builder for the number of servings recommended for the corresponding calorie level (Figure 5.3).

TABLE 5.1
Perfect Meal Plan: 1400–1700 Calorie Level

Fueling Times	Meal Option 1	Meal Option 2
Breakfast	– ½ cup oatmeal cooked – two eggs with ¼ medium avocado – one banana	– one slice whole-wheat toast with 1 tbsp natural peanut butter – 1 cup low-fat yogurt with 1 cup mixed berries
After workout	– shake with CHO and PRO	– 2:1 CHO:PRO ratio
Snack	– one small apple – seven walnuts	– ½ banana with 1 tbsp natural peanut butter
Lunch	– ⅓ cup brown rice with 1½ tsp olive oil – 1 cup raw spinach – ½ cup cooked zucchini and ½ cup cooked bell peppers – 3 oz chicken breast and ½ cup watermelon	– two slices whole-wheat bread with 3 oz turkey, lettuce, tomato, and bell peppers – ¼ medium avocado
Snack	– five whole grain crackers with 1 tbsp almond butter	– one granola bar and 2 tbsp sunflower seeds – one tortilla (6 inch) – ½ cup beans
Dinner	– ½ baked potato – 3 oz salmon – 1½ cup salad with spinach, carrots, and broccoli, 3 tbsp low-fat salad dressing	– 3 oz ground turkey with ½ cup lettuce, ½ cup tomato, ¼ medium avocado, and salsa
Snack	– ½ cup cottage cheese with 1 cup strawberries	– ½ oz raw almonds – one small pear

TABLE 5.2

Perfect Meal Plan: 1700–2000 Calorie Level

Fueling Times	Meal Option 1	Meal Option 2
Breakfast	– two slices whole-wheat toast with 1 tbsp natural peanut butter each – two scrambled eggs – ½ cup fruit salad	– 1 cup oatmeal cooked with one sliced banana – eight chopped pecans – 1 cup low-fat milk
After workout	– shake with CHO and PRO	– 2:1 CHO:PRO ratio
Snack	– one banana with 1 tbsp almond butter	– one small kiwi and seven walnut halves
Lunch	– 1 cup sweet potato wedges with 1½ tsp olive oil – 3 oz grilled chicken breast – 3 cups steamed vegetables (broccoli, cauliflower, carrots, and green beans)	– ⅔ cup rice, cooked with stir-fried shrimp (3 oz) – 2 cups vegetable salad and 3 tbsp salad dressing – 14 grapes and 1 cup carrots
Snack	– one Kashi granola bar – 2 tbsp seeds and ¾ cup pineapple	– five whole wheat crackers with 1 tbsp natural peanut butter – one medium orange
Dinner	– one medium ear of corn – 3 oz pork with 2 cups salad – ¼ medium avocado with 3 tbsp salad dressing	– 1 cup baked sweet potato – 3 oz lean beef – ½ cup steamed broccoli and ½ cup cauliflower with 1½ tsp olive oil and seasonings. – one whole wheat roll
Snack	– two string cheese sticks – small apple	– 6 oz low-fat yogurt with ½ cup berries and 11 almonds

TABLE 5.3
Perfect Meal Plan: 2300–2600 Calorie Level

Fueling Times	Meal Option 1	Meal Option 2
Breakfast	– 1 cup high fiber cereal with 8 oz low-fat milk and ½ cup sliced strawberries and berries – ½ banana and 1 tbsp peanut butter	– two slices whole-wheat toast, – two eggs with 1 cup cooked spinach, onions, avocado, and salsa – 1 cup melon
After workout	– shake with CHO and PRO	– 2:1 CHO:PRO ratio
Snack	– 2 tbsp dried fruit and 11 almonds	– one banana and 1 tbsp almond butter
Lunch	– 1 cup grits cooked – 3 oz lean pork – ½ cup peas – 1 cup spinach salad and 1 cup cucumber with 3 tbsp low-fat dressing – ¼ cup watermelon	– one baked sweet potato – 6 oz grilled tuna – 2 cups steamed vegetables – 1 cup salad with 3 tbsp low-fat dressing – one medium orange
Snack	– one slice whole-wheat toast with 1 tbsp natural peanut butter	– one meal replacement bar and a small apple
Dinner	– 9 oz baked potato – 6 oz salmon – 1 cup salad with 3 tbsp low-fat dressing	– 1 cup brown rice – 6 oz grilled lean beef – 2 cups grilled vegetables – ½ cup avocado

TABLE 5.4

Perfect Meal Plan: 2600–3000 Calorie Level

Fueling time	Meal Option 1	Meal Option 2
Breakfast	– 1 cup oatmeal, cooked – two eggs scrambled with 2 oz cheese – 6 oz orange juice – one banana	– ½ whole-wheat bagel – one egg and 3 oz ham – one large banana with 1 tbsp peanut butter – 8 oz nonfat milk
After workout	– shake with CHO and PRO	– 2:1 CHO:PRO ratio
Snack	– ¼ cup trail mix with ¾ cup pretzels	– one slice whole-wheat bread with 1 tbsp natural peanut butter – ½ banana
Lunch	– 1 cup whole-wheat pasta – 6 oz turkey meatballs in ½ cup marinara sauce – 1 cup steamed broccoli and 1 oz parmesan cheese – 1 cup chopped fruit, seven walnut halves, and 12 cherries	– chicken caesar wrap: one large wrap with 6 oz grilled chicken – 1 cup steamed vegetables (broccoli, asparagus, sugar snaps) – 1 oz parmesan cheese – ½ cup lettuce, 3 tbsp low-fat Caesar dressing – one banana
Snack	– ½ cup Greek yogurt – ½ cup granola – seven chopped walnut halves	– 3 oz tuna with 2 tsp low-fat mayo – one slice crisp rye bread
Dinner	– fish taco: 6 oz grilled white fish, ½ cup sautéed onions, and ½ cup bell peppers with 3 tbsp guacamole and 3 tbsp salsa served on one whole-wheat tortilla (6 inch) – ¼ cup quinoa, cooked – ½ cup soy beans	– 6 oz lamb on one whole-wheat pita flatbread with 1 tbsp hummus, ½ cup tomato, ½ cup cucumber, ½ cup spinach – 11 toasted almonds – 8 oz 1% milk
Snack	– 8 oz milk – one large banana	– ½ cup Greek yogurt – ½ slice banana and ¾ cup blueberries

TABLE 5.5
Perfect Meal Plan: 3100–3400 Calorie Level

Fueling Times	Meal Option 1	Meal Option 2
Breakfast	– three slices whole-wheat toast with 2 tbsp peanut butter – two eggs scrambled – 6 oz orange juice – one banana	– two whole-wheat pancakes with 1 tbsp natural maple syrup – two boiled eggs – one slice whole-wheat toast and 1 tbsp natural peanut butter – 8 oz milk – one banana and 1 cup honeydew (cubed)
After workout	– shake with CHO and PRO	– 2:1 CHO:PRO ratio
Snack	– ½ cup oatmeal cooked with 1¼ cup sliced strawberries – 2 tbsp pumpkin seeds – seven walnut halves	– ½ small whole-wheat bagel with 3 tbsp low-fat cream cheese – 11 almonds – one small apple
Lunch	– club sandwich: three slices whole-wheat bread with 2 tsp low-fat mayo, 3 oz grilled chicken, 3 oz lean ham, and 1 cup tomato sliced – 1 cup raw spinach salad 3 tbsp low fat dressing – one large tangerine	– 6 oz stir-fried steak, 1 cup brown rice cooked, 2 cups diced vegetables (carrots, broccoli, cauliflower) – ½ cup raw green bell peppers and 6 tbsp ranch dressing – one individual bag baked Sunchips
Snack	– 3 cups light popcorn – one Kashi Granola Bar – one small apple	– 14 grapes – 2.5 cup pretzels – ¼ cup watermelon
Dinner	– 6 oz grilled chicken – one small wheat roll – one medium ear of corn – 1 cup mashed potatoes with 2 tsp butter – 2 cups raspberries and blackberries – one scoop low-fat ice cream	– 6 oz grilled sirloin – 5 oz roasted sweet-potato fries – ½ cup EACH: roasted cherry tomatoes, cooked asparagus, and cabbage – 1 cup nonfat yogurt with ¾ cup pineapple – one whole wheat roll with 2 tsp butter – one small apple
Snack	– 1 tbsp natural peanut butter and 1 tbsp jelly on two slices of whole-wheat bread – one plum	– ½ whole-wheat bagel with 3 tbsp low-fat cream cheese – one pear – eight pecan halves

TABLE 5.6

Perfect Meal Plan: 3500–4000 Calorie Level

Fueling times	Meal Option 1	Meal Option 2
Breakfast	– two slices whole-wheat toast with 2 tbsp peanut butter – one whole-wheat bagel – two eggs – 8 oz low-fat milk – one large banana – 6 oz orange juice	– 1 cup cooked oatmeal with ¾ cup blueberries – two slices whole-wheat toast with 2 tsp butter – 8 oz milk – 1 cup Greek yogurt with 1¼ cup sliced strawberry – one banana
After workout	– shake with CHO and PRO	– 2:1 CHO:PRO ratio
Snack	– two slices whole-wheat bread with 2 tbsp peanut butter – one banana	
Lunch	– 6 oz grilled chicken on 6-inch toasted multigrain hoagie roll with ¼ cup sliced tomato and ¼ cup spinach, and two slices low-fat cheese – 1 cup raw vegetables with hummus dip – 1 cup fruit – two Fig Newtons – 6 oz vegetable juice	– four 6-inch whole-wheat tortilla, 3 oz ground lean beef, 4 oz low-fat refried beans, 2 oz grated cheese, ½ cup diced tomato – 1 cup cooked green pepper and ⅓ cups cooked onions – 1 cup raw spinach – one banana
Snack	– ½ pita bread with 4 oz hummus – 11 almonds	– 12 whole-wheat tortilla chips with 3 tbsp guacamole – eight pecan halves
Dinner	– 6 oz grilled salmon – 1 cup brown rice cooked – 1 cup steamed vegetables – one medium orange – ¾ cup blueberries – 1 cup green salad with 3 tbsp low-fat lemon vinaigrette – one small whole wheat roll with 1 tbsp butter (whipped)	– 6 oz grilled buffalo burger on one large whole wheat bun with two slices low-fat cheese – ½ cup cooked sweet potato – ½ cup cooked carrots and ½ cup cooked broccoli – 16 animal crackers – ½ cup applesauce – 12 cherries
Snack	– 1 cup nonfat yogurt with ½ cup Greek yogurt – 1 cup whole grain cereal with ¾ cup blueberries – seven walnut halves	– 3 oz ham and one slice low-fat cheese sandwich on two slices of rye bread with 2 tsp low-fat mayo – 1 cup raspberries

1400–1700	Fueling times					
	Breakfast	Snack	Lunch	Snack	Dinner	Snack
Grains	1	**	1–2	1	1–2	**
Protein/Dairy	1	**	1	**	1	1
Fruits	1–2	1	1–2	**	**	1
Veggies			3		3	
Fats	1	1	1	1	1	**
or						
Meal replacement bar/shake	**	1	**	1	**	1
Total calories	280–340	140–170	350–425	140–170	350–425	140–170

(A)

1700–2000	Fueling times					
	Breakfast	Snack	Lunch	Snack	Dinner	Snack
Grains	1–2	**	2–3	1	2–3	**
Protein/Dairy	1	**	1	**	1	1
Fruits	1–2	1–2	**	1	**	1
Veggies			3		3	
Fats	1–2	1	1–2	1	1–2	1
or						
Meal replacement bar/shake	**	1	**	1	**	1
Total calories	340–400	170–200	425–500	170–200	425–500	170–200

(B)

2000–2300	Fueling times					
	Breakfast	Snack	Lunch	Snack	Dinner	Snack
Grains	1–2	**	1–2	1–2	1–2	**
Protein/Dairy	1	**	1–2	**	1–2	1
Fruits	1–2	1	1	**	**	1
Veggies			3		3	
Fats	1–2	1	2	1–2	1–2	**
or						
Meal replacement bar/shake		1		1		1
Total calories	360–460	180–230	450–575	180–230	450–575	180–230

(C)

FIGURE 5.3 Athletes' Performance, Inc., meal builder systems for (A) 1400–1700, (B) 1700–2000, (C) 2000–2300, (D) 2300–2600, (E) 2600–3000, (F) 3100–3400, and (G) 3500–4000 calorie level (Courtesy of Athletes' Performance, Inc., 2010).

2300–2600	Fueling times					
	Breakfast	Snack	Lunch	Snack	Dinner	Snack
Grains	2	**	2–3	1	2–3	**
Protein/Dairy	1 to 2	**	2	**	2	1
Fruits	1 to 2	1 to 2	1	**	**	1 to 2
Veggies			3		3	
Fats	1 to 2	1	1 to 2	1	2	**
or						
Meal replacement bar/shake		1 + fruit		1 + fruit		1 + fruit
Total calories	460–520	230–260	575–650	230–260	575–650	250–260

(D)

2600–3000	Fueling times					
	Breakfast	Snack	Lunch	Snack	Dinner	Snack
Grains	2–3	1	2–3	1	2–3	**
Protein/Dairy	2	**	2	1	2	1
Fruits	2–3	1	2	**	**	2
Veggies			3		3	
Fats	2	1	2	1	2	**
or						
Meal replacement bar/shake		1 + 2 fruit		1 + 2 fruit		1 + 2 fruit
Total calories	520–600	260–300	650–750	260–300	650–750	260–300

(E)

3100–3400	Fueling times					
	Breakfast	Snack	Lunch	Snack	Dinner	Snack
Grains	3–4	1	3–4	2	3–4	2
Protein/Dairy	2	**	2	**	2	1
Fruits	3	1	1	**	2	1
Veggies			3		3	
Fats	2	2	1–2	1	2	1–2
or						
Meal replacement bar/shake		1 + 2 fruit + 1 fat		1 + 2 fruit + 1 fat		1 + 2 fruit + 1 fat
Total calories	600–680	300–340	750–850	300–340	750–850	300–340

(F)

FIGURE 5.3 Continued

3500–4000	Fueling times					
	Breakfast	Snack	Lunch	Snack	Dinner	Snack
Grains	4–5	1–2	4–5	1	4–5	2–3
Protein/Dairy	2	**	2	**	2	1
Fruits	3–4	1–2	1–3	**	2	1
Veggies			3		3	
Fats	2–3	2–3	2–3	2	2	2–3
or						
Meal replacement bar/shake		1		1		1
Total calories	680–800	340–400	850–1000	340–400	850–1000	340–400

(G)

FIGURE 5.3 Continued

5.6 SPECIAL CONSIDERATIONS WHEN WORKING WITH ATHLETES

5.6.1 EATING DISORDERS AND DISORDERED EATING

Involvement in organized sports and general athletic activities offers many positive benefits on both physical and mental health; however, the pressure of athletic competition compounds an existing cultural emphasis on thinness. The result is an increased risk for athletes to develop disordered eating patterns and possibly even an eating disorder (McArdle et al. 2005; Sundgot-Borgen and Torstveit 2004). A study evaluating Norwegian athletes found that 13.5% of athletes studied had subclinical or clinical eating disorders in comparison with 4.6% of the general population controls (Sundgot-Borgen and Torstveit 2004).

Athletes in many sports face a paradox because the behavior necessary to achieve a body weight for success in their sport (semi-starvation, purging, compulsive exercising) adversely affects health, fuel reserves, physiologic and mental function, and most importantly the ability to train and compete at the level they desire. Reduced carbohydrate intake will affect the body's fuel stores and a decrease in protein intake may lead to a decrease in lean tissue. An overall lack of micronutrients resulting from a low energy intake may make growth, repair, and recovery from exercise difficult and also put the athlete at an increased risk for injury (McArdle et al. 2005).

Eating disorders are traditionally associated with female sports, but disordered eating patterns and eating disorders do occur in male athletes as well, specifically those with an aesthetic component or sports that require the athlete to make weight or have an emphasis on being small and lean. Men currently represent 6%–10% of individuals with eating disorders (Baum 2006; Glazer 2008; McArdle et al. 2005).

In male athletes, 22% of the eating disorders are in those participating in antigravitation sports, like diving, gymnastics, high jump, and pole vaulting; 9% are in endurance sports; and 5% are in ball game sports. In female athletes, 42% of the eating disorders were found in athletes competing in aesthetic sports, 24% were in endurance sports, 17% were in technical sports, and 16% were in ball game sports (Sundgot-Borgen and Torstveit 2004). An additional study on the prevalence of eating disorders among males found that 52% of 25 lower weight category collegiate wrestlers and 59% of lightweight rowers reported bingeing; 8% of the rowers and 16% of the wrestlers showed pathologic eating disorder index profiles (Thiel 1993).

This particular study is consistent with the remainder of the literature, where estimates of the prevalence of eating disorders range between 15% and 62% among female athletes, with the greatest prevalence among athletes in aesthetic sports such as ballet, bodybuilding, diving, figure skating, cheerleading, and gymnastics, secondary to the fact that success in those sports is often associated with leanness (McArdle et al. 2005).

Eating disorders are classified in the Diagnostic and Statistical Manual of Mental Disorders, on the basis of the groupings of symptoms that they present. An eating disorder can be classified as anorexia nervosa, bulimia nervosa, or an eating disorder not otherwise specified; however, many of those with a diagnosis in one category demonstrate behaviors across the diagnosis continuum. There is a fine but solid line between eating disorders and disordered eating, because they are not the same thing. An eating disorder is a serious mental illness that interferes with an athlete's normal daily activities while disordered eating represents a temporary or mild change in an athlete's eating behaviors. Disordered eating patterns can arise if an athlete is trying to make a weight goal, is under stress, or is intending to change their appearance or performance through dietary changes. As long as these patterns are short lived and do not persist, these behaviors need to be monitored but not necessarily treated by a psychiatrist and/or psychologist. It is important to note the behavior because prolonged disordered eating patterns can lead to a full-blown eating disorder (Dionne and Yeudall 2005).

It is critical that the appropriate referrals to a medical professional and registered dietitian be taken when working with an athlete with an eating disorder. It is also important to reach out to more qualified professionals in cases of an eating disorder and lend support to their proposed treatment plan. The complexity, time intensiveness, and expense of managing eating disorders necessitates an interdisciplinary approach representing medicine, nutrition, mental health, athletic training, and athletics administration in order to facilitate early detection and treatment, make it easier for symptomatic athletes to ask for help, and enhance their potential for full recovery (Becker et al. 2008; Dionne and Yeudall 2005).

5.6.2 Female Athlete Triad

In 2007, the American College of Sports Medicine released their updated position stand on the female athlete triad (Nattiv et al. 2007). The female athlete triad refers to the interrelationship among energy availability, menstrual function, and bone mineral density. Female athletes can be found all along a spectrum between health and disease, with those in the danger zone not exhibiting all of the clinical conditions at the same time. Low energy availability (with or without eating disorders), amenorrhea, and osteoporosis alone or in combination pose significant health risks to physically active girls and women. Traditionally body fat percentage has been linked to the female athlete triad, whereas now low energy availability seems to be the triggering cause of the female athlete triad. Some athletes reduce energy availability by increasing energy expenditure more than energy intake, and others practice abnormal eating patterns using one or a combination of the inappropriate compensatory behaviors outlined above.

Sustained low energy availability can impair both mental and physical health. All of the following are consequences of sustained low energy availability:

- Low self-esteem
- Depression
- Anxiety disorders
- Cardiovascular complications
- Endocrine complications
- Reproductive complications
- Skeletal complications
- Gastrointestinal complications
- Renal complications
- Central nervous complications

As the number of missed menstrual cycles accumulates secondary to sustained low energy intake, bone mineral density (BMD) declines, the loss of BMD may not be fully reversible, and the risk for stress fractures increases.

Finally, athletic administrators and the entire team of professionals working with female athletes should aim for triad prevention through education. Young female athletes often do not see that the actions they take to enhance performance may result in future problems with bone density and fertility (Nattiv et al. 2007).

5.7 CONCLUSIONS

The practice of sports nutrition is somewhere between science and art. Getting athletes to change the way they eat can positively impact performance, although creating behavior change is very difficult to do. An integrated and systematic approach assessment, evaluation of needs, intervention/education, and then building deep relationships with the athlete during the monitoring phase of your work with them will set the athlete up for success (Figure 5.4). Integrating meal planning, nutrition education, and creating an environment that supports great nutrition as a training partner and performance enhancer will help the athlete perform at their best and also give them the knowledge and tools to live a high-performance life through great nutrition well after their playing days are done.

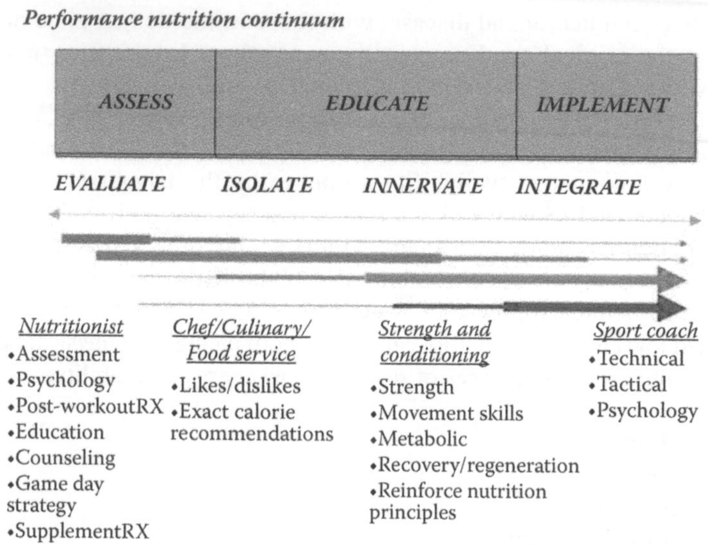

Performance nutrition continuum

FIGURE 5.4   Athletes' Performance, Inc.: performance nutrition continuum.

REFERENCES

American Dietetic Association. 2008. *ADA's Job Descriptions: Models for the Dietetics Profession*. Chicago, IL: American Dietetic Association.

American Dietetic Association. 2009. Position of the American Dietetic Association, Dietitians of Canada and the American College of Sports Medicine: Nutrition and athletic performance. *J Am Dietetic Assoc* 109: 509-527

Baum, A. 2006. Eating disorders in male athletes. *Sports Med* 36: 1–6.

Becker, C., S. Bull, K. Schaumberg, A. Cauble, and A. Franco. 2008. Effectiveness of peer-led eating disorder prevention: A replication trial. *J Clin Psych* 76: 347–354.

Bernardi, E., S. A. Delussu, F. M. Quattrini, A. Rodio, and M. Bernardi. 2007. Energy balance and dietary habits of America's Cup Sailors. *J Sports Sci* 25: 1153–1160.

Burke, L. M., G. R. Cox, N. K. Cummings, and B. Desbrow. 2001. Guidelines for daily carbohydrate intake: Do athletes achieve them? *Sports Med* 31: 267–299.

Casa, D., L. Armstrong, S. K. Hillman, S. J. Montain, R. V. Reiff, B. S. Rich, W. O. Roberts, and J. A. Stone. 2000. National Athletic Trainers' Association position statement: Fluid replacement for athletes. *J Athletic Train* 35: 212–224.

Clark, K. 1999. Sports nutrition counseling: Documentation of performance. *Topics in Clin Nutr* 9: 64–69.

Cole, C., G. Salvaterra, J. E. Davis, M. E. Borja, L. M. Powell, E. C. Dubbs, and P. L. Bordi. 2005. Evaluation of dietary practices of National Collegiate Athletic Association Division I football players. *J Strength Cond Res* 19: 490–494.

Dandoval, W., K. Heller, W. H. Wiese, and D. A. Childs. 1994. Stages of change model for nutritional counseling. *Topics Clin Nutr* 9: 64–69.

Dionne, M., and F. Yeudall. 2005. Monitoring of weight in weight loss programs: A double-edged sword. *J Nutr Educ Behav* 37: 315–318.

Gibson, K., R. Touger-Decker, D. Rigassio-Radler, and J. Parrot. 2010. Demographic and professional characteristics, sports nutrition knowledge, practices and perceived educational needs of Minnesota state high school league varsity athletic coaches. *J Am Dietetic Assoc* 110: A108.

Glazer, J. 2008. Eating disorders among male athletes. *Curr Sports Med Report* 6: 332–337.

Heaney, S., H. O'Connor, J. Gifford, and G. Naughton. 2010. Comparison of strategies for assessing nutritional adequacy in elite female athletes' dietary intake. *Int J Sport Nutr Exerc Metabol* 20: 245–256.

Jacobson, B. H., C. Sobonya, and J. Ransone. 2001. Nutrition practices and knowledge of college varsity athletes: A follow-up. *J Strength Cond Res* 15: 63–68.

Jonnalagadda, S., C. Rosenbloom, and R. Skinner. 2001. Dietary practices, attitudes and physiological status of collegiate freshman football players. *J Strength Cond Res* 15: 507–513.

Karp, J. R., J. D. Johnston, S. Tecklenburg, T. D. Mickleborough, A. D. Fly, and J. M. Stager. 2006. Chocolate milk as a post-exercise recovery aid. *Int J Sport Nutr Exerc Metabol* 16: 78–91.

Kerksick, C., T. Harvey, J. Stout, B. Campbell, C. Wilborn, R. Kreider, D. Kalman, T. Ziegenfuss, H. Lopez, J. Landis, J. L. Ivy, and J. Antonio. 2008. International society of sports nutrition position stand: Nutrient timing. *J Int Soc Sports Nutr* 5: 18.

Kreider, R. B., C. D. Wilborn, L. Taylor, B. Campbell, A. L. Almada, R. Collins, M. Cooke, 2010. ISSN exercise and sport nutrition review: Research and recommendations. *J Int Soc Sports Nutr* 7: 1–43.

Lacey, K., and E. Pritchett. 2003. Nutrition Care Process model: ADA adopts roadmap to quality care and outcomes management. *J Am Dietetic Assoc* 103: 1061–1072.

McArdle, W., F. I. Katch, and V. L Katch. 2005. *Sports and Exercise Nutrition*, pp. 492–525. Baltimore, MD: Lippincott, Williams & Wilkins.

Michael, P., and E. Pritchett. 2002. Complying with Health Insurance Portability and Accountability Act: What it means to dietetics and practitioners. *J Am Dietetic Assoc* 102: 1402–1403.

Nattiv, A., A. Loucks, M. M. Manore, C. Sanborn, J. Sundgot-Borgen, and M. Warren. 2007. American College of Sports Medicine position stand: The female athlete triad. *Med Sci Sports Exerc* 39: 1867–1882.

Phillips, S. 2006. Dietary protein for athletes. *Appl Physiol Nutr Metab* 31: 647–654.

Prochaska, J., J. Norcross, and C. C. DiClemente. 1994. *Changing for Good*. New York: William Morrow and Company.

Rosenbloom, C. 2005. Sports nutrition: Applying ADA's Nutrition Care Process and model to achieve quality care and outcomes for athletes. *SCAN Pulse* 24: 10–17.

Rosenbloom, C. 2007. Sports nutrition: Applying the science. *Nutr Today* 42: 248–254.

Santana, J. C., J. Dawes, J. Antonio, and D. S. Kalman. 2007. The role of the fitness professional in providing sports/exercise nutrition advice. *Nat Strength Cond J* 29: 69–71.

Steinmuller, P. L., N. L. Meyer, L. J. Kruskall, M. M. Manore, N. R. Rodriguez, M. Macedonio, R. L. Bird, and J. R. Berning. 2009. American Dietetic Association standards of practice and standards of professional performance for registered dietitians in sports dietetics. *J Am Dietetic Assoc* 109: 544–552.

Sundgot-Borgen, J., and M. K. Torstveit. 2004. Prevalence of eating disorders in elite athletes is higher than in the general population. *Clin J Sport Med* 14: 25–32.

Taramella, L., and D. Kemler. 1996. Principles of sports nutrition: Does nutrition education enhance athletes' knowledge. *J Am Dietetic Assoc* 96: A88.

Thiel, A. 1993. Subclinical eating disorders in male athletes: A study of the low weight category of rowers and wrestlers. *Acta Psychiatry Scand* 88: 259.

Section II

Role of Individual Nutrients

6 Protein Needs of Athletes

Kristin Dugan and Colin D. Wilborn

CONTENTS

6.1 INTRODUCTION

Protein has long been considered by athletes to be the dietary key to strength gains and lean mass acquisition. Although this is not entirely true, it is reality that, without adequate amino acid availability, protein accretion is not possible. Protein accretion, or positive protein balance, is necessary to increase lean muscle mass. Although it may be assumed that "big muscles" are not necessary for all athletes, it is a myth that strong lean muscles have to make an athlete bulky. The truth is that lean muscle is necessary for a positive metabolism, explosiveness, speed, quickness, and strength. Most would agree that these are favorable characteristics of most all athletes.

There has been much debate over the years on just how much protein is enough protein. The real issue is that we do not store amino acids in the body. The only form of amino acid storage is a transient pool of amino acids available for us to draw from if need be. Given that this pool is transient and easily depleted, we must have adequate protein intake in our diet to replenish this pool. Research studies have found that, with dietary protein or amino acid supplementation, the muscle protein synthesis rate is increased (Biolo et al. 1997; Tipton et al. 1999). This increase in protein synthesis has been seen in the administration of protein (Willoughby et al. 2007), mixed amino acids (Tipton et al. 1999), essential amino acids (Borsheim et al. 2002), branched chain amino acids (Louard et al. 1990), and even leucine alone (Crowe et al. 2006).

Although it has become apparent in recent years that the protein needs of athletes are higher than their sedentary counterparts, there is still some debate as to frequency, quantity, type, and specific athlete need. A review and position stand by the International Society of Sports Nutrition (Campbell et al. 2007) concluded that all of these factors come into play when considering the protein needs of athletes.

6.2   PROTEIN BALANCE

The body is always undulating between a *catabolic* and an *anabolic* state, which is determined by the ratio of protein synthesis versus protein breakdown. When the body is in a catabolic state, protein breakdown exceeds that of protein synthesis, which most commonly results in skeletal-muscle and tissue breakdown. Various methods are capable of reversing this condition by producing an anabolic state in the body, where protein synthesis exceeds protein breakdown, which allows tissue building to occur. The body tends to favor catabolism, which is potentially detrimental to both the training ability of active individuals and the quality of life in sedentary individuals. Because the body is in a continuous state of protein turnover, it is essential to achieve *protein balance*, which refers to the optimal ratio of protein synthesis to protein breakdown. Protein balance is a very important concept, particularly for athletes and active individuals, because proper protein intake can determine the amount of strength and muscle gains retained after each workout. As old proteins are destroyed, new ones are synthesized; therefore skeletal muscle growth only occurs when protein synthesis exceeds that of its breakdown (anabolism). It is thus desirable for those attempting to achieve performance and strength gains to stimulate the synthesis of contractile proteins in skeletal muscle to a rate greater than that of degradation. When this occurs, the net result is a positive protein balance or, more specifically, myofibrillar hypertrophy.

Many studies have been conducted with the ultimate purpose of discovering the methods by which to establish a positive protein balance, especially for those participating in sport and regular physical activity. The most popular approach to the maintenance of a positive protein balance involves protein supplementation, which has been consistently affirmed by empirical research to enhance muscle and strength gains across a variety of populations. It is the amount, type, and timing of such supplementation, however, that continues a decades-long debate among scientists and athletes concerning the proper administration of protein. Although this debate is yet to be resolved, the effect of exercise on protein turnover has been effectively established. The concrete conclusions derived from the effect of exercise can then be interpreted by various populations to understand the potential need for protein supplementation. It has been consistently found that the rate of protein turnover, amino-acid transport, and protein degradation all increase above baseline values after a single bout of resistance training (Biolo et al. 1995; Phillips et al. 1999; Rennie et al. 2004) in both fed (Phillips et al. 2002) and fasted (Biolo et al. 1995; Phillips et al. 1999) subjects, however by different amounts. These studies found an increase in protein synthesis by approximately 100% above baseline levels after exercise, whereas degradation only increased by 50%. Although the fractional synthesis rate of protein was significantly greater after exercise, the results indicated that a negative protein balance occurred despite the slowing of protein turnover (Phillips et al. 1999; Pitkanen et al. 2003), an effect that shifts the protein balance towards neutral as training continues (Phillips et al. 1999). These findings may encourage active individuals to increase their protein availability to working muscles via increased protein intake in order to fuel the increased demand for protein synthesis post-exercise.

A potential training effect must be taken into consideration when investigating the effect of exercise on protein balance. A study by Phillips et al. (2002) found that the acute exercise-induced increases in muscle protein synthesis were gradually reduced after eight weeks of resistance training. These findings are consistent with those observed in chronically resistance-trained individuals (Phillips et al. 1999). In the latter study, when the researchers compared the responses of untrained subjects and subjects with five years of resistance training, it was found that the post-training protein turnover rate was greater in the untrained subjects. This indicates that the body tends to become more efficient in regard to protein turnover as it adapts to regular bouts of resistance training over a prolonged period of time. Although the rate of protein turnover was depressed in trained subjects, eight weeks of resistance training did indeed result in chronic resting protein synthesis (a positive muscle protein status), and a single bout of heavy resistance exercise can increase muscle protein synthesis for up to 24 hours post-exercise (Chesley et al. 1992). Muscle protein synthesis increases rapidly, stays elevated for 24 hours following a heavy bout of resistance training, and then declines to about 14% above baseline at 36 hours (MacDougall et al. 1995). This demonstrates the effectiveness of inducing an increase in protein synthesis by resistance training and suggests the possibility that protein supplementation may need to occur not only around the exercise bout, but additionally during the 24–36 hours after the training session.

6.3 RECOMMENDED DAILY PROTEIN INTAKE

There are 20 amino acids found in protein; humans are able to synthesize 11 of these in the body (nonessential amino acids) and the remaining nine must come from the diet (essential amino acids). A list of the essential and nonessential amino acids appears in Table 6.1.

The ingestion of amino acids is essential to sustain necessary biological processes, and the importance of amino acid supplementation extends far beyond weight training purposes, as outlined in Table 6.2. Consequently, the U.S. Food and Nutrition Board has established various guidelines regarding daily nutrient intake in an effort to prevent nutrient deficiencies and disease among the American population. As a result, the recommended dietary allowance (RDA) was instituted to indicate a minimum daily amount of nutrients required to maintain a healthy lifestyle. Although not an absolute prescription for optimal protein intake to be adopted by all active individuals, the RDA does provide a rough baseline to begin with.

TABLE 6.1
Essential and Nonessential Amino Acids

Essential Amino Acids	Nonessential Amino Acids
– Histidine	– Alanine
– Isoleucine	– Arginine
– Leucine	– Asparagine
– Lysine	– Aspartate
– Methionine	– Cysteine
– Phenylalanine	– Glutamate
– Threonine	– Glutamine
– Tryptophan	– Glycine
– Valine	– Proline
	– Serine
	– Tyrosine

The recommended amount of daily protein intake is generally based on data from nitrogen balance studies, and ranges worldwide from 0.8 to 1.2 g/kg. Protein consumption in America is normally well in excess of the RDA, averaging about 80–100 g per day compared to the recommended 50 g/day (10%–35% daily energy intake) for adults. Unfortunately, the recommendation was established from studies involving sedentary individuals, which does not recognize any potential increase in protein needs for the physically active. Therefore applying the RDA of protein to an active population evokes both speculation and criticism. It has even been suggested that high-protein diets may negatively affect kidney function, but this has not been substantiated (Topic Box 6.1). The next section will discuss the possible adjustments to protein intake advisable for both strength and endurance athletes.

TABLE 6.2
Purposes of Amino Acid Intake

Role of Amino Acid Supplementation

- Metabolism of many organs and tissues
- Synthesis of body proteins
- Metabolic mediators
- Regulatory biological activity (e.g., neurotransmitters, hormones, DNA, RNA)
- Provide structure to all cells
- Prevention of diseases caused by lack of protein
  - *Kwashiorkor*: a pure protein deficiency that occurs primarily in children and is characterized by a bloated belly
  - *Marasmus*: a protein deficiency resulting from a total dietary energy deficiency and characterized by extreme muscle wasting

Source: Adapted from Jeukendrup, A. E., and M. Gleeson. 2010. *Sport nutrition: An introduction to energy production and performance*, 2nd Ed. Champaign, IL: Human Kinetics.

TOPIC BOX 6.1   IS IT POSSIBLE TO CONSUME TOO MUCH PROTEIN?

The body is unable to store excess protein like it does with fat or carbohydrates. Therefore any extra protein consumed that the body does not need is merely excreted. Protein intake above the RDA can cause gastrointestinal discomfort in those not used to such a high dose, so any increase in protein intake should be taken with caution. It has sometimes been suggested that long-term consumption of a high-protein diet may result in impaired kidney function. Such a condition exists only in theory, however, because evidence of it is nonexistent. A high-protein diet may impair kidney function in those with a pre-existing kidney condition or kidney disease (Jeukendrup and Gleeson 2010), however, so individuals with such a condition should seek medical advice from a physician before attempting a high-protein diet.

6.4   PROTEIN RECOMMENDATIONS FOR ATHLETES

Many organizations acknowledge the possibility that strenuous daily activity may increase protein needs in active individuals; however, not all experts agree. Those expending more calories per day tend to consume larger amounts of food to meet the energy demands. As a result of the greater daily caloric intake, larger amounts of protein tend to be consumed each day. According to laboratory measures, daily protein intake is increased by as much as 100% compared to the RDA requirement for a sedentary population (1.6–1.8 versus 0.8 g/kg of body weight), which is much less than the daily protein intake reported by most athletes (Lemon 2000). Several studies have since been conducted with the purpose of investigating the various protein needs of athletes in an array of sports. The external validity of these studies (primarily using a nitrogen balance approach) is questionable, however, because the results may not be directly applicable to exercise performance as laboratory measures instead of applied. Furthermore, it is possible that even if an increased protein requirement was not realized according to nitrogen balance, exercise performance might still be potentially enhanced by a greater protein intake. The extra protein, although not considered to be significant by nitrogen balance standards, might alter a metabolic process or enhance energy utilization during endurance performance or could stimulate anabolism and result in larger muscle mass and strength gains (Lemon 2000). It is thus possible that the recommended protein intake could be suboptimal for a physically active population, even if already dismissed scientifically by the nitrogen balance studies. The results of a substantial amount of research conducted on physically active individuals recently established that regular physical activity can, in fact, increase protein needs in this population. As a result, the adjusted RDA recommendations of protein intake for the physically active remain conflicted and debatable among academics and athletes alike.

The debate over the proper modifications to the RDA for an athletic population tends to revolve around two schools of thought: 1) the belief that participation in exercise and sport increases the nutritional requirement for protein resolutely and 2) the belief that because of training adaptations, the efficiency of protein utilization increases and, therefore, protein requirements for the physically active can always be satisfied by the requirements for sedentary individuals. Unfortunately, there is a web of factors that tends to complicate the two arguments (e.g., energy intake; carbohydrate availability; exercise intensity, duration, and type; dietary-protein quality; training history; gender; age; and timing of nutrient intake). In lieu of the current census of data pertaining to the subject, a substantial amount of studies indicate that the current RDA of protein should indeed be adjusted upward to compensate for the increase in physical activity. The data offer a compromise to the two battling theories, however, by acknowledging not only an upward adjustment needed for the RDA of athletes, but also the prospect that an athlete's diet can compensate for the adjustment without deliberate protein supplementation (Lemon 2000).

There still remains strong empirical evidence for both arguments, and it is understood that amino acids can be oxidized during exercise and that acute endurance exercise has been shown to result in an increased oxidation of various branched chain amino acids (e.g., leucine, isoleucine, and valine). These essential amino acids cannot be synthesized within the body, indicating that they must come from the breakdown of proteins obtained from the diet, thus increasing the daily protein requirement. Even several nitrogen balance studies have confirmed these findings; however, these studies estimate that during prolonged exercise, the relative contribution of protein to energy expenditure is marginal compared to the 5%–15% it provides for the energy expenditure at rest (Jeukendrup and Gleeson 2010). Research has also found that not all amino acids are oxidized to the same degree, suggesting that the estimated protein oxidation rates based on leucine oxidation are overestimated (Koopman et al. 2004). Furthermore, it has been shown that the body adapts to training and becomes more efficient with protein oxidation (Butterfield and Calloway 1984; Phillips et al. 1999). Protein turnover decreases after training, and less net protein degradation occurs, meaning that after an exercise bout, athletes are more efficient and "waste" less protein (Butterfield and Calloway 1984). A study by Lamont et al. (1999) showed that branched-chain amino-acid oxidation was the same in both trained and untrained individuals at the same relative workload, indicating that although protein requirements may increase initially, after training adaptations occur, this increased RDA requirement seems to disappear.

The argument continues as the potential protein requirement of athletes is pondered. Nitrogen balance studies suggest that resistance athletes need approximately 1.5 g/kg of body weight/day; however, this number has been questioned because the studies that concluded this amount are typically short in duration, and a steady state is not always achieved during testing (Rennie and Tipton 2000). A study conducted by Gontzea et al. (1975) demonstrated that the negative nitrogen balance found by many experiments indicative of an increase in protein requirement tends to disappear after about 12 days of training. This principle does tend to fade when training load increases though, because other studies have found that the protein requirement escalates with training load. It is thus maintained that, despite possible evidence to the contrary, strength athletes should ingest about 1.6–1.7 g/kg each day, which is easily achieved with a well-balanced, normal diet without the inclusion

TOPIC BOX 6.2   WHAT ABOUT CREATINE?

Although strength athletes can increase muscle growth with protein supplements, this effect tends to plateau at protein intakes (1.4 g/kg) far below the intakes of experienced body builders (Tarnopolsky et al. 1992). This indicates a possible ceiling effect of protein supplementation, which is potentially raised with the addition of creatine supplementation. Creatine is present in meat and fish, but one would have to consume 4–5 kg of meat/day to equal the creatine intake of supplement studies demonstrating ergogenic effects. For this reason, creatine is most commonly available in powder form to be included with protein powder as an ergogenic supplement. The amount of creatine needed to enhance performance varies among individuals; even modest creatine supplementation (3 g/day) can maintain long-term skeletal muscle gains in strength athletes similar to that of heavy creatine dosages (20 g/day) (Hultman et al. 1996). It is thought that the intake of creatine in combination with large amino-acid intake can potentially explain how a strength athlete can gain mass and strength with protein intakes far exceeding where laboratory studies show no further gains (Lemon 2000).

of extra protein supplementation (Jeukendrup and Gleeson 2010). Furthermore, a 2004 review concluded that the needs of endurance athletes range from 1.0 to 1.6 g/kg of body weight in the case of top sport endurance athletes (Tarnopolsky 2004). The previously discussed research has shown that the increased amino-acid oxidation during exercise might indicate a need for increased protein intake. In fact, many studies have suggested that protein needs may be greater in endurance athletes (Lemon 2000; Meredith et al. 1989) (Topic Box 6.2).

6.5   INFLUENCING FACTORS

As discussed earlier, there are several theories concerning the protein needs of strength athletes, with each argument supported by a body of empirical evidence. Regardless of the debate, the current adjusted recommendation for protein intake for resistance athletes is 1.6–1.7 g/kg of body weight each day. Several factors appear to affect this number. The exact recommendation for the endurance athlete is less clear. However, it has been suggested that their protein needs are similar to the strength athlete (Lemon 2000). In a 2007 review (Campbell et al.), it was concluded that the protein needs of endurance athletes are as high as 1.6 g/kg of body weight where the strength athlete may be 2.0 g/kg of body weight on a daily basis.

6.5.1   ENERGY (FOOD) INTAKE

Inadequate energy intake results in a greater amount of the dietary protein that is required from the diet (Munro 1951), which is most likely due to the diversion of protein to be utilized for energy rather than for functional (enzymatic) and structural (tissue) synthesis (Lemon 2000). This effect is replicated when the energy deficit is caused by an increase in energy expenditure from exercise (Goranzon and Forsum 1985; Walberg et al. 1988), especially in those who are physically active. Protein needs are most likely already increased among strength athletes in order to maintain a higher rate of protein synthesis in the presence of greater absolute tissue. Interestingly, female strength athletes are better able to preserve functional tissue than males during an energy deficit. As a result, females have consistently demonstrated a better ability to maintain body mass at energy intakes below the point where their male counterparts lose a significant percentage of their lean mass (Cortright et al. 1993, 1996, 1997; Pitts 1984; Pitts and Ball 1977). The biological mechanism responsible for this effect may occur via some form of down-regulation of metabolism in females; however, this concept requires much more study.

6.5.2 Carbohydrate Content

The ingestion of amino acids increases its blood concentrations both at rest and post-exercise (Biolo et al. 1997), and these concentrations can be further enhanced by simultaneous carbohydrate intake (Borsheim et al. 2004; Tipton et al. 1999). Carbohydrate availability in exercising muscle is necessary for an intense muscle contraction because of its production of more ATP per unit of oxygen than either fat or protein. Because the body's carbohydrate stores can be relatively easily depleted, even by a single exercise bout, the role of carbohydrate in all forms of exercise has been a topic of interest for decades. An inverse relationship between carbohydrate availability in working muscle and the rate of exercise protein catabolism has been discovered (Lemon and Mullen 1980), which is an idea of great interest. Universal findings suggest that adding some combination of carbohydrate (50–75 g) to a protein source (20–75 g) during heavy resistance training facilitates an increase in the lean mass and overall improvements in body fat percent (Kerksick et al. 2008).

Although the optimal dosage and ratio of amino acids (PRO) to carbohydrates (CHO) required to optimize protein balance is not currently known, a popular approach is to consume a CHO and PRO supplement in a 3:1 or 4:1 ratio within 30 minutes following exercise (Kerksick et al. 2008). Practically, this is the equivalent of consuming 1.2–1.5 g/kg of body weight of simple CHO (such as dextrose or sucrose) with 0.3–0.5 g/kg of body weight of a quality PRO (Borsheim et al. 2002; Rasmussen et al. 2000; Tipton et al. 1999). This practical approach is the most common theory to achieving a desirable protein balance; however, this concept and the details of protein supplementation will be discussed further in the sections to follow.

6.5.3 Protein Quality

Humans only synthesize about half of the necessary amino acids that make up the proteins in the body, so if essential amino acids are not consumed in adequate amounts, normal protein synthesis is compromised. The metabolism of all amino acids is integrated, so it is essential that all 20 amino acids be obtained from the diet. The quality of a protein relates to the degree to which that protein contributes to daily protein requirements and is determined by its essential amino-acid content (Henley and Kuster 1994). Complete proteins (high-quality proteins) contain all of the essential amino acids and typically consist of animal proteins (e.g., dairy products, eggs, meat, and fish). Incomplete proteins (low quality proteins) are deficient in one or more of the essential amino acids and are therefore unable to support human life and growth alone and consist of grains, vegetables, and fruits. There is no significant difference in benefit to protein balance between an essential amino acid–only supplement and a mixed amino-acid supplement (Tipton et al. 1999), so it can be concluded that amino-acid supplementation elicits a positive protein balance response post-exercise regardless of amino acid type.

The most common method to determine protein quality is the Protein Digestibility Corrected Amino Acid Score (PDCAAS), which evaluates protein and assigns each source a ranking determined by comparing the amino-acid profile of the specific food against a standard amino acid profile (Schaafsma 2000) (Table 6.3). The maximum score on the PDCAAS scale is 1.0, which means that after digestion, the protein provides 100% of the essential amino acids required per unit of protein. It must be realized, however, that individuals rarely eat a single protein source at a time, so knowing the individual scores of various protein sources is not always helpful. Most common proteins have scores of 1.0 even though they have different amino acid profiles, so the usefulness of a PDCAAS score can sometimes be fairly limited in its practicality (Jeukendrup and Gleeson 2010).

An appropriate selection of plant protein sources can sufficiently provide the amino acids necessary, but if the right foods are not coordinated together, the individual's dietary protein intake is at risk of being inadequate (Topic Box 6.3). It has been demonstrated that in males between the ages of 50 and 60, strength training produced greater gains in muscle mass in those with a meat-containing diet than those with a lactovegetarian diet (Campbell et al. 1999). This suggests that the type of protein may also play an important role in muscle growth with strength training.

TABLE 6.3
Protein Digestibility Corrected Amino Acid Score (PDCAAS) for Common Foods

Food Source	PDCAAS Value (0.0–1.0)
Whey protein	1.0
Egg-white protein	1.0
Casein protein	1.0
Milk protein	1.0
Soy protein isolate	1.0
Beef	0.92
Soybean	0.91
Kidney beans	0.68
Rye	0.68
Whole wheat	0.54

TOPIC BOX 6.3   HOW DOES VEGETARIANISM MEASURE UP?

Vegetarians are potentially at risk for inadequate protein intake because meat and fish are the most abundant sources of proteins, and animal proteins are generally of higher quality than plant proteins. The quality of protein depends on the kinds of amino acids present in the protein, so animal protein is higher quality not only because all of the essential amino acids are present but also because they are present in larger quantities and in proper proportion. The lack of meat can be balanced by eating more grains and legumes, which are both excellent sources of protein, but these sources are not high-quality proteins. Grains lack lysine, and legumes lack methionine. It is suggested then that vegetarians opt to eat well-processed soybean protein because it is a high-quality protein comparable with that of animal sources.

6.5.4 PROTEIN TYPE

The type of protein ingested, such as whey versus casein protein, may be an important consideration to protein supplementation. Both proteins are derived from milk; however, they differ in their timing of release into the bloodstream. Whey protein exhibits a faster kinetic digestive pattern when compared to casein protein (Boirie et al. 1997; Dangin et al. 2001) and is also responsible for a greater increase in protein synthesis upon ingestion with little to no impact on protein breakdown. The most popular forms of whey protein supplements are available as whey isolates and hydrolyzed whey peptides, which are both preferred among strength athletes, most likely because of their high bioavailability and their inclusion of several critical amino acids (e.g., glutamine, leucine, isoleucine, and valine) (Lemon 2000). Although whey protein has a faster amino-acid release in the body and is sometimes thought to be preferable to any other protein source, casein protein is also a highly effective protein supplement and acts almost in a balance with whey protein supplementation. Casein protein releases amino acids into the blood stream at a slower rate, resulting in little control over protein synthesis, however, with a powerful attenuation of protein breakdown (Kerksick et al. 2008). Numerous studies have investigated the two forms of protein and their effectiveness as ergogenic aids during strength training. Most of the results find that both proteins elicit significant gains in strength and body composition in both male and female strength athletes; however, the two protein types are significantly different from each other in their benefits (Appicelli et al. 1995; Candow et al. 2006; Tipton et al. 2004; Wilborn et al. 2010). Sometimes results suggest that casein may provide a greater overall improvement in protein balance when compared to whey (Boirie et al. 1997; Dangin et al. 2001); however, it is typically advisable to use both whey and casein in conjunction with each other when supplementing the diet with protein. It is generally recommended that individuals consume casein upon waking in the morning and/or before retiring to bed in the evening and to also consume whey protein immediately before and/or immediately after the bout of resistance training. The timing of protein supplementation is also debated, however, and will be discussed next.

6.5.5 PROTEIN TIMING

As mentioned earlier in this chapter, carbohydrate intake can be beneficial to protein supplementation for strength athletes, but this cosupplementation must be timed correctly. Carbohydrate intake immediately following glycogen-depleting exercise can enhance subsequent muscle glycogen resynthesis (Ivy et al. 1988); similarly, it is possible to stimulate muscle growth by minimizing degradation and by maximizing synthesis with carbohydrate and amino-acid ingestion following a bout of strength exercise (Roy et al. 1997; Tipton et al. 1999). This phenomenon is most likely attributed to insulin-stimulated (Farrell et al. 1998; Rasmussen et al. 2000) changes in muscle amino-acid uptake and protein synthesis (Rasmussen et al. 2000).

It has already been established that strength training affects both muscle protein degradation and synthesis, but the magnitude and timing is yet to be perfected (MacDougall et al. 1995; Phillips et al. 1997). Once these two factors have been investigated and refined, it will be a lot easier to provide more precise recommendations to maximize strength gains in not only athletes, but even those who have experienced a loss in motor function caused by disease or disuse, which would be critical in improving quality of life. Researchers have begun to explore the nature of protein and protein plus carbohydrate supplement timing in conjunction with resistance exercise in order to progress towards this goal.

In 2001, Tipton et al. investigated the ingestion of a CHO and PRO (35 g of CHO and 6 g of essential amino acids) supplement consumed either before or immediately after a single bout of resistance exercise performed at 80% of one-repetition maximum (1RM) capability. It was concluded that the effect on net protein balance was greater when the supplement was consumed just prior to exercise and speculated that the increased serum amino-acid levels were most likely the stimulus of the positive protein balance (Tipton et al. 2001). Interestingly, when Tipton et al. replicated their 2001 study with a supplement containing whey protein only instead of a PRO and CHO blend, the authors found a pro-anabolic response when the whey protein was ingested both before and after resistance exercise but with no significant difference between the two administration times (Tipton et al. 2004). These results suggest that a PRO and CHO blend may be more sensitive to time measures surrounding a resistance training bout than when consuming a whey protein supplement alone.

This is consistent with the variable results from an array of studies comparing pre- and post-exercise whey protein supplementation. Some studies demonstrated that pre-exercise ingestion of protein provided better strength gains (Coburn et al. 2006; Tipton et al. 2001; Willoughby et al. 2007), whereas a majority of other research found that post-exercise protein consumption exhibited a larger effect on strength performance and positive protein balance (Borsheim et al. 2002; Cribb et al. 2007a; Cribb et al. 2007b; Hartman et al. 2007; Kerksick et al. 2006, 2007; Kreider et al. 2007; Levenhagen et al. 2001; Miller et al. 2003; Pitkanen et al. 2003; Tarnopolsky et al. 2001; Tipton and Wolfe 2001; Wilkinson et al. 2007), and even additional studies found both timings to have a significant effect but with no significant difference in gains between the two (Cribb and Hayes 2006).

This leads us to the generalization that protein supplementation administered immediately before or immediately after a bout of resistance exercise enhances strength gains (e.g., body composition, 1RM strength, and type II muscle fiber cross-sectional area). In summary, the ingestion of amino acids, either alone or in combination with carbohydrate intake, in close temporal proximity to a bout of resistance training, appears to significantly increase muscle protein synthesis (Tipton et al. 2001, 2004) and to result in greater increases of 1RM strength and leaner body composition (Candow et al. 2006; Coburn et al. 2006; Cribb and Hayes 2006; Kraemer et al. 2007; Willoughby et al. 2007).

6.5.6 TRAINING HISTORY

Amino-acid oxidation tends to increase with regular endurance training (Dohm et al. 1977; Henderson et al. 1985; Layman et al. 1994), which is most likely due to changes in branched-chain oxoacid dehydrogenase activity (Layman et al. 1994). More research is needed to explore this concept, however, because there is no apparent explanation for contradictory observations that fail to support this data (Hood and Terjung 1987). Furthermore, there is additional confusion as to how training status affects protein turnover in strength athletes. It was initially indicated that protein requirements for supporting the increased muscle growth at the beginning of a body-building program might exceed those necessary to maintain the greater muscle mass later in training (Tarnopolsky et al. 1988); however, other research findings suggest that the need for protein remains at similar levels for experienced strength athletes (Lemon et al. 1992; Tarnopolsky et al. 1992). Although muscle protein synthesis can be stimulated by an acute bout of strength exercise in both resistance-trained and untrained subjects, protein breakdown was greater in untrained individuals (Phillips et al. 1999). This provides mechanistic support for the initial observation that a single eccentric bout reduces subsequent muscle damage and pain (Newham et al. 1987) and may also imply that the initial increase in protein needs at the beginning of strength training are reduced with training experience (Lemon 2000).

6.5.7 AGE

Sarcopenia, or muscle wasting because of the aging process, becomes the primary concern for protein balance as one gets older. Although partially caused by a decline in physical activity level, muscle loss is also the result of a 30% reduction in myofibrillar protein synthesis that tends to occur in individuals over 60 years of age (Welle et al. 1993). Muscle performance and function can improve with strength training even into the tenth decade of life (Fiatarone et al. 1990), however, which means sarcopenia can be partially reversed. After three months of regular strength training, the frail and elderly can experience an increase in mixed muscle protein synthesis (Yarasheski et al. 1999), but nutrient intake must be taken into consideration with these gains, because diet tends to be less than ideal in the elderly. Although short-term energy and protein supplementation can enhance protein synthesis and fat-free mass in 60–90-year-old individuals (Bos et al. 2000), it is possible for nutritional supplementation to enhance further muscle growth as strength training continues. It has been observed that a 360-calorie supplement containing 60% carbohydrate, 23% fat, and 17% protein, taken by 72–98-year-old men and women in conjunction with a 10-week strength training program, significantly increased both muscle strength and size more than the same training without supplementation (Singh et al. 1999). In contrast, acute protein intake of 0.6, 1.2, or 2.4 g/kg of body weight did not affect myofibrillar protein synthesis following a 3-week knee extension regimen (Welle and Thornton 1998). These implications seem to be produced by a complex series of concepts not yet understood in the scientific community (Lemon 2000).

The younger population is also of interest, because the dietary protein needs are thought to be greater because of growth (U.S. Food and Nutrition Board 1989). This area still requires more research, however, because it is possible that regular physical activity could further increase protein requirements for the growing population (Roemmich and Sinning 1996, 1997a, 1997b).

6.6 CONCLUSION

The protein needs of individuals who are not physically active can generally be met by ingesting 0.8–1.0 g/kg/day of protein. On the other hand, it is recommended that athletes involved in moderate amounts of intense training consume 1–1.5 g/kg/day of protein, whereas athletes involved in high volume intense training consume 1.5–2.0 g/kg/day of protein (Kreider 2007; Kreider et al. 2010). In addition, proper timing and type of protein must be considered. There does appear to be sufficient evidence to support the use of protein in sport as a safe and effective aid. Protein needs can usually be met by eating protein at every meal. The best food sources of protein come from lean meat and dairy. Chicken, fish, and eggs provide the best options of lean protein, while lean cuts of beef may also be consumed in moderation. Dairy such as fortified skim milk and 2% cheeses can also add protein to the diet while providing other valuable vitamins. Nuts, legumes, and soy can add variety to the diet and are good sources of additional protein. From a training-table perspective, the daily food choices should reflect these ideal sources of protein to adequately meet the needs of athletes, and the needs of the athletes should be individualized based on multiple factors (i.e., goals of the athlete, season, sport/position, etc.).

The International Society of Sports Nutrition has adopted a position stand on protein that highlights the following points (Campbell et al. 2007):

- Exercising individuals need approximately 1.4–2.0 g of protein/kg of body weight/day.
- Concerns that protein intake within this range is unhealthy are unfounded in healthy, exercising individuals.
- An attempt should be made to obtain protein requirements from whole foods, but supplemental protein is a safe and convenient method of ingesting high-quality dietary protein.
- The timing of protein intake in the time period encompassing the exercise session has several benefits including improved recovery and greater gains in fat-free mass.
- Protein residues such as branched-chain amino acids have been shown to be beneficial for the exercising individual, including increasing the rates of

protein synthesis, decreasing the rate of protein degradation, and possibly aiding in recovery from exercise.

- Exercising individuals need more dietary protein than their sedentary counterparts.

REFERENCES

Appicelli, P., T. Ziegenfuss, L. Lowery, K. Carson, M. Rogers, G. Hodsden, and P. Lemon. 1995. Does type of dietary protein supplementation affect muscle strength/size gains in adult bodybuilders? *Can J Appl Physiol* 20(Suppl): 1.

Biolo, G., S. Maggi, and B. Williams. 1995. Increased rates of muscle protein turnover and amino acid transport after resistance exercise in humans. *Am J Physiol* 268: E514–E520.

Biolo, G., K. D. Tipton, and S. Klein. 1997. An abundant supply of amino acids enhances the metabolic effect of exercise on muscle protein. *Am J Physiol* 273: E122–E129.

Boirie, Y., M. Dangin, P. Gachon, M. P. Vasson, J. L. Maubois, and B. Beaufrere. 1997. Slow and fast dietary proteins differently modulate postprandial protein accretion. *Proc Natl Acad Sci USA* 94: 14930–14935.

Borsheim, E., M. G. Cree, K. D. Tipton, T. A. Elliott, A. Aarsland, and R. R. Wolfe. 2004. Effect of carbohydrate intake on net muscle protein synthesis during recovery from resistance exercise. *J Appl Physiol* 96: 674–678.

Borsheim, E., K. D. Tipton, S. E. Wolf, and R. R. Wolfe. 2002. Essential amino acids and muscle protein recovery from resistance exercise. *Am J Physiol Endocrinol Metab* 283: E648–E657.

Bos, C., R. Benamouzig, A. Bruhat, C. Roux, S. Mahé, P. Valensi, C. Gaudichon, F. Ferrière, J. Rauturea, and D. Tomé. 2000. Short-term protein and energy supplementation activates nitrogen kinetics and accretion in poorly nourished elderly subjects. *Am J Clin Nutr* 71: 1129–1137.

Butterfield, G. E., and D. H. Calloway. 1984. Physical activity improves protein utilization in young men. *Brit J Nutr* 51: 171–184.

Campbell, B., R. B. Kreider, T. Ziegenfuss, P. La Bounty, M. Roberts, D. Burke, J. Landis, H. Lopez, and J. Antonio. 2007. International Society of Sports Nutrition position stand: Protein and exercise. *J Inter Soc Sports Nutr* 4: 8.

Campbell, W. W., M. L. Barton, Jr., D. Cyr-Campbell, S. L. Davey, J. L. Beard, G. Parise, and W. J. Evans. 1999. Effects of an omnivorous diet compared with a lacto-ovo-vegetarian diet on resistance-training-induced changes in body composition and skeletal muscle in older men. *Am J Clin Nutr* 70: 1032–1039.

Candow, D. G., N. C. Burke, T. Smith-Palmer, and D. G. Burke. 2006. Effect of whey and soy protein supplementation combined with resistance training in young adults. *Int J Sport Nutr Exerc Metab* 16: 233–244.

Chesley, A., J. D. MacDougall, and M. A. Tarnopolsky. 1992. Changes in human muscle protein synthesis after resistance exercise. *J Appl Physiol* 73: 1383–1388.

Coburn, J. W., D. J. Housh, T. J. Housh, M. H. Malek, T. W. Beck, J. T. Cramer, G. O. Johnson, and P. E. Donlin. 2006. Effects of leucine and whey protein supplementation during eight weeks of unilateral resistance training. *J Strength Cond Res* 20: 284–291.

Cortright, R. N., H. L. Collins, M. P. Chandler, P. W. Lemon, and S. E. DiCarlo. 1996. Diabetes reduces growth and body composition more in male than female rats. *Physiol Beh* 60: 1233–1238.

Cortright, R. N., H. L. Collins, M. P. Chandler, P. W. Lemon, and S. E. DiCarlo. 1997. Daily exercise reduces fat, protein, and body mass in male but not female rats. *Physiol Beh* 62: 105–111.

Cortright, R. N., M. E. Rogers, and P. Lemon. 1993. Does protein intake during endurance exercise affect growth, nitrogen balance, or exercise performance? *Can J Appl Physiol* 18: 403P.

Cribb, P. J., and A. Hayes. 2006. Effects of supplement timing and resistance exercise on skeletal muscle hypertrophy. *Med Sci Sports Exerc* 38: 1918–1925.

Cribb, P. J., A. D. Williams, and A. Hayes. 2007a. A creatine-protein-carbohydrate supplement enhances responses to resistance training. *Med Sci Sports Exerc* 39: 1960–1968.

Cribb, P. J., A. D. Williams, C. G. Stathis, M. F. Carey, and A. Hayes. 2007b. Effects of whey isolate, creatine, and resistance training on muscle hypertrophy. *Med Sci Sports Exerc* 39: 298–307.

Crowe, M. J., J. N. Weatherson, and B. F. Bowden. 2006. Effects of dietary leucine supplementation on exercise performance. *Eur J Appl Phys* 97(6): 664–672.

Dangin, M., Y. Boirie, C. Garcia-Rodenas, P. Gachon, J. Fauquant, P. Callier, O. Ballevre, and B. Beaufrere. 2001. The digestion rate of protein is an independent regulating factor of postprandial protein retention. *Am J Physiol Endocrinol Metab* 280: E340–E348.

Dohm, G. L., A. L. Hecker, W. E. Brown, G. J. Klain, F. R. Puente, E. W. Askew, and G. R. Beecher. 1977. Adaptation of protein metabolism to endurance training. *Biochem J* 164: 705–708.

Farrell, P. A., M. J. Fedele, T. C. Vary, S. R. Kimble, and L. S. Jefferson. 1998. Effects of intensity of acute-resistance exercise on rates of protein synthesis in moderately diabetic rats. *J Appl Physiol* 85: 2291–2297.

Fiatarone, M. A., E. C. Marks, N. D. Ryan, C. N. Meredith, L. A. Lipstiz, and W. J. Evans. 1990. High intensity strength training in nonagenarians: Effects on skeletal muscle. *J Am Med Assoc* 263: 3029–3034.

Gontzea, I., M. Suzuki, and S. Dumitracha. 1975. The influence of adaptation to physical effort on nitrogen balance in man. *Nutr Reports Int* 11: 231–236.

Goranzon, H., and E. Forsum. 1985. Effect of reduced energy intake versus increased physical activity on the outcome of nitrogen balance experiments in man. *Am J Clin Nutr* 41: 919–928.

Hartman, J. W., J. E. Tang, S. B. Wilkinson, M. A. Tarnopolsky, R. L. Lawrence, A. V. Fullerton, and S. M. Phillips. 2007. Consumption of fat-free fluid milk after resistance exercise promotes greater lean mass accretion than does consumption of soy or carbohydrate in young, novice, male weightlifters. *Am J Clin Nutr* 86: 373–381.

Henderson, S. A., A. L. Black, and G. A. Brooks. 1985. Leucine turnover in trained rats during exercise. *Am J Physiol* 249: E137–E144.

Henley, E. C., and J. M. Kuster. 1994. Protein quality evaluation by protein digestibility-corrected amino acid scoring. *Food Tech* 48: 74–77.

Hood, D. A., and R. L. Terjung. 1987. Effect of endurance training on leucine oxidation in perfused rat skeletal muscle. *Am J Physiol* 253: E648–E656.

Hultman, E., K. Soderlund, J. Timmons, G. Cederblad, and P. L. Greenhaff. 1996. Muscle creatine loading in man. *J Appl Physiol* 81: 232–237.

Ivy, J. L., A. L. Katz, C. L. Culter, W. M. Sherman, and E. F. Coyle. 1988. Muscle glycogen synthesis after exercise: Effect of time of carbohydrate ingestion. *J Appl Physiol* 64: 1480–1485.

Jeukendrup, A. E., and M. Gleeson. 2010. *Sport nutrition: An introduction to energy production and performance*, 2nd Ed. Champaign, IL: Human Kinetics.

Kerksick, C. M., T. Harvey, J. Stout, B. Campbell, C. Wilborn, R. Kreider, D. Kalman, T. Ziegenfuss, H. Lopez, J. Landis, J. L. Ivy, and J. Antonio. 2008. International society of sport nutrition position stand: Nutrient timing. *J Inter Soc Sports Nutr* 5: 17.

Kerksick, C. M., C. L. Rasmussen, S. L. Lancaster, B. Magu, P. Smith, C. Melton, M. Greenwood, A. L. Almada, C. P. Earnest, and R. B. Kreider. 2006. The effects of protein and amino acid supplementation on performance and training adaptations during ten weeks of resistance training. *J Strength Cond Res* 20: 643–653.

Kerksick, C. M., C. Rasmussen, S. Lancaster, M. Starks, P. Smith, C. Melton, M. Greenwood, A. Almada, and R. Kreider. 2007. Impact of differing protein sources and a creatine containing nutritional formula after 12 weeks of resistance training. *Nutrition* 23: 647–656.

Koopman, R., A. M. Wagenmakers, R. F. Manders, A. G. Zorenc, J. G. Senden, M. Gorselink, H. A. Keizer, and L. J. C. van Loon. 2004. Combined ingestion of protein and free leucine with carbohydrate increases post-exercise muscle protein synthesis in vivo in male subjects. *Am J Physiol Endocrinol Metab* 288: E645–E653.

Kraemer, W. J., D. L. Hatfield, B. A. Spiering, J. L. Vingren, M. S. Fragala, J. Y. Ho, J. S. Volek, J. M. Anderson, and C. M. Maresh. 2007. Effects of a multi-nutrient supplement on exercise performance and hormonal responses to resistance exercise. *Eur J Appl Physiol* 101: 637–646.

Kreider, R. B., C. D. Wilborn, L. Taylor, B. Campbell, A. L. Almada, R. Collins et al. 2010. ISSN exercise & sport nutrition review: Research and recommendations. *J ISSN* 7(7).

Kreider, R. B., C. P. Earnest, J. Lundberg, C. Rasmussen, M. Greenwood, P. Cowan, and A. L. Almada. 2007. Effects of ingesting protein with various forms of carbohydrate following resistance-exercise on substrate availability and markers of anabolism, catabolism, and immunity. *J Int Soc Sports Nutr* 4: 18.

Lamont, L. S., A. J. McCullough, and S. C. Kalhan. 1999. Comparison of leucine kinetics in endurance-trained and sedentary humans. *J Appl Physiol* 86: 320–325.

Layman, D. K., G. L. Paul, and M. H. Olken. 1994. Amino acid metabolism during exercise. *Nutrition in Exercise and Sport*, edited by I. Wolinsky and J. F. Hickson, 2nd Ed., pp. 123–137. Boca Raton, FL: CRC Press.

Lemon, P. R. 2000. Beyond the zone: Protein needs of active individuals. *J Am College Nutr* 5: 513S–521S.

Lemon, P. R., and J. P. Mullin. 1980. Effect of initial muscle glycogen levels on protein catabolism during exercise. *J Appl Physiol* 48: 624–629.

Lemon, P. R., M. A. Tarnopolsky, J. D. MacDougall, and S. A. Atkinson. 1992. Protein requirements and muscle mass/strength changes during intensive training in novice bodybuilders. *J Appl Physiol* 73: 767–775.

Levenhagen, D. K., J. D. Gresham, M. G. Carlson, D. J. Maron, M. J. Borel, and P. J. Flakoll. 2001. Post-exercise nutrient intake timing in humans is critical to recovery of leg glucose and protein homeostasis. *Am J Physiol Endocrinol Metab* 280: E982–E993.

Louard, R. J., Barrett E. J., and R. A. Gelfand. 1990. Effect of infused branched-chain amino acids on muscle and whole-body amino acid metabolism in man. *Clin Sci* 79: 457–466.

MacDougall, J. D., M. J. Gibala, and M. A. Tarnopolsky. 1995. The time course for elevated muscle protein synthesis following heavy resistance exercise. *Can J Appl Physiol* 20: 480–486.

Meredith, C. N., M. J. Zackin, W. R. Frontera, and W. J. Evans. 1989. Dietary protein requirements and body protein metabolism in endurance-trained men. *J Appl Physiol* 66: 2850–2856.

Miller, S. L., K. D. Tipton, D. L. Chinkes, S. E. Wolf, and R. R. Wolfe. 2003. Independent and combined effects of amino acids and glucose after resistance exercise. *Med Sci Sports Exerc* 35: 449–455.

Munro, H. N. 1951. Carbohydrate and fat as factors in protein utilization and metabolism. *Physiol Rev* 31: 449–488.

Newham, D. J., D. A. Jones, and P. M. Clarkson. 1987. Repeated high-force eccentric exercise: Effects on muscle pain and damage. *J Appl Physiol* 63: 1381–1386.

Phillips, S. M., G. Parise, and B. D. Roy. 2002. Resistance-training-induced adaptations in skeletal muscle protein turnover in the fed state. *Can J Physiol Pharmacol* 80: 1045–1053.

Phillips, S. M., K. D. Tipton, A. Aarsland, S. E. Wolfe, and R. R. Wolfe. 1997. Mixed muscle protein synthesis and breakdown after resistance exercise in humans. *Am J Physiol* 273: E99–E107.

Phillips, S. M., K. D. Tipton, and A. A. Ferrando. 1999. Resistance training reduces the acute exercise-induced increase in muscle protein turnover. *Am J Physiol* 276: E118–E124.

Pitkanen, H. T., T. Nykanen, J. Knuutinen, K. Lahti, O. Keinanen, M. Alen, P. V. Komi, and A. A. Mero. 2003. Free amino acid pool and muscle protein balance after resistance exercise. *Med Sci Sports Exerc* 35: 784–792.

Pitts, G. C. 1984. Body composition in the rat: interactions of exercise, age, sex, and diet. *Am J Physiol* 246: R495–R501.

Pitts, G. C. and L. S. Ball. 1977. Exercise, dietary obesity and growth in the rat. *Am J Physiol* 232: R38–R44.

Rasmussen, B. B., K. D. Tipton, S. L. Miller, S. E. Wolf, and R. R. Wolfe. 2000. An oral essential amino acid-carbohydrate supplement enhances muscle protein anabolism after resistance exercise. *J Appl Physiol* 88: 386–392.

Rennie, M. J. and K. D. Tipton. 2000. Protein and amino acid metabolism during and after exercise and the effects of nutrition. *Annu Rev Nutr* 20: 457–483.

Rennie, M. J., H. Wackerhage, and E. E. Spangenburg. 2004. Control of the size of the human muscle mass. *Annu Rev Physiol* 66: 799–828.

Roemmich, R. N., and W. E. Sinning. 1996. Sport-seasonal changes in body composition, growth, power, and strength of adolescent wrestlers. *Int J Sports Med* 17: 92–99.

Roemmich, R. N., and W. E. Sinning. 1997a. Weight loss and wrestling training: Effects on nutrition, growth, maturation, body composition, and strength. *J Appl Physiol* 82: 1751–1759.

Roemmich, R. N., and W. E. Sinning. 1997b. Weight loss and wrestling training: Effects on growth-related hormones. *J Appl Physiol* 82: 1760–1764.

Roy, B. D., M. A. Tarnopolsky, J. D. MacDougall, J. Fowles, and K. E. Yarasheski. 1997. Effect of glucose supplement timing on protein metabolism after resistance training. *J Appl Physiol* 82: 1882–1888.

Schaafsma, G. 2000. The protein digestibility corrected amino acid score. *J Nutr* 130(7): 18655–18675.

Singh, M. A., W. Ding, T. J. Manfredi, G. S. Solares, E. F. O'Neill, K. M. Clements, N. D. Ryan, J. J. Kehayias, R. A. Fielding, and W. J. Evans. 1999. Insulin-like growth factor I in skeletal muscle after weight lifting exercise in frail elders. *Am J Physiol* 277: E135–E143.

Tarnopolsky, M. A. 2004. Protein requirements for endurance athletes. *Nutrition* 20: 662–668.

Tarnopolsky, M. A., S. A. Atkinson, J. D. MacDougall, A. Chesley, S. Phillips, and H. Schwarcz. 1992. Evaluation of protein requirements for trained strength athletes. *J Appl Physiol* 73: 1986–1995.

Tarnopolsky, M. A., J. D. MacDougall, and S. A. Atkinson. 1988. Influence of protein intake and training status on nitrogen balance and lean body mass. *J Appl Physiol* 64: 187–193.

Tarnopolsky, M. A., G. Parise, N. J. Yardley, C. S. Ballantyne, S. Olatinji, and S. M. Phillips. 2001. Creatine-dextrose and protein-dextrose induce similar strength gains during training. *Med Sci Sports Exerc* 33: 2044–2052.

Tipton, K. D., T. A. Elliott, and M. G. Cree. 2004. Ingestion of casein and whey proteins results in muscle anabolism after resistance exercise. *Med Sci Sports Exerc* 36: 2073–2081.

Tipton, K. D., A. A. Ferrando, and S. M. Phillips. 1999. Post-exercise net protein synthesis in human muscle from orally administered amino acids. *Am J Physiol* 276: E628–E634.

Tipton, K. D., B. B. Rasmussen, S. L. Miller, S. E. Wolf, S. K. Owens-Stovall, B. E. Petrini, and R. R. Wolfe. 2001. Timing of amino acid-carbohydrate ingestion alters anabolic response of muscle to resistance exercise. *Am J Physiol Endocrinol Metab* 281: E197–E206.

Tipton, K. D., and R. R. Wolfe. 2001. Exercise, protein metabolism, and muscle growth. *Int J Sport Nutr Exerc Metab* 11: 109–132.

U.S. Food and Nutrition Board. 1989. *Recommended Dietary Allowances*. Washington, D.C.: National Academy Press.

Walberg, J. L., M. K. Leidy, D. J. Sturgill, D. E. Hinkle, S. J. Richey, and D. R. Sebolt. 1988. Macronutrient content of a hypoenergy diet affects nitrogen retention and muscle function in weight lifters. *Int J Sport Nutr* 9: 261–266.

Welle, S., and C. A. Thornton. 1998. High protein meals do not enhance myofibrillar synthesis after resistance exercise in 62–75-yr-old men and women. *Am J Physiol* 274: E677–E683.

Welle, S., C. Thornton, R. Jozefowicz, and M. Statt. 1993. Myofibrillar protein synthesis in young and old men. *Am J Physiol* 264: E693–E698.

Wilborn, C. D., L.W. Taylor, C. A. Foster, M., B. Campbell, M. McAdams, K. Dugan, M. Lewing, T. Jones, C. Woodall, and A. White. 2010. The effects of pre- and post-exercise whey versus casein protein consumption on body composition and performance measures in collegiate female athletes. *Med Sci Sports Exerc* 42: S2855.

Wilkinson, S. B., M. A. Tarnopolsky, M. J. Macdonald, J. R. Macdonald, D. Armstrong, and S. M. Phillips. 2007. Consumption of fluid skim milk promotes greater muscle protein accretion after resistance exercise than does consumption of an isonitrogenous and isoenergetic soy-protein beverage. *Am J Clin Nutr* 85:1031–1040.

Willoughby, D. S., J. R. Stout, and C. D. Wilborn. 2007. Effects of resistance training and protein plus amino acid supplementation on muscle anabolic, mass, and strength. *Amino Acids* 32: 467–477.

Yarasheski, K. E., J. Pak-Loduca, D. L. Hasten, K. A. Obert, M. B. Brown, and D. R. Sinacore. 1999. Resistance exercise training increases mixed muscle protein synthesis rate in frail men and women 76 yr old. *Am J Physiol* 277: E118–E125.

7 Carbohydrate Needs of Athletes

Christopher J. Rasmussen

CONTENTS

7.1 INTRODUCTION

Athletes have special nutritional needs that go above and beyond those of the normal sedentary individual. To optimize performance, athletes need a solid foundation that includes proper training and nutrition. Proper training should be based on the principles of training and largely depends on the goals of the individual athlete and the point in time within the training cycle (pre-season, in-season, and post-season). Proper nutrition should focus on a variety of whole foods that adequately meet the demands of the athlete, and this nutritional approach will vary depending on the athlete's "season" and individual goals (hypertrophy versus strength gains, etc.). This chapter largely addresses the specific nutritional needs of athletes and more specifically the carbohydrate needs of athletes.

Numerous studies have documented that athletes can improve their training sessions and performance with a quality nutritional plan that includes the correct amount of carbohydrates (Coyle 1995; Haff et al. 2003; Haub et al. 2003). To gain a better understanding of how carbohydrate intake can improve performance for the athlete, it is important to realize what drives their performance. Therefore, the chapter begins with a description of the factors associated with optimal performance of the athlete and the factors that limit their performance. The second section emphasizes how carbohydrates in the everyday diet serve as the foundation of the training-table concept. The third section focuses on pre-exercise carbohydrate intake of the athlete and different forms of carbohydrate loading. The fourth section discusses carbohydrate supplementation during exercise and the differences between solid and liquid supplementation. The fifth section looks into how post-exercise carbohydrate supplementation is vital during the short window immediately following exercise. Finally, the last section briefly discusses immune system considerations. A concise summary then reviews the most important points of the chapter and brings it to a close to provide some take-home and practical issues for the reader.

7.2   FACTORS LIMITING ATHLETIC PERFORMANCE

Manipulating the principles of training depending on the overall goals while coinciding with the respective training season helps optimize training and subsequent performance. Prior to discussing the specific carbohydrate needs of athletes, it is important to understand a few of the factors that limit athletic performance along with one popular scapegoat that may not be responsible for all the ills for which it is blamed. Dehydration, the depletion of muscle glycogen and limited blood glucose availability can all play a role in fatigue during athletic training and/or competition.

7.2.1   DEHYDRATION

The body transfers heat to the environment through conduction, convection, radiation, evaporation, or a combination of these methods. Evaporation is the primary avenue for heat dissipation during exercise, accounting for roughly 80% of the total heat loss during exercise. With prolonged exercise or exercise in a hot and humid environment, blood volume is reduced by a loss of water through sweat. As exercise continues in a hot, humid environment, a redistribution of blood from the core to the periphery takes place to cool the body. Cardiac filling is reduced as the total blood volume gradually decreases with an increase in the duration of exercise. This leads to a decrease in venous return to the right side of the heart. Subsequently, stroke volume is reduced. The heart rate then tries to compensate for the decreased stroke volume by increasing its effort to maintain cardiac output. Collectively, these alterations are referred to as the cardiovascular drift.

The benefit of cardiovascular drift is that one is able to continue exercising at a low to moderate intensity. The drawback is that the body is unable to compensate fully for the decreased stroke volume at high exercise intensities because the heart rate attains its maximum value at much lower exercise intensities. A loss of body fluid equal to 1% of body weight (approximately 2.0 pounds for a 200-pound athlete) can significantly reduce blood volume, cause undue stress on the cardiovascular system, and limit physical performance (Coyle and Montain 1992). When dehydration reaches 4%, athletes can experience heat cramps and heat exhaustion (Armstrong et al. 1985), and when it reaches upwards of 6%, there may be cessation of sweating, a rise in body temperature, and eventually heat stroke (Sutton and Bar-Or 1980).

7.2.2 Muscle Glycogen/Blood Glucose Depletion

Collectively, the depletion of muscle glycogen and the decline in blood glucose can also put a damper on athletic performance. Carbohydrates serve as a very limited energy source compared to the energy stored as protein and triglyceride. The average carbohydrate stores represent approximately 2000 kcal of energy, comprising only 1%–2% of the total bodily energy stores (Goodman 1988). Carbohydrate is stored in skeletal muscle (79% of total carbohydrate) and liver (14% of total carbohydrate) in the form of glycogen and in the blood (7% of the total carbohydrate) in the form of glucose (Sherman 1995). Plasma fatty acids and muscle triglycerides are able to supply the needed energy during low-intensity exercise (i.e., 25% VO_{2max}) (Coyle 1995). Carbohydrate use is relatively low and is derived from blood glucose.

Exercise at lower intensities can be maintained for several hours because the liver is able to continually supply glucose to the working muscles. As the intensity of exercise increases, the amount of carbohydrate necessary to keep pace with the increased demand also increases. A combination of blood glucose and muscle glycogen contributes a large percentage of the energy requirements at moderate exercise intensities (i.e., 65% VO_{2max}) (Coyle 1995). At the beginning of exercise, muscle glycogen is the preferred fuel source, but as these levels decline there is increased dependence on blood glucose by the exercising muscles and other tissues in the body that prefer glucose as a fuel source (i.e., nervous system).

Higher-intensity exercise (85% VO_{2max}) is performed at a level that promotes an even higher rate of muscle glycogen breakdown and carbohydrate oxidation (Coyle 1995), which results in an accelerated rate of lactic acid production and ultimately accumulation in muscle and blood. Higher-intensity exercise represents the highest level an athlete can maintain for approximately 60 minutes. At these high intensities, carbohydrate oxidation accounts for more than two-thirds of the required energy, with the remainder coming from a combination of plasma fatty acids and intramuscular triglycerides. Given the fact that most competitive athletes often train and compete at a high intensity, it is easy to reason why the depletion of muscle glycogen and the subsequent decline in blood glucose can be such a deterrent to athletic performance. Maintaining adequate hydration and energy supplies is therefore essential to the performance of the athlete, which creates the basic rationale for the consumption of sports drinks during training or competition.

7.2.3 LACTIC ACID AND LACTATE

Contrary to popular belief, lactic acid and lactate are not responsible for all the ills for which they are blamed. Lactic acid and lactate are not the same compound. Lactate is any salt of lactic acid that enters the blood during high-intensity efforts. Recall that lactic acid is a by-product of glycolysis or carbohydrate breakdown during anaerobic conditions. Although most people believe that it is responsible for muscle soreness and exhaustion during all types of exercise, lactic acid accumulates in muscle fibers only during relatively brief high-intensity efforts and is also a constant substrate that is taken up by the liver and converted to glucose to provide a constant flux of glucose into the blood, which is free to be taken up in the working muscle.

Athletes have been told for years that the primary reason they cannot "push" any longer during intense exercise is that lactic acid has built up in their muscles. This is not entirely true, and there is evidence to disprove it. It is possible to experience muscle fatigue while the lactic-acid concentration in the muscle remains low. Marathon runners, for example, may have near-resting lactic-acid levels at the end of a race, despite their exhaustion (Thibault 2006). Conversely, there can be an absence of fatigue when the lactic-acid concentration in the muscle is high. Exhausting isometric efforts with the quadriceps, for example, can cause fatigue and ultimately terminate the exercise. Minutes after completion, the athlete can once again produce the initial force despite the fact that the degree of acidity in the muscles decreases to normal rather slowly. Therefore, it is difficult to accept the idea that an increase in lactic acid in the muscle causes fatigue because a high degree of acidity without fatigue can be observed.

Lactate can also serve as an important fuel source by other tissues by converting it to pyruvate and oxidizing it in the mitochondria. For example, during exercise lactate serves as a significant fuel source for the cardiac muscle of the working heart (Thibault 2006). Therefore, the fatigue experienced by the athlete is largely caused by a combination of dehydration and inadequate energy supplies, not excess lactic acid. It is imperative to consider these factors before we proceed with discussions on the carbohydrate needs of athletes.

7.3 CARBOHYDRATES IN THE EVERYDAY DIET

The daily approach to nutrition forms the foundation of the training-table concept. Nutrition not only plays a role in athletic performance but can also influence our general health, well being, appearance, behavior, and mood. Nutrients in the diet aid with growth and development, regulate metabolism, and provide energy. Carbohydrates contain 4 calories/g and are classified as a macronutrient along with the other calorie containing nutrients fat (9 kcal/g) and protein (4 kcal/g). Alcohol also contains calories (7 kcal/g), but these are often referred to as empty calories because they are of little to no nutritional value. Carbohydrates are the leading nutrient fuel for working muscles and are utilized more readily than fats and protein. In addition, they can be broken down to glucose to be used by the brain and nervous system for energy. Glucose is also converted to glycogen for storage in the liver and muscle.

7.3.1 Carbohydrate Structure and Classification

From a structural point of view, carbohydrates have traditionally been classified as simple and complex. Simple carbohydrates are formed from individual glucose, sucrose, or fructose molecules, whereas complex carbohydrates are formed from chains of glucose molecules. More specifically, there are two types of simple carbohydrates, monosaccharides and disaccharides. Monosaccharides are made up of glucose, fructose, and galactose, and disaccharides are made up of sucrose, lactose, and maltose. Complex carbohydrates are known as polysaccharides and include starch, glycogen, and cellulose (an indigestible fiber).

7.3.2 Glycemic Index and Glycemic Load

Recently the glycemic index (GI) and glycemic load (GL) have been used more readily to classify carbohydrates. The GI is a ranking of foods based on their actual postprandial blood glucose response compared with a reference food, either glucose or white bread. Foods are ranked on a scale of 0 to 100 with 0 representing the lowest GI and 100 representing the highest. The GI concept was first developed in 1981 by a team of scientists led by Dr. David Jenkins, a professor of nutrition at the University of Toronto, Canada, to help determine which foods were best for people with diabetes (Brand-Miller et al. 1999).

At that time, the diet for people with diabetes was based on a system of carbohydrate exchanges or portions, which was complicated and not very logical. The carbohydrate-exchange systems assumed that all starchy foods produce the same effect on blood-sugar levels, even though some earlier studies had already proven that this was not correct. Jenkins was one of the first researchers to question this assumption and to investigate how real foods behave in the bodies of real people (Brand-Miller et al. 1999). The GI of a food is based on several factors including: the physical form of the food, the amylase-to-amylopectin ratio (two different types of starch), sugar content, fiber content, fat content, and the acidity of the food (Brand-Miller et al. 1999). The index consists of a scale from 0 to 100 with 0 (water) representing the lowest ranking and 100 (pure glucose) representing the highest ranking. The GI of a carbohydrate has a profound effect on subsequent glucose and insulin responses:

- High-GI carbohydrates (i.e., dextrose and maltose) produce large increases in glucose and insulin levels.
- Moderate-GI carbohydrates (i.e., sucrose and lactose) produce modest increases in glucose and insulin levels.
- Low-GI carbohydrates (i.e., fructose and maltodextrin) produce small increases in glucose and insulin levels.

It has been suggested that manipulating the GI of a sports supplement may optimize carbohydrate availability for exercise, particularly prolonged intense exercise. Caution should be used, however, with applying the GI to whole foods that contain several ingredients. The GI is more accurate for individually packed foods/supplements because of the minimal number of ingredients and the standardization that exists with the processing of these snacks/supplements. The GI is not applicable to whole foods/meals and has not been established for many of these whole foods/meals.

Thus, Harvard researchers created the GL in the late 1990s to take into account the amount of carbohydrate in a given serving of a food (Salmeron et al. 1997). These researchers reported that the GL is an independent predictor of an individual's risk for developing Type 2 diabetes (Salmeron et al. 1997) and coronary heart disease (Liu et al. 2000). The GL is based on not only the glycemic index of a particular food but also the grams of carbohydrate in that given food (GL = [GI × the amount of carbohydrate]/100). It also has a scale with 10 or less representing a low GL, 11–19 representing a medium GL, and 20 or greater representing a high GL. It is a variable that represents the quality and quantity of a carbohydrate (Salmeron et al. 1997). The higher the GL for the carbohydrate, the greater the expected increase in blood glucose. Subsequently, this would lead to a significantly greater increase in circulating insulin (Foster-Powell et al. 2002; Ludwig 2003). The GL therefore provides a more useful measure that is applicable to food in the everyday diet. In addition, it can be a helpful tool for athletes looking to lose, maintain, or gain weight. Table 7.1 lists many foods and their respective glycemic-index and glycemic-load rankings.

7.3.3 CARBOHYDRATE RECOMMENDATIONS

It is recommended that the nonexercising individual consume approximately 55% of their total calories from carbohydrates. Considering that daily energy expenditure for athletes is approximately 1.5 to 3 times higher than for the average individual, it is imperative to maintain the balance between energy intake and expenditure. Carbohydrate intake requirements vary depending on the type of athlete, with the recommended intake for those athletes engaged in endurance events (ultramarathons, marathons, stage cycling, triathlons, etc.) set at approximately 60%–65% of total calories or 7–9 g/kg/day (Sherman 1995; Sherman and Wimer 1991). The high recommendation is because carbohydrates are the preferred fuel source and are needed for long continuous activity. The recommended carbohydrate intake for those athletes engaged in strength/power type of events (power lifting, Olympic lifting, football, rugby, etc.) is slightly lower than that of the endurance athlete or approximately 55% of total calories or 5–6 g/kg/day (Lambert et al. 2004). This level of carbohydrate intake seems to be crucial in order to maintain high-intensity resistance-training workouts.

Finally, the recommended carbohydrate intake for those athletes engaged in physique type of events (body building, fitness/figure competition, etc.) varies and largely depends on where the athlete is in their training/competition cycle. These athletes are somewhat unique in that they are perhaps the only class of athlete that is judged solely on appearance (muscle hypertrophy, symmetry, definition, etc.). The total carbohydrate intake for these athletes tends to decrease as a competition nears. During training, or the "building phase" as it is commonly known, carbohydrate intake largely mirrors that of other strength/power athletes (55%–60% of total calories). As competition nears, the carbohydrate intake is reduced to 40%–45% of total calories or 2–3 g/kg/day. This is commonly referred to the "cutting phase" where

TABLE 7.1

Glycemic Index (GI) and Glycemic Loads (GL) of Various Foods using White Bread (GI = 100) as the Standard

Food	GI	GL	Food	GI	GL
Bakery products			Fruits (continued)		
Angel food cake	95	19	Peaches	60	5
Croissant	96	17	Pears	47	4
Doughnut (cake)	108	17	Pineapples	94	6
Bran muffin	85	15	Plums	34	3
Scones	131	7	Watermelon	103	4
Beverages			Legumes		
Coca-Cola	76	14	Baked beans	69	7
Gatorade	111	12	Chickpeas	47	10
Orange juice	71	13	Kidney beans	41	7
Smoothie, raspberry	48	14	Lentils	41	5
Breads			Pasta and noodles		
Bagel	103	25	Linguine	65	22
Baguette (French)	136	15	Macaroni	67	23
Pita bread	82	10	Spaghetti	59	20
Rye bread	58	5	Snack foods		
Breakfast cereals			Corn chips	103	18
All-Bran	54	9	Jelly beans	112	22
Corn flakes	130	24	M & Ms (peanut)	47	6
Grapenuts	107	16	Peanuts	21	1
Life	94	14	Popcorn	103	8
Special K	98	14	Potato chips	77	11
Cereal grains and pasta			Powerbar (chocolate)	79	24
Barley	36	11	Pretzels	119	16
Brown rice	79	18	Skittles	100	32
Cracked wheat	68	12	Snickers bar	78	19
White rice (long grain)	80	24	Sugars		
Dairy foods			Fructose	27	2
Ice cream	87	8	Glucose	141	10
Ice cream (low fat)	71	3	Honey	78	10
Milk (full fat)	38	3	Lactose	66	5
Milk (skim)	46	4	Maltose	150	11
Yogurt (artificial sweetener)	20	2	Sucrose	97	7
Fruits			Vegetables		
Apples	52	6	Corn	78	9
Banana	74	12	Carrots	131	5
Cherries	32	3	Peas	68	3
Grapefruit	36	3	Potato (baked)	121	26
Grapes	62	7	Sweet potato	87	17
Oranges	60	5	Yam	53	13

carbohydrates are largely replaced with protein and quality fats. The majority of these athletes know that replacing carbohydrate with protein and unsaturated fat is an effective way to promote significant losses of fat mass while sparing lean body mass. Numerous studies have demonstrated this in the research setting and have attributed it to possible increased insulin sensitivity and the thermogenic properties involved in digesting different macronutrients (Baba et al. 1999; Parker et al. 2002; Slov 1999).

It is important to remember that these guidelines should always consider individual total energy needs, the specificity of training, and individual performance. For example, if there is inadequate carbohydrate intake between endurance and/or high-repetition strength-training sessions, the quality of strength training could potentially be less than desired. This could very well result in less than optimal strength and power development over the course of a training cycle.

7.4 PRE-EXERCISE CARBOHYDRATE INTAKE

Pre-exercise nutrition traditionally focuses specifically on carbohydrate intake especially for athletes engaging in endurance type of events or those lasting in excess of 60 minutes. Years of research have demonstrated that as exercise intensity increases, there is a greater reliance on muscle glycogen as the primary energy source. Furthermore, the perception of fatigue during prolonged strenuous exercise coincides with the decrease in muscle glycogen concentration (Ahlborg et al. 1967; Hermansen et al. 1967).

7.4.1 CARBOHYDRATE LOADING

Carbohydrate-loading techniques have been investigated for years in attempts to maximize pre-exercise glycogen levels. According to Ivy (2008), muscle glycogen stores normally range between 90 and 100 $\mu mol \cdot g^{-1}$ wet muscle weight. Endurance training can increase the average muscle glycogen concentration to 120–130 $\mu mol \cdot g^{-1}$ wet muscle weight, and consuming a high-carbohydrate diet can elevate the glycogen stores to 140–150 $\mu mol \cdot g^{-1}$ wet muscle weight during training.

7.4.1.1 Traditional Model

Early investigations by Bergstrom et al. (1967) discovered that the most effective method of increasing muscle glycogen stores was by first depleting these stores with intense exercise. Also, a diet high in protein and fat and void of carbohydrate was to be followed for three days in an attempt to maintain a low glycogen concentration. Finally, a second intense exercise session was conducted in an attempt to lower muscle glycogen stores even more followed immediately by a high carbohydrate diet for three days. This traditional approach was found to double the normal levels of muscle glycogen stores, thus providing a significantly increased amount of available stored fuel during competitive endurance events. Despite its effectiveness, the two glycogen-depleting exercise sessions combined with the three-day diet between proved quite challenging for many athletes and oftentimes resulted in unwanted fatigue and lethargy leading up to their event.

7.4.1.2 Modified Model

In an attempt to refine the traditional carbohydrate-loading technique, Sherman (1995) tried to develop a less extreme and/or more modern method. Their protocol began with a similar glycogen-depleting exercise session followed immediately by a three-day mixed diet comprised of 45%–50% carbohydrate. This mirrored the natural training taper often exhibited by endurance athletes prior to a major event. The training taper was continued for the next three days while the carbohydrate intake was increased to nearly 70% of total calories. This method was found to increase muscle glycogen levels to nearly 200 $\mu mol \cdot g^{-1}$ wet muscle weight, which was similar to that found with the traditional method proposed by Bergstrom et al. (1967).

The highlight of this more modern method was the fact that the carbohydrate-loading technique was more attuned with the normal training schedules used by endurance athletes prior to competition. Further attempts have been made to simplify the carbohydrate-loading techniques even more by decreasing the time needed to maximize muscle glycogen stores. Recent research has demonstrated that highly trained athletes can increase muscle glycogen stores within a 24-hour period by performing only three minutes of supramaximal exercise followed by a high-carbohydrate diet (Fairchild et al. 2002). This method begins with a short, intense exercise session, followed by a rest period and subsequent high-carbohydrate diet. In addition, Bussau et al. (2002) reported that trained athletes could increase their muscle glycogen stores to 180 $\mu mol \cdot g^{-1}$ wet muscle weight in 24 hours after glycogen-depleting exercise if they remained inactive during recovery and ingested 10 g of carbohydrate/kg of body weight. These abbreviated methods could prove beneficial for those endurance athletes engaged in multiple competitions within the same week (track meets, staged cycling, etc.).

7.4.2 Carbohydrate Intake Immediately Prior to Exercise

As the event nears, pre-exercise carbohydrate intake should consist largely of moderate- to low-GI foods/supplements that provide the slow, sustained release of carbohydrates and protein necessary to fuel a workout. It generally takes about 2–4 hours for dietary carbohydrate to be digested and begin to be stored as muscle and liver glycogen. Thus, pre-exercise meals should be consumed about 4–6 hours before exercise (Kreider et al. 1998). Putting this into an average everyday scenario means that if an athlete trains in the afternoon, breakfast is the most important meal to top off muscle and liver glycogen levels. If the athlete trains first thing in the morning, the meal the evening before is vital.

The benefit/purposes of the precompetition meal are to

- Super compensate muscle and liver glycogen levels
- Decrease the rate of lipolysis and fatty acid oxidation
- Increase the reliance of blood glucose at the onset of exercise
- Fully hydrate
- Delay the onset of fatigue
- Improve performance

The selection of foods/supplements is largely up to the individual athlete and their personal preferences. It is recommended that the athlete consume something familiar on the day of competition as opposed to experimenting with a novel food/supplement.

Recent research has indicated that ingesting a light carbohydrate and protein snack 30–60 minutes before exercise (e.g., 50 g of carbohydrate and 5–10 g of protein) serves to further increase carbohydrate availability toward the end of an intense exercise bout because of the slight increase in glucose and insulin levels (Cade 1997; Carli 1992). This can serve to increase the availability of amino acids and decrease exercise-induced catabolism (Cade 1997; Carli 1992; Kreider et al. 1998). Insulin inhibits protein degradation and apparently offsets the catabolic effects of other hormones, namely cortisol (Komi 1992). Anabolic actions of insulin seem to be related to its nitrogen-sparing effects and promotion of nitrogen retention (Komi 1992). In addition, resistance training in combination with immediate amino-acid administration has been shown to augment protein synthesis acutely. One would thus expect more pronounced muscle hypertrophy over a prolonged period (Table 7.2).

A limited number of investigators have administered a carbohydrate-protein supplement before a strength/power workout. Tipton et al. (2001), put six subjects through two random trials to determine whether an oral essential amino acid-carbohydrate (EAC) supplement would be a more effective stimulator of muscle protein anabolism if given immediately before or immediately after a ~45-minute lower-body resistance-exercise bout. Ingestion of EAC changed net muscle protein balance from negative values, i.e., net release, to positive net uptake in both trials. However, the total response to the consumption of EAC immediately before exercise was greater than the response when EAC was consumed immediately after exercise. Total net phenylalanine uptake, an indicator of muscle protein synthesis, across the leg over three hours was greater when the supplement was administered before exercise as opposed to when the supplement was administered after exercise. Furthermore, the authors concluded that the change from a catabolic state in the muscle to an anabolic state seemed to be primarily attributable to an increase in muscle protein synthesis.

TABLE 7.2

Ideal Pre-exercise Meals (4–6 Hours Prior) and Snacks (30–60 Minutes Prior)

Meals (200–300 g of carbohydrate and 30–40 g of protein)	Snacks (30–50 g of carbohydrate and 5–10 g of protein)
• Oatmeal with protein powder and toast with peanut butter	• Ready-to-drink protein supplement shake and energy bar
• Tuna sandwich with fruit	• Half a bagel with peanut butter
• Salad with chicken breast and steamed vegetables	• Sports drink with protein
• Extra lean hamburger with cheese on a whole wheat bun with baked sweet potato fries	• Glucose-electrolyte solution with protein bar
• Meal replacement shake with fruit	• ½ cup cottage cheese and banana

---

This was likely the result of an elevated blood flow during exercise that maximizes delivery to the muscle. This study demonstrated that the acute effects of EAC supplementation on muscle anabolism are even greater if the EAC is ingested before the training bout.

7.5 CARBOHYDRATE SUPPLEMENTATION DURING EXERCISE

Nutrition during an intense training session can aid in the quality of the workout, especially if the workout exceeds 60–90 minutes. Nutrition during exercise for the majority of athletes usually centers on supplementation more so than pre- and post-exercise nutrition if for no other reason than the convenience supplements provide. Convenience supplements may include any of the following:

- Glucose-electrolyte solutions or "sports drinks"
- Meal replacement powders
- Ready-to-drink supplements
- Energy bars
- Energy gels or "Gu" packs
- Fitness waters

These supplements are typically fortified with differing amounts of vitamins and minerals and differ in the amount of carbohydrate, protein, and fat they contain. It is now well established that with prolonged continuous exercise, time to fatigue at moderate, submaximal exercise intensities is related to pre-exercise muscle glycogen concentrations, thus highlighting the importance of everyday nutrition along with pre-exercise nutrition (Bergstrom et al. 1967).

In addition, a glucose-electrolyte solution has been the recommended supplement of choice for decades during exercise in order to preserve muscle glycogen and maintain blood-glucose levels to provide a constant exogenous fuel source to the working muscles. The beneficial effects of solid and liquid carbohydrate/protein supplements are similar when thermal stress is not a factor. Liquid supplements do provide the added benefits of aiding rehydration and tend to be digested more easily for most athletes while exercising. Cyclists, for example, can generally empty from the stomach up to 1000 mL of fluid/hour, and therefore 40–60 grams of carbohydrate can be easily ingested while consuming a large volume of fluid (Coyle and Montain 1992). On the other hand, runners generally consume less than 500 mL of fluid/hour (Noakes et al. 1991). This is because of the difficulty of drinking on the run and the potential discomfort of running with a full stomach. Therefore, runners tend to use more concentrated solutions than do cyclists in order to consume adequate amounts of carbohydrates. For cyclists, a carbohydrate solution of 4%–6% is generally sufficient when fluid replacement is important. For runners, this concentration may have to be 8%–10% to provide adequate carbohydrate. Glucose concentrations in excess of 10% seem to delay gastric emptying and compromise fluid replacement (Figure 7.1).

Carbohydrate availability is especially important during a workout in order to maintain energy levels and training intensity. Thus, supplements with high GI

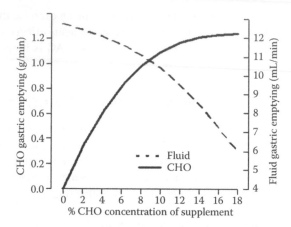

FIGURE 7.1 The effect of carbohydrate concentration on the rate of gastric emptying of fluids and carbohydrate during exercise from the stomach. Carbohydrate concentrations of 8%–10% maximize carbohydrate gastric emptying without substantially reducing fluid delivery (From McConell et al. *Med Sci Sports Exerc* 28: 1300–1304.)

sources should make up the majority of supplements ingested during an intense workout. The athlete should experiment with different formulations to find the one that works best for them prior to competition. The three macronutrients all have the potential to provide calories to drive muscular contraction. However, the body prefers to burn carbohydrates during exercise and, depending on the exercise intensity and duration, will burn carbohydrates at a very quick rate during an intense training session.

At low exercise intensities, the energy needed is provided primarily from the oxidation of plasma fatty acids that are broken down from stored triglycerides in adipose tissue (Coyle 1995). As exercise intensity increases, plasma fatty-acid turnover does not increase, and the additional energy is obtained by the utilization of muscle glycogen, blood glucose, and intramuscular triglycerides. Further increases in exercise intensity are fueled mostly by increases in muscle glycogen utilization with some additional increase in blood glucose oxidation (Coyle 1995). Recently, glycogenolysis has been demonstrated to be an important energy supplier during high-intensity, intermittent exercises, such as resistance training. Resistance training that centers on higher-repetition schemes (8–12 repetitions) and moderate loads may have an even greater effect on muscle glycogen concentration than those of lower-repetition schemes (Haff et al. 2003). Fluids and electrolytes can be lost especially in hot and humid conditions.

7.5.1 Long Duration Exercise

When a training session lasts more than one hour, the athletes should ingest a glucose-electrolyte solution in order to maintain blood-glucose levels, spare muscle glycogen, help prevent dehydration, and reduce the immunosuppressive effects of intense exercise (Burke 1997; Maughan and Noakes 1991; Nieman 1998; Nieman and Pedersen 1999; Sherman et al. 1998). Many athletes do not replenish fluids and

TABLE 7.3
Ideal Nutrient Composition for a Sports Drink during Exercise

Nutrient Objectives	Ideal Composition (per 12 oz water)
• Replace fluids and electrolytes • Preserve muscle glycogen • Maintain blood-glucose levels • Minimize cortisol increases • Set the stage for a faster recovery	• High-glycemic carbohydrates, such as glucose, sucrose, and maltodextrin: 20–26 g • Whey protein: 5–6 g • Vitamin C: 30–120 g • Vitamin E: 20–60 IU • Sodium: 100–250 mg • Potassium: 60–120 mg • Magnesium: 60–120 mg

carbohydrates at a fast enough rate during exercise for several reasons: lack of accessibility, personal preference, and the gastrointestinal discomfort that nutrient ingestion can cause during exercise can discourage supplementation. In addition, intense training often suppresses appetite and/or alters hunger patterns so that many athletes do not feel like eating (Berning 1998). However, supplementation during a training session can have a profound effect on performance, especially if the workout is longer than 60 minutes. Table 7.3 gives an example of the ideal nutrient composition for a sports drink during exercise. A sports drink such as that shown in Table 7.3 should be ingested at minimum every 20 minutes during a training session to help improve performance and reduce muscle protein breakdown during prolonged bouts of moderate to high intensity exercise (>90 minutes).

Sucrose, starches, and maltodextrins, when taken separately or in combination, seem to have similar effects on performance and exhibit similar metabolic effects to glucose (Coggan and Coyle 1987; Coyle et al. 1986; Goodpaster et al. 1996). It is recommended that fructose be avoided because fructose is absorbed in the small intestine half as fast as glucose, and fructose produces a lower blood glucose and insulin response than glucose (Cori 1926; Levine et al. 1983). Consuming large concentrations of fructose during exercise can result in gastrointestinal discomfort, diarrhea, and an inadequate rate of glucose availability.

7.5.2 SHORT DURATION EXERCISE

With short-term, high-intensity exercise, the relation between the availability of muscle glycogen and performance is less clear. One study that utilized 15 high-intensity, 6-second bouts on a cycle ergometer concluded that a higher-carbohydrate regimen over 48 hours helped subjects maintain a higher power output compared with the exercise and dietary regimen that included the low-carbohydrate content (Balsom et al. 1999). This study demonstrated the importance of a high-carbohydrate diet in relation to short-term, high-intensity exercise.

However, Haub et al. (2003) found that carbohydrate ingestion after maximal exercise does not seem to influence subsequent short-duration, maximal-effort exercise in competitive cyclists. Significant changes between treatments for plasma glucose did exist because the levels significantly decreased during a 60-minute recovery for the placebo group. The lack of performance difference supports the rationale that results gained from the investigations using moderately trained subjects (Haub et al. 1999) and non-sport-specific protocols (Bangsbo et al. 1992) cannot be generalized to competitive athletes. The authors concluded that trained cyclists are likely to rely on factors other than the bioavailability of circulating fuels to influence subsequent short-duration, high-intensity exercise, such as changes in the central nervous system (McConell et al. 1996).

7.6   POST-EXERCISE CARBOHYDRATE INTAKE

Post-exercise nutrition for the competitive athlete is vital to restore muscle glycogen stores, enhance skeletal muscle fiber repair and growth, and maintain overall health and wellness. This is especially important for those athletes engaged in prolonged training or competition sessions on the same or successive days. Multiple training sessions on the same day have now become the norm more than the exception for the elite athlete because of the ever-increasing level of competition and pressure to perform at optimal levels. An example could be a bodybuilder working one muscle group in the morning and an opposing muscle group that evening or triathletes performing an 8-mile run in the morning followed by a mile swim and a 30-mile bike ride after lunch. In addition, athletes involved with team sports (e.g., football, basketball, and soccer) that hold multiple practices throughout the day and week are especially susceptible to nutrient deficiencies and performance decrements if proper post-exercise nutrition guidelines are not followed.

Although it is unlikely that muscle glycogen stores can be completely resynthesized within a few hours by nutritional supplementation alone, it would behoove all competitive athletes to maximize the rate of muscle glycogen storage after exercise. This will ultimately result in faster recovery from training, thus possibly allowing for a greater training volume (Haff et al. 2003), which could result in additive adaptations that may translate into improved performance. Both during and after an intense exercise bout, the body is in a catabolic state, and thus key stored nutrients are being broken down to supply available fuel sources to the working muscle. However, the opportunity exists to alter the catabolic state into a more anabolic hormonal profile in which the athlete actually begins to rebuild muscle and thus initiate a much faster recovery. Exercise that results in glycogen depletion will activate glycogen synthase, the enzyme responsible for controlling the transfer of glucose from UDP-glucose to an amylase chain. This also happens to be the rate-limiting step of glycogen formation. The degree of glycogen synthase activation is influenced by the extent of glycogen depletion. The complete resynthesis of muscle glycogen, however, is ultimately dependent on adequate carbohydrate intake.

Carbohydrates composed of glucose or glucose polymers are the most effective for replenishment of muscle glycogen, whereas fructose is the most beneficial for the replenishment of liver glycogen. Glucose and fructose are metabolized differently and have different gastric emptying rates; thus their appearance into the bloodstream occurs at different rates. Furthermore, the insulin response to a glucose supplement is generally much greater than that of a fructose supplement. The fact that approximately 79% and 14% of total carbohydrate is stored in skeletal muscle and the liver, respectively, is further indication of the importance of consuming glucose or glucose polymers post-exercise.

Blom et al. (1987) found that ingestion of glucose and sucrose was twice as effective as fructose for restoration of muscle glycogen. The maximal stimulatory effect of oral glucose intake on post-exercise muscle glycogen synthesis was reached at a dose of 0.70 g/kg taken every second hour after exercise in which the muscle glycogen concentration was reduced by an average of 80%. In addition, the rate of post-exercise muscle glycogen synthesis increases with increasing oral glucose intake, up to a maximum rate of approximately 6 mmol/kg/hour. Blom et al. indicated that the differences between glucose and fructose supplementation were a result of the way the body metabolized these sugars. Fructose metabolism takes place predominantly in the liver, whereas the majority of glucose seems to bypass the liver and be stored or oxidized by the muscle (Ivy 1998).

Subsequent research by Burke et al. (1993) found that the intake of high-GI carbohydrate foods after prolonged exercise produces significantly greater glycogen storage than consumption of low GI carbohydrate foods 24 hours post-exercise. Although the meal immediately after exercise elicited exaggerated blood glucose and plasma insulin responses that were similar for the low-GI and high-GI meals, for the remainder of the 24 hours, the low-GI meals elicited lower glucose and insulin responses that the high-GI meals. Costill et al. (1981) reported that a diet of simple carbohydrates (glucose/fructose/sucrose) was as effective in restoring muscle glycogen levels 24 hours after exercise depletion as a diet based on "starch" or complex-carbohydrate foods. However, after 48 hours, the complex-carbohydrate diet resulted in greater muscle glycogen gains than the simple carbohydrate diet. It can be theorized that simple-carbohydrate foods (high GI) are absorbed quickly and may be useful as an immediate substrate in the early stages of glycogen restoration. They tend to be less useful in the later stages when they may be stored as fat rather than glycogen. Complex-carbohydrate foods (low GI) are absorbed more slowly and thus are more valuable during the latter stages of glycogen storage.

The underlying theme is that one should not wait to take full advantage of the post-exercise window of opportunity. Figure 7.2 clearly shows this to be the case. This chart summarizes the effects of delayed nutrient supplementation on muscle anabolic activities. As is clearly shown, nearly every important anabolic process is reduced after three hours.

7.7 TRAINING TABLE: CARBOHYDRATES

The term "training table" often refers to a dining hall or room where athletes in training eat supervised meals. These have become more popular within both male and female professional and collegiate sports over the last decade as the pressure to perform at high levels continues to increase. A majority of both professional and collegiate teams have hired full-time sports nutritionists to oversee the training table and counsel athletes on their diets. This can be a challenging feat for the sports nutrition staff, depending on whether the athlete is aiming to gain weight, lose weight,

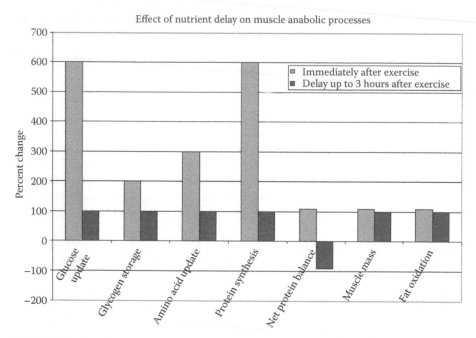

FIGURE 7.2   An illustration of the effect of nutrient delay on muscle anabolic processes. A delay in nutrient supplementation of up to 3 hours can dramatically decrease important anabolic activities including glycogen storage and protein balance. (Adapted from Tipton, K. D., B. B. Rasmussen, S. L. Miller, S. E. Wolf, S. K. Owens-Stovall, B. E. Petrini, and R. R. Wolfe. 2001. *Am J Physiol Endocrinol Metabol* 281: E197–E206.)

or even redistribute weight in hopes of achieving a competitive advantage in regards to a certain physical-fitness parameter. To make matters worse, the typical student athlete or even professional athlete leads a rushed lifestyle and rarely wakes up in time for breakfast. On top of that they hurry through the middle of their day without much regard for lunch aside from an occasional trip to a fast-food restaurant. By the time dinner rolls around, they are so hungry they gorge on anything and everything in sight, setting up a cycle that can be devastating to their training goals and hard to derail.

Because carbohydrates are the leading nutrient fuel for working muscles, they obviously play a major role within the daily menus. Meals should ideally be equally spaced throughout the day depending on training, practice, and games. Small frequent meals and snacks provide a gradual release of nutrients to the working muscles without extreme fluctuations in blood-sugar levels. To encourage this type of lifestyle, especially in regards to nutrition, the training table rarely closes and permits the athlete to take snacks (apple, banana, milk, protein bar, etc.) with them after a meal. Moderate- to high-carbohydrate meals and snacks based on low- to moderate-GI and -GL foods should form the foundation of every athlete's diet. Carbohydrate foods higher in fiber are generally recommended over carbohydrate foods high in sugar, especially prior to competition. However, it is important for each individual athlete to find some common carbohydrate choices that work for them and stick with them if possible. It is never a good idea to experiment with a new food combination the day of a game. In addition, it is important not to forget that the training or game time often dictates the timing of meals.

As was mentioned previously, pre-exercise or pre-game meals should be consumed 4–6 hours prior to the advent of activity. If practice is scheduled for the early morning, the meal the evening prior is the most important meal. If practice is scheduled for noon, breakfast becomes the most important meal, and if the game starts at 7 p.m., lunch serves as the pre-game meal. In addition, a light snack is recommended 30–60 minutes prior to the workout or game in order to top off muscle glycogen levels. It is important to be mindful and consider these guidelines when contemplating carbohydrate choices within the training table. Doing so will form the foundation of a successful nutritional strategy.

7.8 THE IMMUNE SYSTEM AND ATHLETIC PERFORMANCE

Athletes engaged in intense training run the risk of overtraining. Overtraining is usually encountered after several days of intense training and is generally associated with muscle fatigue. During the training period, transient signs and symptoms may occur including changes in the profile of mood state, where tension, depression, anger, fatigue, and confusion may be present. Other signs include depleted muscle glycogen stores, increased resting heart rate, increased cortisol secretion, decreased appetite, sleep disturbances, head colds, and immunosuppression. Most of the symptoms that result from overtraining, collectively referred to as overtraining syndrome, are subjective and identifiable only after the individual's performance has suffered. Unfortunately, these symptoms can be highly individualized, which can make it difficult for athletes, trainers, and coaches to recognize that performance decrements are brought on by overtraining. The first indication of overtraining syndrome is a decline in physical performance. The athlete can sense a loss in muscle strength, coordination, and maximal working capacity.

The immune system provides a line of defense against invading bacteria, parasites, viruses, and tumor cells. The system depends on the actions of specialized cells and antibodies. Unfortunately, one of the most serious consequences of overtraining is the negative effect it has on the body's immune system. Recent studies confirm that excessive training suppresses normal immune functions, increasing the overtrained athlete's susceptibility to infections (Mackinnon 1989; McCarthy and Dale 1988). Numerous studies show that short bouts of intense exercise can temporarily impair the immune response, and successive days of heavy training can amplify this suppression (Brahmi et al. 1985). Several investigators have reported an increased incidence of illness following a single, exhaustive exercise bout.

Intense exercise during illness might also decrease one's ability to fight off infection and increase the risk of even greater complications. In some cases, supplementation may help attenuate the immunosuppression typically seen with overtraining and in doing so may help prevent overtraining. To bolster the first line of defense, the athlete must ensure that adequate calories are being consumed. Athletes maintaining heavy-volume training often do not consume enough calories to keep up with energy demands because of the suppressive effect exercise can have on the appetite (Berning

1998) . This point can be especially concerning for competitive athletes engaged in prolonged training or competition sessions on the same or successive days.

Multiple training sessions on the same day have now become the norm more than the exception for the elite athlete owing to the ever-increasing level of competition and the pressure to perform at optimal levels. An example for the endurance athlete is performing a long, slow, distance run in the morning followed up by a circuit weight-training session that evening. The strength–power athlete may target one body part in a strength-training session in the morning and follow up with a second strength-training session targeting another body part in the evening.

To demonstrate the importance of macronutrient timing, Flakoll et al. (2001) provided either a placebo, carbohydrate, or carbohydrate/protein supplement to U.S. Marine recruits immediately after exercise during 54 days of basic training to test the long-term impact of post-exercise carbohydrate/protein supplementation on variables such as health, muscle soreness, and function. Compared to the placebo and carbohydrate groups, the combined carbohydrate/protein group had 33% fewer total medical visits, 28% fewer visits for bacterial/viral infections, 37% fewer visits for muscle and joint problems, and 83% fewer visits for heat exhaustion. Muscle soreness was also reduced immediately after exercise by the carbohydrate/protein supplement. The authors postulated that post-exercise carbohydrate protein supplementation not only may enhance muscle protein deposition but also have significant potential to affect health, muscle soreness, and tissue hydration positively during prolonged intense exercise training.

This suggests a potential therapeutic approach for the prevention of health problems in severely stressed exercising populations. Hence, it is essential for the athlete who trains regularly to consume an adequate balance of macronutrients and micronutrients at the proper times throughout the day, especially during periods of heavy training. Athletes involved in intense training not only have greater macronutrient needs but, more specifically, greater dietary carbohydrate and protein needs than individuals who do not train.

7.9   CONCLUSION

Proper training, maintaining a positive energy balance, adhering to proper nutrient timing, and obtaining adequate rest and recovery form the foundation for optimal performance. To optimize performance, athletes need a solid foundation that includes proper training and nutrition. Training for all athletes should be based on the proper utilization of the principles of training depending on individual goals and the training season (pre-season, in-season, and post-season). It has been well documented that athletes have special nutritional needs that go above and beyond those of the normal sedentary individual.

The daily approach to nutrition forms the foundation of the training-table concept. The nutritional base should focus on an everyday diet that emphasizes whole foods. The types of macronutrients selected are of the utmost importance for developing a well-refined everyday diet. Pre-exercise carbohydrate intake helps top off glycogen stores prior to exercise, setting the stage for a successful workout. Carbohydrate supplementation during exercise helps to maintain energy supplies and subsequent exercise intensity. Post-exercise carbohydrate intake speeds recovery and prepares the body for future exercise. Carbohydrate supplements that research has shown can help improve energy availability (e.g., sports drinks, carbohydrate) and/or promote recovery (carbohydrate, protein) can provide additional benefits in certain situations. Following these training and nutritional recommendations can serve as the foundation for a successful athlete.

REFERENCES

Ahlborg, B., J. Bergstrom, L. G. Ekelund, and E. Hultman. 1967. Muscle glycogen and muscle electrolytes during prolonged physical exercise. *Acta Physiol Scand* 70: 129–142.

Armstrong, L. E., D. L. Costill, and W. J. Fink. 1985. Influence of diuretic-induced dehydration on competitive running performance. *Med Sci Sports Ex* 17: 456–461.

Baba, N. H., S. Sawaya, N. Torbay, Z. Habbal, S. Azar, and S. A. Hashim. 1999. High protein vs high carbohydrate hypoenergetic diet for the treatment of obese hyperinsulinemic subjects. *Int J Obesity Related Metab Disorders* 23: 1202–1206.

Balsom, P. D., G. C. Gaitanos, K. Soderlund, and B. Ekblom. 1999. High-intensity exercise and muscle glycogen availability in humans. *Acta Physiol Scand* 165: 337–345.

Bangsbo, J., T. E. Graham, B. Kiens, and B. Saltin. 1992. Elevated muscle glycogen and anaerobic energy production during exhaustive exercise in man. *J Physiol* 451: 205–227.

Bergstrom, J., L. Hermansen, E. Hultman, and B. Saltin. 1967. Diet, muscle glycogen and physical performance. *Acta Physiol Scand* 71: 140–150.

Berning, J. R. 1998. Energy intake, diet and muscle wasting. In *Overtraining in Sport*, edited by R. B. Kreider, A. C. Fry, and M. L. O'Toole, pp. 275–288. Champaign, IL: Human Kinetics.

Blom, P., A. Hostmark, O. Vaage, K. Kardel, and S. Maehlum. 1987. Effects of different post-exercise sugar diets on the rate of muscle glycogen synthesis. *Med Sci Sports Exerc* 19: 491–496.

Brahmi, Z., J. E. Thomas, M. Park, and I. R. G. Dowdeswell. 1985. The effect of acute exercise on natural killer cell activity of trained and sedentary subjects. *J Clin Immunol* 5: 321–328.

Brand-Miller, J., T. M. S. Wolever, S. Colagiuri, and K. Foster-Powell, eds. 1999. *The Glucose Revolution*. New York: Marlowe & Company.

Burke, L. M. 1997. Nutrition for post-exercise recovery. *Austral J Sci Med Sport* 29: 3–10.

Burke, L., G. Collier, and M. Hargreaves. 1993. Muscle glycogen storage after prolonged exercise: Effect of the glycemic index of carbohydrate feedings. *J Appl Physiol* 75: 1019–1023.

Bussau, V. A., T. J. Fairchild, A. Rao, P. Steele, and P. A. Fournier. 2002. Carbohydrate loading in human muscle: An improved 1 day protocol. *Eur J Appl Physiol* 87: 290–295.

Cade, J. R. 1997. Dietary intervention and training in swimmers. *Eur J Physiol Occup Physiol* 63: 210–215.

Carli, G. 1992. Changes in the exercise-induced hormone response to branched chain amino acid administration. *Eur J Physiol Occup Physiol* 64: 272–277.

Coggan, A. R., and E. F. Coyle. 1987. Reversal of fatigue during prolonged exercise by carbohydrate infusion or ingestion. *J Appl Physiol* 63: 2388–2395.

Cori, C. F. 1926. The fate of sugar in the animal body: III. The rate of glycogen formation in the liver of normal and insulinized rats during the absorption of glucose, fructose, and galactose. *J Biol Chem* 70: 577–589.

Costill, D., W. M. Sherman, W. J. Fink, C. Maresh, M. Witten, and J. Jiller. 1981. The role of dietary carbohydrates in muscle glycogen synthesis after strenuous running. *Am J Clin Nutr* 34: 1821–1836.

Coyle, E. F. 1995. Substrate utilization during exercise in active people. *Am J Clin Nutr* 61(suppl): 968S–979S.

Coyle, E. F., A. R. Coggan, M. K. Hemmert, and J. L. Ivy. 1986. Muscle glycogen utilization during prolonged strenuous exercise when fed carbohydrate. *J Appl Physiol* 61: 165–172.

Coyle, E. F., and Montain S. J. 1992. Carbohydrate and fluid ingestion during exercise: Are there trade-offs? *Med Sci Sports Exerc* 24: 671–678.

Fairchild, T. J., S. Flectcher, P. Steele, C. Goodman, B. Dawson, and P. A. Fournier. 2002. Rapid carbohydrate loading after a short bout of near maximal-intensity exercise. *Med Sci Sports Exerc* 34: 980–986.

Flakoll, P. J., T. Judy, K. Flinn, C. Carr, and S. Flinn. 2001. Postexercise protein supplementation improves health and muscle soreness during basic military training in marine recruits. *J Appl Physiol* 96: 951–956.

Foster-Powell, K., S. H. Holt, and J. Brand-Miller. 2002. International table of glycemic index and glycemic load values. *Am J Clin Nutr* 76: 5–56.

Goodman, M. N. 1988. Amino acid and protein metabolism. In *Exercise, Nutrition, and Energy Metabolism*, edited by R. L. Terjung and E.S. Horton, pp. 89–99. New York: Macmillan.

Goodpaster, B. H., D. Costill, W. J. Fink, T. A. Trappe, A. C. Jozsi, R. D. Starling, and S. W. Trappe. 1996. The effects of pre-exercise starch ingestion on endurane performance. *Int J Sports Med* 17: 366–372.

Haff, G. G., M. J. Lehmkuhl, L. B. McCoy, and M. H. Stone. 2003. Carbohydrate supplementation and resistance training. *J Strength Cond Res* 7: 187–196.

Haub, M. D., G. G. Haff, and J. A. Potteiger. 2003. The effect of liquid carbohydrate ingestion on repeated maximal effort exercise in competitive cyclists. *J Strength Cond Res* 17: 20–25.

Haub, M. D., J. A. Potteiger, D. J. Jacobsen, K. L. Nau, L. A. Magee, and M. J. Comeau. 1999. Glycogen replenishment and repeated maximal effort exercise: Effect of liquid carbohydrate. *Int J Sport Nutr* 9: 406–415.

Hermansen, L., E. Hultman, and B. Saltin. 1967. Muscle glycogen during prolonged severe exercise. *Acta Physiol Scand* 71: 129–139.

Ivy, J. L. 1998. Glycogen resynthesis after exercise: Effect of carbohydrate intake. *Int J Sports Med* 19: S142–S145.

Ivy, J. L. 2008. Nutrition before, during and after exercise for the endurance athlete. In *Essentials of Sports Nutrition and Supplements*, edited by J. Antonio, D. Kalman, J. Stout, M. Greenwood, D. Willoughby, and G. G. Haff, pp. 621–646. New York: Humana Press.

Komi, P. V., ed. 1992. Strength and power in sport [Hormonal mechanisms related to the expression of muscular strength and power]. Cambridge, MA: Blackwell Scientific.

Kreider, R., A. C. Fry, and M. L. O'Toole, eds. 1998. *Overtraining in Sport*. Champaign, IL: Human Kinetics.

Lambert, C. P., L. L. Frank, and W. J. Evans. 2004. Macronutrient considerations for the sport of bodybuilding. *Sports Med* 34: 317–327.

Levine, C., W. J. Evans, B. S. Cadarett, E. C. Fisher, and B. A. Bullen. 1983. Fructose and glucose ingestion and muscle glycogen use during submaximal exercise. *J Appl Physiol* 55: 1761–1771.

Liu, S., W. C. Willett, and J. J. Stampfer. 2000. A prospective study of dietary glycemic load, carbohydrate intake, and risk of coronary heart disease in US women. *Am J Clin Nutr* 71: 1455–1461.

Ludwig, D. S. 2003. Glycemic load comes of age. *J Nutr* 133: 2695–2696.

Mackinnon, L. T. 1989. Exercise and natural killer cells: What is the relationship? *Sports Med* 7: 141–149.

Maughan, R. J., and R. D. Noakes. 1991. Fluid replacement and exercise stress: A brief review of studies on fluid replacement and some guidelines for the athlete. *Sports Med* 12: 16–31.

McCarthy, D. A., and M. M. Dale. 1988. The leucocytosis of exercise: A review and model. *Sports Med* 6: 333–363.

McConell, G., K. Kloot, and M. Hargreaves. 1996. Effect of timing of carbohydrate ingestion on endurance exercise performance. *Med Sci Sports Exerc* 28: 1300–1304.

Nieman, D. C. 1998. Influence of carbohydrate on the immune response to intensive, prolonged exercise. *Exerc Immunol Rev* 4: 64–76.

Nieman, D. C., O. R. Fagoaga, D. E. Butterworth, B. J. Warren, A. Utter, J. M. Davis, D. A. Henson, and S. L. Nehlsen-Cannarella. 1997. Carbohydrate supplementation affects blood granulocyte and monocyte trafficking but not function after 2.5 h of running. *Am J Clin Nutr* 66: 153–159.

Nieman, D. C., and B. K. Pedersen. 1999. Exercise and immune function: Recent developments. *Sports Med* 27: 73–80.

Noakes, T. D., K. H. Myburgh, J. Du Plessia, L. Lang, M. Lambert, C. van der Riet, and R. Schall. 1991. Metabolic rate, not percent dehydration, predicts rectal temperature in marathon runners. *Med Sci Sports Exerc* 23: 443–449.

Parker, B., M. Noakes, N. Luscombe, and P. Clifton. 2002. Effect of a high-protein, high-monounsaturated fat weight loss diet on glycemic control and lipid levels in type 2 diabetes. *Diabetes Care* 25: 425–430.

Salmeron, J., A. Ascherio, and E. B. Rimm. 1997. Dietary fiber, glycemic load, and risk of NIDDM in men. *Diabetes Care* 20: 545–550.

Sherman, W. M. 1995. Metabolism of sugars and physical performance. *Am J Clin Nutr* 62: S228–S241.

Sherman, W. M., K. A. Jacobs, and N. Leenders. 1998. Carbohydrate metabolism during endurance exercise. In *Overtraining in Sport*, edited by R. B. Kreider, A. C. Fry, and M. L. O'Toole, pp. 289–308. Champaign, IL: Human Kinetics.

Sherman, W. M., and G. S. Wimer. 1991. Insufficient dietary carbohydrate during training: Does it impair athletic performance? *Int J Sport Nutr* 1: 28–44.

Slov, A. R., S. Toubro, B. Rønn, L. Holm, and A. Astrup. 1999. Randomized trial on protein vs. carbohydrate in ad libitum fat reduced diet for the treatment of obesity. *Int J Obesity Rel Metabol Disorders* 23: 528–536.

Sutton, J. R., and O. Bar-Or. 1980. Thermal illness in fun running. *Am Heart J* 100: 778–781.

Thibault, G. 2006. Ahead of the pack. *Training Cond* 16: 25–31.

Tipton, K. D., B. B. Rasmussen, S. L. Miller, S. E. Wolf, S. K. Owens-Stovall, B. E. Petrini, and R. R. Wolfe. 2001. Timing of amino acid-carbohydrate ingestion alters anabolic response of muscle to resistance exercise. *Am J Physiol Endocrinol Metabol* 281: E197–E206.

8 Fat Needs of Athletes

*Jonathan M. Oliver, Michelle A. Mardock,
and Justin P. Dobson*

CONTENTS

8.1   INTRODUCTION

Exercising muscle requires a significant amount of energy to do work. Much of the energy required for exercising muscle is provided from stored forms of fat and carbohydrates. Although protein may also provide energy to working muscle, its contribution during exercise is considered negligible under most circumstances. Fat is present in abundance in the human body compared with carbohydrate stores, regardless of fitness level and body-fat percentage. In fact, fat comprises the largest fuel reserve in the body, exceeding that of carbohydrate several fold (Horowitz and Klein 2000). Fat is also the ideal fuel for exercising muscle because it is stored not only in adipose tissue, but in muscle, as intramuscular triglycerides, as well as circulating in the blood carried by protein carriers called lipoproteins. Fat contains more than twice as much energy per gram as carbohydrates and is stored in the absence of water, unlike carbohydrates, making it far more efficient per unit weight than its counterparts for energy during exercise (Jeukendrup et al. 1998b). Taken together, it is easy to see how fat is of great importance to exercising muscle.

The purpose of this chapter is to briefly highlight the different types of fats an athlete can obtain in their diet, provide a brief discussion of fat metabolism as it relates to digestion and absorption of dietary sources, provide an explanation of how fat is utilized during exercise, and finally provide verifiable dietary recommendations for fat intake for athletes of all levels. The guidelines can then be used to begin a training program with an understanding of fat sources or to augment a dietary plan in an effort to maximize performance.

8.2 STRUCTURE AND CLASSIFICATION OF DIETARY FAT

8.2.1 Dietary Fat Structure

The primary source of dietary fat is consumed in the form of triacylglycerols, also called triglycerides. Triglycerides contribute 90%–95% of the total energy derived from fat in the human body (Iqbal and Mahmood-Hussain 2009). Structurally, triglycerides exist as three fatty acid chains attached to a glycerol backbone. As in the diet, triglycerides are also the primary storage depot of fat within the human body. Other forms of dietary fat include phospholipids and sterols. Phospholipids contain phosphate, whereas sterols are complex molecules containing hydrocarbon rings in addition to other structural components. In the body, phospholipids are found on the surface of lipoproteins—macromolecules composed of a variety of lipids and proteins (Ginsberg 1998). One source of phospholipids familiar to most people is in egg yolks. Egg yolks contain phosphotidylcholine, which is a dietary phospholipid. Sterols exist in both plant and animal sources. In animal sources, sterols are referred to as cholesterol, whereas in plants the sterols are referred to simply as plant sterols. Cholesterol serves as a component to cell membranes and as a precursor for several hormones, primarily the "sex" hormones testosterone and estrogen (Ginsberg 1998).

8.2.2 Classification of Dietary Fats

Dietary fats can be classified in a number of ways. One way to delineate between different dietary fats is by their length, or the number of carbons in their fatty acid chains. Short-chain fatty acids have less than 6 carbons, whereas medium-chain fatty acids have 6–12 carbons. Both short- and medium-chain fatty acids are metabolized differently than long-chain fatty acids, which have more than 12 carbons. Most fatty-acid chains that exist in the body are of the long-chain type and typically range from 16 to 20 carbons in length.

Still another way to differentiate between dietary fats is based on their degree of saturation. Saturated fatty acids have hydrogen atoms attached to each carbon

TABLE 8.1

Common Fatty Acids and Their Structures

Symbol	Name	Structure
Saturated fatty acids		
12:0	Lauric acid	$CH_3(CH_2)_{10}COOH$
16:0	Palmitic acid	$CH_3(CH_2)_{14}COOH$
Monounsaturated fatty acids		
16:1n-7	Palmitoleic acid	$CH_3(CH_2)_5CH=CH(CH_2)_7COOH$
18:1n-9	Oleic acid	$CH_3(CH_2)_7CH=CH(CH_2)_7COOH$
Polyunsaturated fatty acids		
20:5n-3	Eicosapentaenoic acid	$CH_3CH_2(CH=CHCH_2)_5(CH_2)_2COOH$
22:6n-3	Docosohexenoic acid	$CH_3CH_2(CH=CHCH_2)_6CH_2COOH$

Source: LipidBank (http://www.lipidbank.jp)

atom in a hydrocarbon chain, whereas unsaturated fatty acids are missing at least one pair of hydrogen atoms attached to a carbon; thus the chain contains at least one carbon-to-carbon double bond. Monounsaturated fats contain one double bond, whereas polyunsaturated fats have two or more double bonds (White 2009). Omega-6 and omega-3 fatty acids are polyunsaturated fatty acids where the first double bond occurs on the sixth carbon for the former and on the third carbon for the latter.

Table 8.1 provides some common fatty acids along with their symbol, name, and structure. The symbol gives the number of fatty acids in the chain followed by number of double bonds. Monounsaturated fatty acids only contain one double bond, whereas the notation for polyunsaturated fatty acids describes more than one double bond. The notation "n-x" for fatty acids indicates the position of the last double bond in the fatty acid counting from the terminal end. Both eicosapentaenoic acid (EPA) and docosahexaenoic acid (DHA) are omega-3 fatty acids.

Trans fatty acids, which are predominantly produced during a process called hydrogenation, have double bonds arranged in a trans configuration. During hydrogenation, some unsaturated fatty acids are converted to saturated fatty acids. The unsaturated fatty acids are changed from a cis to trans configuration. Trans fatty acids produced this way are referred to as "synthetic" or "industrial" trans fatty acids.

8.2.3 Dietary Fat Structure Impacts Health

The degree of saturation is not only a way to differentiate dietary fats, it has also been shown to have important health effects associated with their consumption. Saturated fatty acids have been shown to have a detrimental effect on cholesterol levels, primarily increasing low-density lipoprotein (LDL) cholesterol levels (White 2009). An increased level of LDL cholesterol has been linked to an increased risk of coronary heart disease (CHD) and, thus, intake of saturated fatty acids has been associated with this increased risk (Hu et al. 2001). Trans fatty-acid intake has also been linked to CHD. Trans fatty acids exert a negative effect on serum lipids by increasing LDL cholesterol and triglyceride levels and reducing high-density lipoprotein (HDL) levels (White 2009).

Increased dietary intakes of monounsaturated fatty acids, on the other hand, have been shown to decrease the risk of CHD (Wahrburg 2004; White 2009). Consumption of monounsaturated fatty acids has been shown to lower total cholesterol and LDL (Hu et al. 2001; White 2009). The National Cholesterol Education Panel has suggested up to 20% of total calories may be consumed in the form of monounsaturated fats as part of a therapeutic lifestyle change diet due to their cholesterol lowering effects (Executive Summary of the Third Report of the National Cholesterol Education Program Expert Panel on Detection, Evaluation, and Treatment of High Blood Cholesterol in Adults 2001).

Polyunsaturated fatty acids have also been shown to have cholesterol-lowering effects as well. In particular, they have been shown to lower LDL cholesterol (Rodriguez-Cruz et al. 2005). Omega-6 and omega-3 fatty acids are polyunsaturated fatty acids, which are also considered essential fatty acids because of the body's inability to make them. Omega-6 fatty acids have been shown to lower total and LDL cholesterol significantly when consumed instead of saturated fatty acids. Omega-3 fatty acids have also been shown to have significant impact on CHD prevention. In particular, EPA and DHA have been shown to have a lowering effect on serum triglycerides. Omega-3 fatty acids also play a role in maintaining endothelial function. Endothelial dysfunction is a major factor in atherogenesis (Wahrburg 2004).

8.3 FAT METABOLISM

8.3.1 DIGESTION AND ABSORPTION

Metabolism of dietary fats involves several steps in the digestive process, with the process of digestion beginning when fats enter the mouth. This occurs when the salivary glands of the mouth secrete a lingual lipase that combines with the food in the oral cavity, and through chewing, the food is ground into smaller pieces for passage into the stomach (Carey et al. 1983; Hamosh and Burns 1977). The acidic pH of the stomach helps the lingual lipase work more efficiently. While in the stomach, the food is emulsified with the help of the peristaltic contractions of the stomach muscle.

Upon ingestion of a meal high in fat, the gall bladder contracts, emptying its contents into the small intestine. The pH of the intestine is favorable to further break down fats from a fat-rich meal (Carey et al. 1983; Go 1973; Go et al. 1970). The contents of the gall bladder help to further break down fat, combined with several enzymes secreted by the pancreas, including pancreatic lipase and bile acids that help break down the fats into individual fatty acids to be transported and subsequently stored (Carey et al. 1983). At this point in the digestive process, the majority of fats have been absorbed (Carey et al. 1983), however, only about 30% of dietary cholesterol has been absorbed (Grundy 1983). Several mechanisms are responsible for the less than optimal state of cholesterol absorption. However, the body has the ability to increase production of cholesterol when dietary cholesterol is low or decrease production when dietary cholesterol is high (Grundy 1983).

8.3.2 TRANSPORT AND STORAGE

The different types of triglycerides described earlier are transported differently. Depending on the chain length and level of saturation, smaller and less-saturated fatty acids can enter directly into the circulatory system for transport. Larger chain fatty acids (i.e., more than 12 carbons in length) require protein carriers, called lipoproteins. The four major classes of lipoproteins are chylomicrons, very low-density lipoproteins (VLDL), LDL, and HDL (Ginsberg 1998). The primary transporters of fatty acids following a meal include chylomicrons and VLDLs, which are taken up in the lymphatic system from the small intestine. These lipoproteins can transport the digested fats through the lymphatic system into the bloodstream to their target tissues, which could include adipose tissue, muscle tissue, and the liver.

Once absorbed in the intestine, these longer-chain fatty acids are packaged into chylomicrons to facilitate transport. After secretion from the intestine, the chylomicrons enter into the lymphatic system where several changes occur. Apoproteins are added to allow for these longer chain fatty acids to be transported via the blood to their final destination of storage (Ginsberg 1994). Lipoprotein lipase (LPL) will catalyze the hydrolysis of the triglycerides from the chylomicrons to allow them to be taken up by tissues to be stored as potential energy, primarily adipose tissue and muscle (Illingworth 1993). What remains after the hydrolysis by LPL are small particles of the chylomicrons that include cholesterol, phospholipids, apolipoproteins, and very little triglyceride. The remaining particles can then be integrated into HDL or be catabolized by the liver. Because of the long process described previously, the appearance of fats in the circulation after a high fat meal is slow. This is due to the rate of transport as well as the ability of fat to slow gastric emptying (Jeukendrup et al. 1998a). A meal that is high in fat can slow gastric emptying for up to six hours and in some cases even longer if the concentration of fat is significantly high in a particular meal.

8.3.3 FATTY-ACID TRANSPORT

Before fatty acids can be used for energy, they must first be transported into the muscle cell. This occurs actively through protein transporters, which transport the fatty acid across the muscle-cell membrane into the cytoplasm of the muscle cell. Conversion of fatty acids into energy for use in the muscle occurs in the mitochondria of the cell. Prior to entry into the mitochondria for conversion into energy, the fatty acid must be activated. Activation occurs outside of the mitochondria by means of an enzyme called acyl-coenzyme A (CoA) synthetase. Once this occurs, the activated fatty acid must then be transported over the mitochondrial membrane. This occurs by means of two transferases: carnitine palmitoyl transferases I and II. The exact mechanisms by which these two transferases translocate the activated fatty acid are outside of the scope of this chapter. A more detailed description can be found in the work of Jeukendup et al. (1998b).

8.3.4   FATTY-ACID OXIDATION

In order to convert the transported fatty acids into energy, the fatty acids must go through a stepwise process known as beta-oxidation. Beta-oxidation is a process whereby the fatty acid is degraded to an acetyl-CoA and an acyl-CoA unit. The acetyl-CoA can then enter into the tricarboxylic acid (TCA) cycle to be converted into energy for use in the muscle. The acyl-CoA unit acts again as a substrate for the beta-oxidation cycle until it is completely oxidized, and the resulting acetyl-CoA units are used in the TCA cycle to produce intermediates that can produce adenosine triphosphate (ATP) in the electron transport chain through aerobic pathways. The number of carbons and the degree of saturation has been shown to affect the rate at which fatty acids are oxidized, with medium-chain fatty acids being more quickly oxidized than their long-chain counterparts (Jeukendrup et al. 1998b).

8.4   FAT METABOLISM DURING EXERCISE

When an athlete is at rest, particularly in the fasting state, fat is the primary fuel source of choice for the body. The levels of circulating hormones in the body at times of fasting stimulate lipolysis, the breakdown of fats, in adipose tissue, which releases fatty acids into the bloodstream for delivery to other tissues for energy requirements (Horowitz and Klein 2000). If the levels of fatty acids in the body during these times exceed what is demanded by the body's working tissues, they are re-esterified and stored again in adipose tissue. The majority of fat released from adipose tissue during these times is in fact re-esterified. This is different than what occurs in the fed state. In the fed state, particularly after a meal high in carbohydrates, fat becomes less of a fuel source even at rest. This is due to the different circulating levels of hormones after a meal, particularly insulin, because of its promotion of nutrient storage (i.e., fatty acids, glucose, and amino acids). Insulin has an inhibitory effect on the breakdown of fat from adipose tissue (Horowitz and Klein 2000; Jeukendrup et al. 1998b), thus effecting the fuel utilization at that time in the body.

Whether at rest or during exercise, fat is able to be used for conversion into energy through a process called beta-oxidation. This occurs in the mitochondria of working cells. The energy created by fat for use by working muscle is greater than any other fuel that is provided by the body. However, the process of fat delivery, beta-oxidation, and ultimate conversion of fat to energy for use is a complex process involving a number of steps (Jeukendrup et al. 1998b), which is the reason that fat is considered a "slow" fuel source in the body.

During exercise, skeletal muscles require fuel to function. Although the muscle has several stored forms of energy, the energy stored within the muscle in the form of fat (intramuscular triglyceride), is small compared with stores within adipose tissue. We have already discussed how much more energy can be produced from the breakdown of fats, so now we need to determine where fat is stored and how fat is delivered to the working muscle during exercise to provide a fuel source required for working muscles to synthesize ATP.

8.4.1 ADIPOSE TISSUE

Adipose tissue contains the largest reservoir of fats for use for working muscle. As an example, a 180-pound (82-kg) man with 12% body fat would have about 22 pounds (10 kg) of total body fat. This represents almost 90,000 calories of stored energy in the form of fat. Although not all of this can be used for energy, it still represents a considerable amount of energy for a man with a relatively low body-fat percentage. Before these stored fats can be used for energy, they must be broken down into fatty acids and transferred to the muscle.

Lipolysis is the pathway that is responsible for the breakdown of stored triglycerides into fatty acids and glycerol. In adipose tissue, this is performed by hormone-sensitive lipase and monoacylglycerol lipase, which are tightly regulated under a second messenger system following hormonal stimulation. The major stimulatory factor that affects hormone-sensitive lipase is circulating epinephrine, whereas insulin is the major inhibitory factor that can turn off the activation of hormone-sensitive lipase. Other hormones that have been shown to stimulate lipolysis include glucocorticoids, thyroid-stimulating hormone, and growth hormone (Jeukendrup et al. 1998b), of which the glucocorticoids and growth hormone are known to increase as both exercise intensity and duration of exercise increase.

At the onset of exercise, the activation of the sympathetic nervous system causes increases in circulating catecholamines, primarily epinephrine, which stimulate the activity of hormone-sensitive lipase and lipolysis in adipose tissue. This stimulates the release of fatty acids from the adipose tissue that must then be passively or actively transported across the cell membrane of the fat cell with the help of membrane-associated proteins. Once this occurs, they are transported in the circulation bound to protein, primarily albumin, in which they can travel to target tissues or in this case active skeletal muscle. These fatty acids are eventually released from the albumin and actively transported across the muscle membrane into the cytoplasm of the muscle cell and further into the mitochondria where they can be used for energy.

While lipolysis is stimulated at the onset of exercise, the rate of appearance of fatty acids in the blood actually declines. This is due to the increase in fatty acid uptake by the muscle, in an attempt to increase the number of fuel sources in the active muscle to meet the metabolic demands from the exercise. Lipolysis eventually catches up, and the concentration of fatty acids in the blood increases above the rate of disappearance. The reverse can occur at the cessation of exercise with an increase in concentration of fatty acids in the blood. This can be regarded as positive, because these fatty acids can be used to replenish intramuscular triglyceride stores. Fatty acids not taken up into the muscle can be re-esterified and subsequently stored in adipose tissue.

At intensities greater than 80%, the reliance on fat as fuel from adipose tissue is decreased. Even though high levels of epinephrine have been shown to stimulate lipolysis from adipose tissue, the increase in glycolytic flux, combined with the increased levels of circulating lactate, may reduce lipolysis, thereby increasing re-esterification at these intensities (Jeukendrup et al. 1998b). Additionally, at these intensities, the increased blood flow to muscles reduces the available blood flow to adipose tissue, which has been shown to reduce fatty-acid removal from adipose tissue (Horowitz and Klein 2000), thus reducing the availability of circulating fatty acids.

8.4.2 CIRCULATING FATTY ACIDS

Fatty acids also circulate in the blood bound to lipoproteins, primarily VLDL and chylomicrons. These triglycerides bound to lipoproteins are unable to cross into the muscle cell for use as energy without being released from the lipoprotein carrier. LPL is responsible for hydrolyzing the triglyceride from the lipoprotein so the fatty acid can be transported into the muscle cell. The activity of this lipase has been shown to be tissue-specific, especially during times of fasting and exercise. For instance, during fasting and exercise, LPL's activity has been shown to increase in the heart and skeletal muscle while concomitantly decreasing in adipose tissue (Jeukendrup et al. 1998b). To what degree circulating lipoproteins contribute to overall fat oxidation during exercise has been difficult to quantify, but studies report they appear to be very small (Horowitz and Klein 2000).

8.4.3 INTRAMUSCULAR TRIGLYCERIDE

Fat is also stored inside muscle as intramuscular triglycerides. The extent of intramuscular triglyceride varies by type of muscle fiber, nutritional status, and training status of the individual. To what extent intramuscular triglyceride accounts for overall fat oxidation during exercise has been disputed, ranging from 15 to 50%, depending on aforementioned variables affecting intramuscular triglycerides along with the intensity and duration of said exercise (Martin et al. 1993; Romijn et al. 1993, 1995). However, it is well known that intramuscular triglyceride does contribute because the overall rate of fat oxidation cannot be accounted for solely based on the oxidation from fat from adipose stores (Jeukendrup et al. 1998b). Studies have shown increased reliance on intramuscular triglycerides when performing long durations of exercise (Horowitz and Klein 2000; Phillips et al. 1996). Chronic endurance training can lead to increased mitochondrial content (Morgan et al. 1971) and total intramuscular triglyceride stores (Morgan et al. 1969). Moreover, some researchers have shown increased intramuscular triglyceride oxidation following endurance activities (Hurley et al. 1984; Martin et al. 1993). This increased oxidation, along with increased amounts of total intramuscular triglycerides and overall mitochondria, would benefit endurance athletes tremendously because they could tap into a larger amount of immediate energy compared to an untrained individual.

8.5 EXERCISE EFFECTS

8.5.1 EFFECT OF EXERCISE ON FAT METABOLISM

Endurance training has been shown to have a marked improvement in performance, as well as a shift in substrate utilization. The changes in substrate utilization present as an enhancement of oxidative potential. Oxidation of fat at the same absolute and relative intensity has been shown to increase after training. The mechanisms responsible for this improvement are not completely understood; however, several physiological adaptations have been proposed to he responsible for this increase in fat utilization. Endurance training increases both the size and number of mitochondria within the muscles. This also results in an increase in the oxidative enzymes responsible for the oxidation of fats, including those responsible for transfer of fatty acids into the mitochondria. An increase in capillary density has also been shown as a result of endurance training, providing a better means to transport fatty acids to the working muscle. The increase in capillary density has also been proposed to increase blood flow to adipose tissue, thereby increasing the rate at which fatty acids can be removed from adipose tissue (Horowitz and Klein 2000).

The increase in fatty-acid oxidation cannot be completely accounted for from fatty acids provided by adipose tissue. Therefore, some studies have reported higher intramuscular triglyceride reliance after training. Thus, it appears that training does increase the depot of intramuscular triglyceride and oxidation at the same absolute intensity (Jeukendrup et al. 1998c).

8.5.2 EFFECT OF EXERCISE ON CHOLESTEROL

Endurance training (i.e., jogging, running, cycling, swimming, etc.) has been shown to have positive effects on LDL cholesterol and total cholesterol, reducing LDL cholesterol by approximately 5% and total cholesterol by 1% (Leon and Sanchez 2001). There appears to be a dose-response effect, suggesting that increasing aerobic exercise has a greater benefit (Williams 2009). Athletes who participate in more high-intensity intermittent exercise, such as football, baseball, and softball, may not observe these benefits unless they incorporate more aerobic-based exercise into their training (Williams 2009). This is particularly true for larger athletes who have a high-percent body fat or a higher body mass index (Buell et al. 2008). Weight loss that may occur as a result of exercise training and/or caloric restriction has also been shown to have positive benefits on blood-lipid profiles (Cziraky 2004; Hausenloy and Yellon 2008).

The effects of exercise on HDL cholesterol are not as clear-cut as with LDL cholesterol. Several factors play into whether or not HDL cholesterol changes with a particular exercise regime. Individuals with a low body mass index (27–30 kg/m² or lower) have been reported to have better improvements in HDL cholesterols that those with a high body mass index following an exercise program (Kodama et al. 2007; Nicklas et al. 1997; Schwartz 1987). This holds true as well for high body-fat percentage, in that there is some metabolic dysfunction that attenuates the benefits of exercise on HDL cholesterol (Coon et al. 1989; Durstine et al. 2001). Additionally, studies have shown that having low baseline levels of HDL cholesterol prior to starting exercise training will not illicit as strong a response (if any) to the exercise stimulus as compared with elevated levels after training in those who had HDL cholesterol levels of 37 mg/dl or greater (Durstine et al. 2001; Nicklas et al. 1997; Zmuda et al. 1998). Kodama et al. (2007) performed a meta-analysis and found that duration of an exercise session was essential to elevating levels of HDL cholesterol, whereas frequency and/or intensity were not as important. They noted that every 10-minute addition to an exercise session correlated with a 1.4-mg/dL increase in HDL cholesterol levels (Kodama et al. 2007).

8.6 DIETARY RECOMMENDATIONS

Dietary fat is a necessary and essential part of a well-balanced diet. Dietary fat provides fuel for resting and working muscles, provides essential fatty acids that our bodies are unable to produce, and assists in the metabolism of fat-soluble vitamins (Nutrition and Athletic Performance 2009). Essential fatty acids are important precursors to regulatory compounds that take part in a variety of physiological reactions. Additionally, fat-soluble vitamins (A, D, E, and K) are required for many metabolic processes. Having energy to fuel working muscles is of greater importance to athletes than for the general population.

The established acceptable range of total fat intake in adults is around 20%–35% of total energy intake (U.S. Department of Agriculture 2005). Although this level of fat intake is appropriate for athletes, an increase of up to 50% of caloric intake can be safely ingested by athletes participating in high-volume training (Kreider et al. 2010; Venkatraman et al. 2000). Interestingly, during times of extensive training, it has been reported that only 17% of male and 40% of female elite athletes followed the recommended guidelines (Economos et al. 1993). This can have a significant impact on performance, particularly for endurance and ultraendurance athletes. Unlike recommendations for protein and carbohydrate, there is no distinction in the recommended levels of fat intake for endurance versus strength/power athletes. For athletes attempting to lose body fat, an intake of 0.5–1.0 g/kg of the athlete's body weight per day is recommended (Kreider et al. 2010). It is important to note that consuming less than 20% of calories as fat can impair immune function and health status in athletes (Burke and Kiens 2006; Loucks 2004, 2007; Venkatraman et al. 2000). Thus, ideal fat intake should be a consideration when planning an athlete's nutritional strategy.

In addition to recommendations for total fat intake, the Dietary Guidelines for Americans recommend consuming less than 10% of energy intake from saturated fatty acids and replacing the remainder with monounsaturated and polyunsaturated fatty acids (U.S. Department of Agriculture 2005). Saturated fats are predominantly found in full-fat dairy products, fatty meats, and foods prepared with butter or lard. By consuming low-fat dairy products, choosing lean protein sources, and preparing foods with oils that are rich in monounsaturated and polyunsaturated fats, saturated fat intake can be greatly reduced. The guidelines also recommend that cholesterol intake be limited to less than 300 mg/day. Cholesterol is present in animal products such as meat, poultry, fish, seafood, egg yolks, high-fat dairy products, and foods prepared with animal fats such as cookies, muffins, and casseroles.

Finally, consumption of trans fatty acids should be minimal to avoid the well-established negative effects to which trans fat consumption is linked (U.S. Department of Agriculture 2005). Trans fatty acids are similar to saturated fatty acids in their promotion of CHD (Institute of Medicine 2005; U.S. Department of Agriculture 2005; Wahrburg 2004). The majority of trans fatty acids are found in processed foods that contain partially hydrogenated oils, although some trans fatty acids are found in meat and milk products produced from grazing animals. It is unknown whether the metabolic effects of natural trans fatty acids differ from synthetic fatty acids (U.S. Department of Agriculture 2005). As in the general population, athletes may benefit from following these dietary guidelines for fat intake. Table 8.2 provides the fat composition of various foods found in a normal diet, such as poultry, meat, dairy, and eggs, as well as oils used in cooking. A brief review of this table allows healthy choices to be made based on the current recommendations.

Unlike carbohydrates and protein, fat provides 9 calories/g, which is more than double the calories provided by carbohydrates and protein on a per gram basis. Therefore, to determine how many grams of fat an athlete should consume, it is important to first look at total caloric requirements, as well as those calories that need to be derived from protein and carbohydrates. For instance, if an athlete is expected to consume 3000 calories/day, this would mean that 900 calories should be obtained from fat sources (30% of 3000 calories is 900 calories). Because fat contains 9 calories/g, the athlete should aim to consume somewhere around 100 grams (900 calories ÷ 9 calories = 100 grams) of fat per day. It is important for athletes to take into account the fats in foods that one would typically not expect. Many athletes and the general population alike do not take into account the fat content of everyday foods. Table 8.2 provides some everyday foods with their fat content. Exceeding 100 g/day is very easy if poor choices are made. With today's increasing reliance on fast foods and the high fat associated with these meal offerings, an athlete could reach 100 grams in just one meal, but this is obviously not a recommended intake practice. Thus, proper selection of food choices for everyday meals and snacks is vital to meeting, and not exceeding, the recommended intake levels for dietary fat.

8.6.1 FAT SOURCES IN THE DIET

Monounsaturated fats are found in high concentrations in plant oils. The best sources of monounsaturated fats include: olive, sunflower, peanut, and sesame oils (see Table 8.2), nuts and seeds, avocados, and olives. Salmon, mackerel, herring, and sardines are also relatively high in monounsaturated fats. Polyunsaturated fats are also abundant in oils from fish and plants. The best sources of omega-3 fatty acids are fatty fish such as mackerel, lake trout, herring, sardines, bluefin and albacore tuna, and salmon. Table 8.3 lists various fish, vegetable, nut, and seed sources that may be used to increase mono- and polyunsaturated fat in the diet. α-Linoleic acid (an omega-6 polyunsaturated fatty acid), is found in the oils of tofu, soybeans, canola, walnut, and flaxseed (Kreider et al. 2010).

Saturated fats are usually solid at room temperature and come almost exclusively from animal sources. Saturated fats are found in relatively high amounts in fatty meats and cheeses, high-fat dairy products, butter, and coconut. Trans fatty acids are found in processed foods such as commercial baked goods and products containing partially hydrogenated vegetable oils. In general, athletes should limit the intake of saturated fats and especially trans fatty acids regardless of training status and volume because of the negative associated health effects and because they do not have a positive effect on exercise performance.

TABLE 8.2

Fat Composition of Common Foods

Food	Serving Size	Total Fat (g)	Saturated Fat (g)	Monounsaturated Fat (g)	Polyunsaturated Fat (g)	Cholesterol (mg)
Fats and oils						
Safflower oil	1 tbsp	13.6	0.8	2	10.2	0
Sunflower oil	1 tbsp	13.6	1.2	7.8	3.9	0
Soybean	1 tbsp	13.6	2	3.2	7.9	0
Corn oil	1 tbsp	13.6	1.7	3.3	8	0
Cottonseed oil	1 tbsp	13.6	3.5	2.4	7.1	0
Olive oil	1 tbsp	13.6	1	8	4	0
Canola oil	1 tbsp	13.6	1.7	3.3	8	0
Peanut oil	1 tbsp	13.6	1.9	5.4	5.7	0
Sesame oil	1 tbsp	13.5	2.3	6.2	4.3	0
Margarine, tub	1 tbsp	6.6	1.2	2.3	2.8	0
Margarine, tub, reduced fat	1 tbsp	5.1	1.4	1.9	1.4	0
Shortening, partially hydrogenated	1 tbsp	9.9	3.2	5.2	1.1	0
Lard	1 tbsp	12.8	5	5.8	1.4	12
Butter, stick	1 tbsp	11.5	7.2	3.3	0.4	30.5
Poultry and meat						
Chicken, breast, no skin, cooked	3 oz	3	0.9	1.1	0.7	72
Chicken, leg, no skin, cooked	3 oz	7.1	1	2.6	1.7	80
Turkey, breast, no skin, cooked	3 oz	0.6	0.2	0.1	0.2	71
Turkey sausage, cooked	2 oz	10.1	2.1	2.9	2.6	90
Turkey sausage, reduced fat, cooked	2 oz	5.9	1.6	2.2	1.5	33
Pork, tenderloin, cooked	3 oz	2.7	0.9	1	0.4	48
Pork chop, boneless, cooked	3 oz	6.5	2.2	2.8	0.8	71

Pork sausage, cooked	2 oz	16	5.3	6.4	2.1	35
Ham, boneless, roasted	3 oz	3.7	1.2	1.7	0.5	45
Beef, ground, 90% lean, broiled	3 oz	10	3.9	4.2	0.4	72
Beef, ground, 70% lean, broiled	3 oz	13.21	5.3	6.4	0.4	66
Beef, top sirloin steak, trimmed, cooked	3 oz	4.9	1.2	1.5	0.1	47
Beef, round, roasted	3 oz	3.5	1.2	1.5	0.1	47
Beef, prime rib, cooked	3 oz	29.7	12.3	12.9	1	73
Beef, hot dog	1 link	16.8	6.7	8.1	0.7	30
Dairy and eggs						
Milk, whole	8 oz	8	4.6	2	0.5	24
Milk, 2%	8 oz	4.9	3	1.4	0.2	20
Milk, skim	8 oz	0.6	0.4	0.2	0.02	5
Cheese, cheddar	1 oz	9.4	6	2.7	0.3	30
Cheese, cheddar, reduced fat	1 oz	2	1.2	0.6	0.6	6
Cheese, mozzarella, part skim	1 oz	5.7	3.1	1.4	0.1	15
Egg, large, boiled	1 each	5.3	1.6	2	0.7	212
Egg white	½ c	0.2	0	0	0	0
Yogurt, whole milk	1 c	8	5.1	2.2	0.2	32
Yogurt, low-fat	1 c	2.6	1.7	0.7	0.08	10
Cottage cheese, 2% fat	½ c	2.8	1.1	0.5	0.08	11
Cottage cheese, 4% fat	½ c	4.5	1.8	0.8	0.1	18
Sour cream	1 tbsp	2.4	1.4	0.6	0.1	6
Sour cream, reduced fat	1 tbsp	1.8	1.1	0.5	0.07	6

TABLE 8.3
Common Foods Containing Mono- and Polyunsaturated Fats

Food	Serving Size	Total Fat (g)	Saturated Fat (g)	Mono-unsaturated Fat (g)	Poly-unsaturated Fat (g)	Cholesterol (mg)
Nuts and seeds						
Macadamia, dry roasted	1 oz	21.7	3.3	17.1	3.4	0
Pecans, dry roasted	1 oz	20.2	1.6	12.6	5	0
Almonds, dry roasted	1 oz	16	1.5	10.4	3.4	0
Cashews, dry roasted	1 oz	13.7	2.8	8.1	2.3	0
Peanuts, dry roasted	1 oz	14	1.9	7	4.4	0
Walnuts, dry roasted	1 oz	17.5	1.6	4	11.1	0
Sunflower seeds, dry roasted	1 oz	14.1	1.5	2.7	9.3	0
Sesame seeds, dry roasted	1 oz	15.5	2.2	5.9	6.8	0
Soybeans, dry roasted	1 oz	7.2	1	1.6	4.1	0
Coconut, flaked, sweetened	½ c	11.9	11.2	0.6	0.9	0
Fruits and vegetables						
Avocado, sliced	½ c	10.7	3.1	14.3	2.7	0
Olives, green	10 each	4.1	0.5	3.1	0.4	0
Fish and shellfish						
Salmon, Atlantic, cooked, dry heat	3 oz	10.5	2.1	3.8	3.8	54
Tuna, bluefin, cooked, dry heat	3 oz	5.3	1.4	1.7	1.6	42
Albacore tuna, cooked, canned in water	3 oz	2.5	0.7	0.7	0.9	36
Trout, cooked, moist heat	3 oz	6.1	1.8	1.8	2	58
Mackerel, cooked, moist heat	3 oz	15.1	3.5	6	3.7	64
Herring, cooked, moist heat	3 oz	9.9	2.2	4.1	2.3	65
Sardines, canned in oil	3 oz	9.8	1.3	3.3	4.4	120
Halibut, cooked, moist heat	3 oz	2.5	0.4	0.8	0.8	35
Shrimp, cooked, moist heat	3 oz	0.9	0.3	0.2	0.4	166
Lobster, Northern, cooked, moist heat	3 oz	0.5	0.9	0.1	0.08	61
Crab, Alaskan, cooked, moist heat	3 oz	1.3	0.11	0.2	0.5	45

8.6.2 HIGH-FAT DIETS AND FAT LOADING

The fact that fat provides more energy than carbohydrates, can be stored in the absence of water, and can fuel exercise at a variety of intensities makes it a desirable option in fueling athletic performance. Because of fat's varied attributes, several studies have investigated the effect of high-fat diets on various issues that could affect athletic performance. Of particular interest is whether high-fat diets can reduce the amount of fuel used from glycogen by shifting the body's fuel preference to fat, therefore delaying fatigue in many of the longer-endurance sports. A high dietary-fat intake has been shown to increase intramuscular triglyceride stores and enzymes responsible for fat breakdown in trained individuals (Hoppeler et al. 1999; Kiens et al. 1987). However, studies investigating high-fat diets have not provided consistent conclusions. Although the long-term ingestion of a high-fat diet results in higher rates of fat oxidation and reduced rates of muscle glycogen use during submaximal exercise compared with an isoenergetic high-carbohydrate diet (Brown et al. 2000; Goedecke et al. 1999; Lambert et al. 1994; Peters 2003), the majority of studies have not demonstrated performance benefits from high-fat diets. Furthermore, methodological and design flaws may limit interpretation of some results (Burke et al. 2004; Burke and Hawley 2002; Jeukendrup et al. 1998c). Additionally, excessive dietary fat intake can increase adipose storage, increasing body weight significantly. This can have a detrimental effect on performance because body composition is usually an important variable in optimal sport performance outcomes. Therefore, at this time, high-fat diets are not recommended in the short or long term for athletes desiring performance improvements (Nutrition and Athletic Performance 2009).

Athletes who are asked to gain weight to increase size may often increase calories through an overconsumption of calories in the form of fat. Although this may increase the size of the individual, consuming more than the recommended caloric percentage in fat calories can have negative effects on an athlete's health (Buell et al. 2008) and, therefore, is not recommended for athletes wanting to gain size. Instead, the focus for these individuals is to increase their consumption of overall calories and shift to a diet with a higher percentage of protein as a fuel source to provide the building blocks to promote muscle hypertrophy.

8.6.3 TRAINING TABLE

Optimizing nutritional intake is an important strategy in maximizing an athlete's performance. A training table should offer a variety of foods containing healthy fat choices from various sources. Lean protein sources like turkey, skinless chicken, fish, shellfish, and "loin" cuts of meats such as pork tenderloin or beef tenderloin should be prepared with heart-healthy oils instead of butter or solid margarines. A variety of nuts, seeds, and low-fat dairy products should be on hand. The majority of an athlete's daily fat calories should come from foods high in monounsaturated and polyunsaturated fats. Intake of foods high in saturated and trans-saturated fats should be limited for both health and performance reasons.

Although there is an established role of carbohydrates and protein for pre-workout and post-workout recovery, the role of fat at each of these time points is undetermined. The need to replenish intramuscular triglycerides after a long bout of aerobic activity would suggest the need to refuel with fats. However, unlike carbohydrates and protein, there are currently no guidelines for fat loading prior to an event or for fat loading immediately following a bout of exercise. Tables 8.2 and 8.3 provide some common foods and their fat content and breakdown. An athlete should strive to consume an appropriate amount of predominantly healthy fats throughout the day. Additionally, care should be given by those athletes who experience gastrointestinal distress following the consumption of higher-fat foods, and changes should be made to ensure that fat intolerance does not hinder performance.

8.7   CONCLUSION

Fueling exercising athletes requires an understanding of the proper macronutrient balance to achieve the best performance. In this chapter, we learned the role fat can play in fueling exercising muscle. It is important for all athletes to strive for a balanced diet and one that helps them achieve their goals of performance. By consuming the proper amount of fat, the diet can provide fuel for exercising muscle, as well as provide the necessary precursors to other important physiological processes within the body.

REFERENCES

Brown, R. C., C. M. Cox, and A. Goulding. 2000. High-carbohydrate versus high-fat diets: Effect on body composition in trained cyclists. *Med Sci Sports Exerc* 32: 690–694.

Buell, J. L., D. Calland, F. Hanks, B. Johnston, B. Pester, R. Sweeney, and R. Thorne. 2008. Presence of metabolic syndrome in football linemen. *J Athl Train* 43: 608–616.

Burke, L. M., and J. A. Hawley. 2002. Effects of short-term fat adaptation on metabolism and performance of prolonged exercise. *Med Sci Sports Exerc* 34: 1492–1498.

Burke, L. M., and B. Kiens. 2006. "Fat adaptation" for athletic performance: The nail in the coffin? *J Appl Physiol* 100: 7–8.

Burke, L. M., B. Kiens, and J. L. Ivy. 2004. Carbohydrates and fat for training and recovery. *J Sports Sci* 22: 15–30.

Carey, M. C., D. M. Small, and C. M. Bliss. 1983. Lipid digestion and absorption. *Annu Rev Physiol* 45: 651–677.

Coon, P. J., E. R. Bleecker, D. T. Drinkwater, D. A. Meyers, and A. P. Goldberg. 1989. Effects of body composition and exercise capacity on glucose tolerance, insulin, and lipoprotein lipids in healthy older men: A cross-sectional and longitudinal intervention study. *Metabol* 38: 1201–1209.

Cziraky, M. J. 2004. Management of dyslipidemia in patients with metabolic syndrome. *J Am Pharm Assoc* 44: 478–490.

Durstine, J. L., P. W. Grandjean, P. G. Davis, M. A. Ferguson, N. L. Alderson, and K. D. DuBose. 2001. Blood lipid and lipoprotein adaptations to exercise: A quantitative analysis. *Sports Med* 31: 1033–1062.

Economos, C. D., S. S. Bortz, and M. E. Nelson. 1993. Nutritional practices of elite athletes: Practical recommendations. *Sports Med* 16: 381–399.

Executive Summary of the Third Report of the National Cholesterol Education Program (NCEP) Expert Panel on Detection, Evaluation, and Treatment of High Blood Cholesterol in Adults (Adult Treatment Panel III). 2001. *JAMA* 285: 2486–2497.

Ginsberg, H. N. 1994. Lipoprotein metabolism and its relationship to athlerosclerosis. *Med Clin North Am* 78: 1–20.

Ginsberg, H. N. 1998. Lipoprotein physiology. *Endocrinol Metabol Clin North Am* 27: 503–519.

Go, V. L. M. 1973. Coordination of the digestive sequence. *Mayo Clin Proc* 48: 613–616.

Go, V. L. M., A. F. Hofmann, and W. H. J. Summerskill. 1970. Pancreozymin bioassay in man based on pancreatice enzyme secretion: Potency of specific amino acids and other digestive products. *J Clin Invest* 49: 1558–1564.

Goedecke, J. H., C. Christie, G. Wilson, S. C. Dennis, T. D. Noakes, W. G. Hopkins, and E. V. Lambert. 1999. Metabolic adaptations to a high-fat diet in endurance cyclists. *Metabolism* 48: 1509–1517.

Grundy, S. M. 1983. Absorption and metabolism of dietary cholesterol. *Annu Rev Nutr* 3: 71–96.

Hamosh, M., and W. A. Burns. 1977. Rat lingual lipase: Factors affecting enzyme activity and secretion. *Am J Physiol* 235: D416–D421.

Hausenloy, D. J., and D. M. Yellon. 2008. Targeting residual cardiovascular risk: Raising high-density lipoprotein cholesterol levels. *Postgrad Med J* 84: 590–598.

Hoppeler, H., R. Billeter, P. J. Horvath, J. J. Leddy, and D. R. Pendergast. 1999. Muscle structure with low- and high-fat diets in well-trained male runners. *Int J Sports Med* 20: 522–526.

Horowitz, J. F., and S. Klein. 2000. Lipid metabolism during endurance exercise. *Am J Clin Nutr* 72(suppl): 558S–563S.

Hu, F. B., J. E. Manson, and W. C. Willett. 2001. Types of dietary fat and risk of coronary heart disease: A critical review. *J Am Coll Nutr* 20: 5–19.

Hurley, B. F., D. R. Seals, J. M. Hagberg, A. C. Goldberg, S. M. Ostrove, J. O. Holloszy, W. G. Wiest, and A. P. Goldberg. 1984. High-density-lipoprotein cholesterol in bodybuilders v powerlifters: Negative effects of androgen use. *JAMA* 252: 504–513.

Illingworth, D. R. 1993. Lipoprotein metabolism. *Am J Kidney Dis* 22: 90–97.

Institute of Medicine. 2005. *Dietary Reference Intakes for Energy, Carbohydrate, Fiber, Fat, Fatty Acids, Cholesterol, Protein, and Amino Acids.* Washington, D.C.: The National Academies Press.

Iqbal, J., and M. Mahmood-Hussain. 2009. Intestinal lipid absorption. *Am J Physiol Endocrinol Metab* 296: E1183–E1194.

Jeukendrup, A. E., W. H. M. Saris, and A. J. M. Wagenmakers. 1998a. Fat metabolism during exercise: A review. Part III: Effects of nutritional interventions. *Int J Sports Med* 19: 371–379.

Jeukendrup, A. E., W. H. M. Saris, and A. J. M. Wagenmakers. 1998b. Fat metabolism during exercise: A review. Part I: Fatty acid mobilization and muscle metabolism. *Int J Sports Med* 19: 231–244.

Jeukendrup, A. E., W. H. M. Saris, and A. J. M. Wagenmakers. 1998c. Fat metabolism during exercise: A review. Part II: Regulation of metabolism and the effects of training. *Int J Sports Med* 19: 293–302.

Kiens, B., B. Essen-Gustavsson, P. Gad, and H. Lithell. 1987. Lipoprotein lipase activity and intramuscular triglyceride stores after long-term high-fat and high-carbohydrate diets in physically trained men. *Clin Physiol* 7: 1–9.

Kodama, S., S. Tanaka, K. Saito, M. Shu, Y. Sone, F. Onitake, E. Suzuki, H. Shimano, S. Yamamoto, K. Kondo, Y. Ohashi, N. Yamada, and H. Sone. 2007. Effect of aerobic exercise training on serum levels of high-density lipoprotein cholesterol: A meta-analysis. *Arch Intern Med* 167: 999–1008.

Kreider, R. B., C. D. Wilborn, L. Taylor, B. Campbell, A. L. Almada, R. Collins, M. Cooke, C. P. Earnest, M. Greenwood, D. S. Kalman, C. M. Kerksick, S. M. Kleiner, B. Leutholtz, H. Lopez, L. M. Lowery, R. Mendel, A. Smith, M. Spano, R. Wildman, D. S. Willoughby, T. N. Ziegenfuss, and J. Antonio. 2010. ISSN exercise & sport nutrition review: Research & recommendations. *J Int Soc Sports Nutr* 7: 7. Retrieved from http://www.jissn.com/content/7/1/7.

Lambert, E. V., D. P. Speechly, S. C. Dennis, and T. D. Noakes. 1994. Enhanced endurance in trained cyclists during moderate intensity exercise following 2 weeks adaptation to a high fat diet. *Eur J Appl Physiol Occup Physiol* 69: 287–293.

Leon, A. S., and O. A. Sanchez. 2001. Response of blood lipids to exercise training alone or combined with dietary interventions. *Med Sci Sports Exerc* 33(6 Suppl): S502–S515.

Loucks, A. B. 2004. Energy balance and body composition in sports and exercise. *J Sports Sci* 22: 1–14.

Loucks, A. B. 2007. Low energy availability in the marathon and other endurance sports. *Sports Med* 37: 348–352.

Martin, W. H., 3rd, G. P. Dalsky, B. F. Hurley, D. E. Matthews, D. M. Bier, J. M. Hagberg, M. A. Rogers, D. S. King, and J. O. Holloszy. 1993. Effect of endurance training on plasma free fatty acid turnover and oxidation during exercise. *Am J Physiol* 265: E708–E714.

Morgan, T. E., L. A. Cobb, F. A. Short, R. Ross, and D. R. Gum. 1971. Effects of long-term exercise on human muscle mitochondria. In *Muscle Metabolism during Exercise*, edited by B. P. B. Saltin. New York: Plenum Press.

Morgan, T. E., F. A. Short, and L. A. Cobb. 1969. Effect of long-term exercise on skeletal muscle lipid composition. *Am J Physiol* 216: 82–86.

Nicklas, B., L. Katzel, J. Busby-Whitehead, and A. P. Goldberg. 1997. Increases in high-density lipoprotein cholesterol with endurance exercise training are blunted in obese compared with lean men. *Metabolism* 46: 566–561.

Peters, E. M. 2003. Nutritional aspects in ultra-endurance exercise. *Curr Opin Clin Nutr Metab Care* 6: 427–434.

Phillips, S. M., H. J. Green, M. A. Tarnopolsky, G. F. Heigenhauser, R. E. Hill, and S. M. Grant. 1996. Effects of training duration on substrate turnover and oxidation during exercise. *J Appl Physiol* 81: 2182–2191.

Rodriguez, N. R., N. M. DiMarco, S. Langley, American Dietetic Association, Dietians of Canada, and American College of Sports Medicine. 2009. Position of the American Dietetic Association, Dietitians of Canada, and the American College of Sports Medicine: Nutrition and athletic performance. *Med Sci Sports Exerc* 109(3): 509–527.

Rodriguez-Cruz, M., A. R. Tovar, M. del Prado, and N. Torres. 2005. Molecular mechanism of ction and health benefits of polyunsaturated fatty acids. *Rev Invest Clin* 57: 457–472.

Romijn, J. A., E. F. Coyle, L. S. Sidossis, A. Gastaldelli, J. F. Horowitz, E. Endert, and J. J. Wolfe. 1993. Regulation of endogenous fat and carbohydrate metabolism in relation to exercise intensity and duration. *Am J Physiol* 265: E380–E391.

Romijn, J. A., E. F. Coyle, L. S. Sidossis, X. J. Zhang, and J. J. Wolfe. 1995. Relationship between fatty acid delivery and fatty acid oxidation during strenuous exercise. *J Appl Physiol* 79: 1939–1945.

Schwartz, R. 1987. The independent effects of dietary weight loss and aerobic training on high density lipoproteins and apolipoprotein A-I concentrations in obese men. *Metabolism* 36: 165–171.

U.S. Department of Agriculture. 2005. *Dietary Guidelines for Americans*. Washington, D.C.: Government Printing Office. Also available online: http://www.cnpp.usda.gov/DGAs2010-PolicyDocument.htm (accessed February 02, 2011).

Venkatraman, J. T., J. Leddy, and D. Pendergast. 2000. Dietary fats and immune status in athletes: Clinical implications. *Med Sci Sports Exerc* 32(7 Suppl): S389–S395.

Wahrburg, U. 2004. What are the health effects of fat? *Eur J Nutr* 43(Suppl 1): 6–11.

White, B. 2009. Dietary fatty acids. *Am Fam Physician* 80: 345–350.

Williams, P. T. 2009. Incident hypercholesterolemia in relation to changes in vigorous physical activity. *Med Sci Sports Exerc* 41: 74–80.

Zmuda, J., S. Yurgalevitch, M. Flynn, L. L. Bausserman, A. Saratelli, D. J. Spannaus-Martin, P. N. Herbert, and P. D. Thompson. 1998. Exercise training has little effect on HDL levels and metabolism in men with initially low HDL cholesterol. *Atherosclerosis* 137: 215–221.

9 Micronutrient Needs of Athletes

Fanny Dufour and Lem W. Taylor IV

CONTENTS

9.1 INTRODUCTION TO MICRONUTRIENTS

Macronutrients (fats, proteins, carbohydrates, and water) are ingested in large quantities in the diet, providing sources of energy required for cellular hydration, fueling, and synthesis of the functional structures used for physical work. Conversely, micronutrients including vitamins and minerals are not direct providers of energy sources to the body and are consumed in relatively small quantities. Micronutrients act as catalysts in the myriad of biologic reactions that process the energy-producing macronutrients that are consumed in the daily diet. They play a vital role in facilitating most aspects of physiological and metabolic functions in the body and provide the foundation for the processes contributing to health and physical performance. Relative to sports performance, micronutrients play key roles in carbohydrate, fat, and protein synthesis and metabolism, oxygen transfer and transport, bone, tissue, and muscle repair and growth, as well as combating oxidative damage from the stress of training.

Most athletes consume diets that provide sufficient amounts of these micronutrients in order to maintain increased performance and training adaptations. Unless it has been established that the athlete is suffering from specific deficiencies, there is no evidence that micronutrient supplementation above the recommended daily allowance (RDA) has a positive impact on performance; thus micronutrients are not typically thought of as ergogenic. On the other hand, athletes competing in weight-dependent sports (i.e., boxing, wrestling), those with notoriously restricted nutrient intakes (i.e., diving, gymnastics), or those choosing to follow vegetarian diets have micronutrient intakes that are typically 70% less than recommended and could benefit from the additional supplementation. The type of sport, season, training conditions, and specific demands can also dictate certain micronutrient needs and solicit potential deficiencies. It is important to understand and appreciate the functions of these vitamins and minerals to ensure that athletes are consuming a diversified and nutritionally dense diet supporting their overall health in an effort to offset any performance decrements associated with low micronutrient intakes. Thus, the concept of the training table would focus on providing this nutritional support through properly selected food choices on a daily basis.

9.2   VITAMINS

Vitamins consist of organic compounds found in limited quantities within the foods that we eat. With the exception of vitamins K and D and some B vitamins, these compounds cannot be synthesized by the body and are therefore considered essential nutrients. Although not a direct source of energy themselves, vitamins are, however, essential for catalyzing the metabolic processes contributing to functional health, growth, and performance. Thirteen compounds have been established as vitamins and are subdivided into two categories: water soluble and fat soluble. The water-soluble vitamins consist of vitamin C (ascorbic acid), B vitamins including B_1 (thiamin), B_2 (riboflavin), B_3 (niacin), B_6 (pyridoxine), B_{12} (cobalamin), folic acid, biotin, and pantothenic acid. Water-soluble vitamins dissolve in water, and unlike fat-soluble vitamins they are not stored in the body, and any excesses are excreted through the urine. These vitamins are also easily destroyed during food storage and preparation (light and heat exposure); therefore foods should be refrigerated, stored in low light conditions, and leftover water from cooking vegetables should be reused because it contains many of the lost nutrients. Fat-soluble vitamins are vitamins A (retinol), D (calciferol), E (tocopherol), and K (menadione). These vitamins are dissolved in fat and absorbed into the bloodstream, and any excesses are stored in the liver for future use by the body. As we will discover in the following sections, water- and fat-soluble vitamins are all critical to proper health and function, although they are each unique in chemical characteristics, function, and kinetics.

9.2.1 Water-Soluble Vitamins

9.2.1.1 Vitamin C

Vitamin C, also known as ascorbic acid, is undoubtedly the most important water-soluble vitamin responsible for supporting metabolic functions directly associated with exercise response and recovery. Vitamin C is a principal contributor to collagen, elastin, and bone-matrix synthesis, assisting in recovery by maintaining healthy cartilage and connective tissue. It is also required in the biological processes involving the production of exercise-responsive hormones such as epinephrine and cortisol. Additionally, vitamin C supports oxidative metabolism from fats because it is a component in synthesizing carnitine, which allows for the transport of fatty acids into the mitochondria for energy. Perhaps some of the most fundamental actions of vitamin C are found in its powerful antioxidant capabilities in detoxifying heavy metals, facilitating endogenous antioxidant activities, and providing protection from environmental and exercise-induced free radicals (see Section 9.4). Dietary sources of vitamin C include oranges, strawberries, mangoes, kale, chard, broccoli, and sweet potatoes (Table 9.1). Adequate intake (AI) is utilized when a specific daily

TABLE 9.1
RDA and Sources for Water-Soluble Vitamins

Vitamin	RDA/AI (Men/Women)	Dietary Sources
C (ascorbic acid)	90 mg/75 mg	Papaya, acerola fruit, pineapple, oranges, kiwi, strawberries, bell peppers, broccoli, leafy greens, potatoes, cabbage, and brussels sprouts
B$_1$ (thiamin)	1.2 mg/1.1 mg	Liver, pork, ham, whole grains, soybeans, peas, legumes, seeds, and nuts
B$_2$ (riboflavin)	1.3 mg/1.1 mg	Dairy, meat, fish, poultry, whole grains, nuts, broccoli, asparagus, and spinach
B$_3$ (niacin)	16 mg/14 mg	Leafy greens, legumes, milk, salmon, meat, and poultry
B$_6$ (pyridoxine)	1.3 mg	Whole grains, nuts, legumes, dairy, eggs, shellfish, fish, meat, and poultry
B$_{12}$ (cobalamin)	2.4 µg	Meat, poultry, fish, liver, eggs, dairy, and fortified cereals
Folic acid	400 µg	Liver, meat, eggs, whole grains, leafy greens, legumes, bananas, peaches, and nuts
Biotin	30 µg	Eggs, meat, fish, milk, whole grains, legumes, nuts, bananas, and mushrooms
Pantothenic acid	5 mg	Eggs, liver, dairy, broccoli, potatoes, legumes, whole grains, and leafy greens

Source: Food and Nutrition Board of the Institute of Medicine. Dietary reference intakes for thiamin, riboflavin, niacin, vitamin B$_6$, folate, vitamin B$_{12}$, pantothenic acid, biotin, and choline. Washington, DC: National Academy Press; 2000.

allowance cannot be established and represents the average daily nutrient intake based on intake estimates within a healthy population assumed to be adequate. The intestinal absorption of vitamin C from supplements or in the diet is generally 500 mg, and there is an inverse relationship between the absorption rate of vitamin C and the quantity consumed (i.e., > dose = < absorption). Therefore, in order to maximize the absorption of vitamin C, it is best consumed in a time-release form or throughout the day. To further enhance the actions of vitamin C, it is commonplace to find mixed formulations, consume it along with other antioxidants (i.e., selenium, vitamin E) or bioflavonoids found in lemons, oranges, and grapefruit (i.e., quercetin, green tea, resveratrol). Vitamin C is also known to facilitate nonheme iron transport and absorption, such that drinking a glass of orange juice can aid in absorbing the iron from fortified cereals and breads. Although physical activity may increase an athlete's vitamin C needs, most consume above the RDA and are rarely found deficient. However, the symptoms of such deficiency could lead to performance decrements resulting from chronic fatigue, reduced recovery and tissue repair, suppressed immunity, and the increased occurrence of injuries (Table 9.2).

TABLE 9.2
Water-Soluble Vitamin Benefits and Deficiency Symptoms

Vitamin	Functions and Benefits	Deficiency
C (ascorbic acid)	Collagen and connective-tissue formation, iron absorption, immune function, steroid and catecholamine synthesis; antioxidant: reduces cellular damage	Fatigue, anemia, loss of appetite, slow wound healing, bruising, joint pain, infection susceptibility
B_1 (thiamin)	Supports carbohydrate and amino-acid metabolism, central nervous system function	Weakness, muscle wasting, decreased endurance, depression, weight loss, and beriberi
B_2 (riboflavin)	Promotes oxidative metabolism and electron transport system and maintains skin health	Altered skin, membrane, and nervous system function, mouth and lip sores
B_3 (niacin)	Supports anaerobic glycolysis, oxidative metabolism, electron transport, and fat synthesis and maintains healthy skin	Fatigue, irritability, loss of appetite, skin lesions, digestive issues, and pellagra
B_6 (pyridoxine)	Promotes amino-acid metabolism, glycogenesis, glycogenolysis, and formation of red blood cells	Dermatitis, anemia, seizures, conjunctivitis, and mouth sores
B_{12} (cobalamin)	Promotes formation of red and white blood cells and maintains nerve, skin, and digestive tissues	Anemia, neurologic and gastrointestinal symptoms, infections, and fatigue
Folic acid	Supports formation of red and white blood cells and maintains digestion	Anemia, weakness, diarrhea, and infections
Biotin	Promotes carbohydrate, fat, and amino-acid metabolism	Weakness, nausea, and skin abnormalities
Pantothenic acid	Promotes oxidative metabolism and fat synthesis	Loss of appetite, fatigue, and depression

9.2.1.2 B-Complex Vitamins

Vitamins B_1, B_2, B_3, and B_6, pantothenic acid, and biotin, also known as the B-complex, are involved in the energy production of both carbohydrate and fats during varying intensities of exercise (Table 9.2). It is important to note that despite their varying forms and functions, they are as a whole indispensable to the energy-producing systems stressed during exercise training.

Vitamin B_1 (thiamin) serves as a coenzyme used in the energy-producing reactions during exercise supporting carbohydrate, fat, and branched chain amino-acid metabolism. With most weight-restricted athletes, B_1 deficiency is of some concern, although supplementation in well-nourished athletes has shown no effect on performance. Because thiamin aids in converting pyruvate to acetyl-coenzyme A for use in the Kreb's cycle, acute thiamin deficiency may lead to an accumulation of pyruvate, which can increase circulating lactate levels, thus inhibiting work output (Woolf and Manore, 2006).

Vitamin B_2 (riboflavin) is an important component of the coenzymes flavin mononucleotide (FMN) and flavin adenine dinucleotide (FAD). These coenzymes are hydrogen acceptors in the mitochondrial electron transport chain, playing an important role in the metabolism of fats, carbohydrate, and proteins via oxidative energy production. Additionally, FMN and FAD are contributors to steroid hormone production and amino-acid metabolism. Riboflavin is also used by the body to convert vitamin B_6 to its active form.

Vitamin B_6 becomes active as pyridoxal phosphate (PLP), which is a cofactor in many of the reactions involved in amino-acid metabolism. Increased protein consumption or protein breakdown resulting from exercise may warrant additional B_6 consumption in some individuals. PLP is also involved in glycogen breakdown as a component in the production of glycogen phosphorylase, the hormone regulating glycogenolysis.

Vitamin B_{12}, available only in meat products within the diet (Table 9.1), supports the production of nucleic acids involved in red and white blood cell formation in bone marrow. Vitamin B_{12} also contains the trace element cobalt, which along with folic acid plays key roles in DNA, RNA, protein, and heme-iron synthesis. Both folate and B_{12} are responsible for the production of red blood cells, tissue repair, and protein synthesis. Folate and vitamin B_6 work synergistically with B_{12} to lower serum homocysteine levels (lowering risk for cardiovascular disease). Strict vegetarians, women, and energy-restricted athletes may be particularly susceptible to deficiencies of vitamin B_{12} because its provenance is primarily from meat (Table 9.1).

Pantothenic acid is a precursor for coenzyme A, the essential component in carbohydrate and fat oxidation. Pantothenic plays a role in the metabolism of fatty and amino acids and is a contributor in the production of fat, cholesterol, steroid hormones, and the neurotransmitter acetylcholine. Biotin is responsible in the support of energy metabolism via the synthesis of fatty acids, the metabolism of branched chain amino acids, and gluconeogenesis (conversion of noncarbohydrate sources to glucose). Although not common, B-complex deficiencies adversely affecting performance can occur in vegetarian athletes; it is therefore advisable to supplement with the RDA for B_{12} (Table 9.1) if not consuming meat products in the diet.

TABLE 9.3

RDA and Sources for Fat-Soluble Vitamins

Vitamin	RDA/AI (Men/Women)	Dietary Sources
A (retinol)	0.9 mg/0.7 mg	Liver, fish, dairy, eggs, carrots, leafy greens, bell peppers, tomatoes, oranges, and sweet potatoes
D (calciferol)	600 mg	UVB rays from sunlight, liver, fish, eggs, fortified dairy, and grain products
E (tocopherol)	15 mg	Vegetable, nut, and seed oils; margarine, butter, and fatty meats
K (menadione)	120 μg/90 μg	Leafy greens, vegetable oils, liver, eggs, and butter

9.2.2 FAT-SOLUBLE VITAMINS

9.2.2.1 Vitamin D

Vitamin D is an important fat-soluble vitamin serving many purposes in the body including the regulation and absorption of calcium, protein synthesis, skeletal development, and bone mineralization. Vitamin D increases the absorption of calcium, which is mainly why milk is fortified with vitamin D. It is not exceptionally prominent in the diet (Table 9.3) and is mostly found in vitamin D-fortified foods. Instead, vitamin D is produced by the skin following exposure to UVB radiation from the sun; in fact, the skin supplies 80%–100% of the body's vitamin D needs. This is why geographic location, season, skin pigmentation, and lifestyle can dramatically affect vitamin D production and can influence supplementation needs. Darker skinned athletes competing indoors or in the northern half of the United States during the fall or winter months are typically at a higher risk of vitamin D deficiency (Cannell, 2009).

9.2.2.2 Vitamins A, E, and K

Vitamin A is derived from two sources: retinol and the carotenoids. α- and β-carotene are known as A pro-vitamins, or precursors to vitamin A production in the body. Vitamin A plays a critical role in maintaining immune function, vision, tissue growth, blood cellular components, and bone production. Carotenoids, in particular β-carotene and lycopene, are most commonly associated with their powerful antioxidative capabilities, which are able to combat oxidative stress and damage from cellular free radicals (see Section 9.4). Vitamin E exists in eight different forms, α-tocopherol being the predominant and most active in human plasma. Pertaining to exercise, α-tocopherol's most important contribution would be as a powerful lipid-soluble antioxidant agent contributing to the decrease in cellular membrane damage associate with high intensity or heavy training loads (see Section 9.4). Vitamin K is a coenzyme in the formation of glycoproteins, is required for the synthesis of blood clotting factors, and is not typically associated with performance in athletes. Table 9.4 outlines some benefits as well as deficiency risks associated with the fat-soluble vitamins.

9.3 MINERALS

Minerals are inorganic compounds found in various foods, and there are approximately 20 deemed as essential nutrients for proper metabolic and physiologic

TABLE 9.4
Fat-Soluble Vitamin Benefits and Deficiency Symptoms

Vitamin	Function and Benefits	Deficiency
A (retinol)	Promotes bone growth and supports immune function, skin tissue, mucous membranes, and pigments of the eye	Infections and impairment of dim-light vision, growth, and wound healing
D (calciferol)	Promotes the absorption of calcium and bone formation	Bone weakness
E (tocopherol)	Antioxidant: protects against free radicals and protects cell membranes	Anemia, muscle degradation, and neurologic damage
K (menadione)	Supports the formation of clotting agents	Hemorrhage and bleeding

function in the body. These compounds can be further separated into two groups: macrominerals and microminerals (or trace elements). These elements are deemed "macro" or "micro" based on the quantities that are recommended to ingest in the diet on a daily basis. The seven macrominerals are sodium, phosphorus, potassium, magnesium, sulfur, chlorine, and calcium, all of which are responsible for catalyzing reactions for muscle contraction, oxygen transport, oxidative metabolism, nerve impulse, bone and heart health, as well as serving as electrolytes and antioxidants. There are 14 trace elements including zinc, selenium, molybdenum, manganese, iron, iodine, fluorine, copper, and chromium. These microminerals are important in maintaining health by supporting antioxidant activities, immune function, oxidative metabolism, bone health, and oxygen transport. The next few sections will address how both macrominerals and trace elements contribute to maintaining optimal athletic performance, as well as the conditions contributing to the need for some athletes to supplement with certain minerals. Specifically, the following section will address the minerals that are most associated and relevant when discussing the needs for athletes and what they need to consume to ensure both health and ideal performance.

9.3.1 MACROMINERALS

9.3.1.1 Magnesium

Magnesium is the cofactor in over 300 major biosynthetic reactions, and most of it is combined with calcium and phosphorus within the bone. Magnesium is essential for normal heart rhythm, DNA, RNA and protein synthesis, bone mineralization, glycogenolysis, fat oxidation, as well as neuromuscular and cellular membrane function. The supplementation of magnesium has shown the ability to improve cardiorespiratory function and endurance capacity during exercise by reducing oxygen uptake and heart rate during endurance exercise (Lukaski 2001). The stress of training could reduce magnesium levels in addition to losses through sweat and urine; therefore, if not consuming adequate magnesium in the diet, an athlete could be at potential risk for deficiency. Despite the benefits of magnesium supplementation on sports performance in deficient athletes, more research is needed to determine any benefits in those with normal levels. As with all vitamins and minerals, the RDA for

TABLE 9.5

Macromineral RDA and Sources

Macromineral	RDA/AI (Men/Women)	Dietary Sources
Sodium	1500 mg	Table salt, snack chips, pickles, processed and canned foods, fish, meat, and bread
Phosphorus	700 mg	Fish, eggs, milk, cheese, meat, whole grains, legumes, nuts, and carbonated beverages
Potassium	4700 mg	Bananas, oranges, avocados, cantaloupes, tomatoes, potatoes, fish, meat, yogurt, and milk
Magnesium	420 mg/320 mg	Soy, legumes, nuts, leafy greens, whole grains, seafood, yogurt, and milk
Chlorine	2300 mg	Table salt, fish, beans, milk, meat, and canned and processed foods
Calcium	1000 mg	Dairy, beans, egg, cauliflower, sesame, and leafy greens

Source: Food and Nutrition Board of the Institute of Medicine. 2010. Dietary reference intakes for calcium and vitamin D. Washington, DC: National Academy Press; and Food and Nutrition Board of the Institute of Medicine. 2004. Dietary reference intakes: water, potassium, sodium, chloride, and sulfate. Washington, DC: National Academy Press.

magnesium (Table 9.5) can be achieved through a well-balanced diet. Sources of magnesium in the diet include dark leafy greens, seafood, milk, nuts, and legumes as listed in Table 9.5 with the other macromineral sources. It should be noted that high-fiber diets and the concomitant intake of phosphate, iron, manganese, and calcium (>2 g) can reduce the absorption of magnesium.

9.3.1.2   Calcium

The most abundant mineral in the human body and the major component of bone and teeth is calcium. Calcium is paramount in nerve conduction and muscle excitation and contraction. In fact, muscular contractions cannot occur without the presence of calcium ions in the muscle fiber to initiate the mechanics of muscle shortening. Calcium helps regulate fuel utilization during exercise by stimulating phosphorylase, a focal enzyme involved in glycogenolysis. Calcium also works in conjunction with vitamin K in promoting blood coagulation and wound healing. Some of the best dietary sources of calcium come from milk and other dairy products (Table 9.5). Many fruits and vegetables are also good sources; however, some contain certain acids (oxalic or phytic acid) that may impede the absorption of the calcium. It should be noted when choosing supplements that the absorption rate of calcium has shown to be maximized when taken in doses of 500 mg or less. As discussed earlier, the absorption of calcium can be enhanced with the cosupplementation of vitamin D.

9.3.1.3   Phosphorus and Potassium

Approximately 85% of phosphorus is found in the bone and is essential to the process of bone mineralization. In addition to being the key component of adenosine triphosphate (ATP), the body's energy source, it is also found in nucleic acids and the

TABLE 9.6
Macromineral Benefits and Deficiency Symptoms

Macromineral	Function and Benefits	Deficiency
Sodium	Maintains blood volume and pressure, promotes nerve impulse transmission, muscle contraction, and acid/base balance	Hyponatremia, muscle cramping, nausea, loss of appetite, seizures, and coma
Phosphorus	Constituent of cell membranes, DNA, RNA, ATP, PCr, NADP, buffer in muscle contraction, and promotes bone formation	Muscle weakness and cramping, brittle bones
Potassium	Supports acid/base balance, membrane potential, and nerve impulse and muscle contraction	Muscle cramping, depression, loss of appetite, heart arrhythmia, hypokalemia
Magnesium	Supports protein synthesis, bone formation, and nervous system function	Loss of appetite, fatigue, muscle cramping, and nausea
Chlorine	Supports nerve impulses and cell membrane function, liver function, and HCl formation in the stomach	Impaired fat metabolism, hypertension, and anemia
Calcium	Supports the growth of bones and teeth, aids in nerve transmission, membrane potential, and muscle contraction	Impaired muscle contraction and cramping, weak bones, and osteoporosis

phospholipids that make up cellular membranes. Phosphate in the form of phosphate salts has been speculated to enhance performance by facilitating oxygen release from red blood cells, but this has yet to be proven consistently. Processed foods and soft drinks provide between 20% and 30% of daily intake for phosphorus; other sources include whole grains, fish, eggs, meat, and dairy products (Table 9.5).

Potassium plays a key role in the process of body fluid regulation via stimulation of the hormone aldosterone. Potassium is responsible for proper nerve impulses and muscle contraction and regulates blood pressure aiding in reducing hypertension. In addition to sodium, potassium serves as one of the most supplemented electrolytes in sports drinks that are used as hydration aids and ergogenic aids during specific types of athletic events (Table 9.6).

9.3.1.4 Sodium

Of the major electrolytes in the body, sodium is among the most abundant, with its highest concentrations found in extracellular fluids. Most processed foods have added copious amounts of sodium, although natural foods contain only small quantities. Considering the Western diet, sodium deficiencies are rare. Daily recommended intake for sodium is 1.5 g, which is equivalent to 1.25 g of table salt. Sodium is responsible for homeostatic fluid maintenance along with both blood and osmotic pressure (Bergeron, 2000). The body is equipped with tightly regulated mechanisms to facilitate fluctuations in sodium loss and dietary intake. Despite this regulation, excess water (hypotonic fluids) intake coupled with prolonged sweat loss during endurance events can result in electrolyte imbalances.

Hyponatremia, which is characterized by low blood sodium levels (<130 mmol/L) is a very serious condition often misdiagnosed as dehydration because of its similar symptoms, such as fatigue and disorientation. Left untreated, this condition can result in blood plasma levels of <120 mmol/L, which may lead to coma, seizures, or death. Sodium is generally lost through sweat at volumes of approximately 1.2 g/L. Sweat can contribute to significant sodium losses considering hourly sweat rates during moderate intensity exercise can range from 1 to 2 L/hour and up to 3.5 L/h for higher intensities or during hot and humid conditions.

Sports drinks consumed during exercise should contain between 20 and 60 mmol/L of sodium to facilitate hydration (promote thirst and fluid retention), increase palatability, and aid in mitigating the risk of hyponatremia. Additionally, it is preferable to include 500–700 mg of sodium/L of water in rehydration beverages following exercise to aid in fluid absorption and retention. For athletes, manipulating sodium intake and timing is an easy way to maintain and promote maximal performance while reducing the risk of dehydration, hyponatremia, and heat-related injuries. A detailed approach to fluid intake for athletes and preventing fluid and electrolyte imbalances is addressed in Chapter 10.

9.3.2 Microminerals

9.3.2.1 Iron

Perhaps the most fundamentally important mineral pertaining to sports performance is iron. It plays a vital role in the entire process of cellular respiration, from oxygen transport to electron transfer. Hemoglobin, myoglobin, and the cytochromes in the electron transport chain are all reliant upon iron for their synthesis and function in oxidative metabolism during prolonged aerobic exercise. Iron is the essential nutrient for the optimal transport and distribution of oxygen through the body by the blood to various tissues. There exist two forms of iron: heme and nonheme. Of the average total dietary consumption of iron, only 10% is actually absorbed, with a distribution of 80% nonheme and 20% heme iron. Despite its lower absorption rate of 2–20%, nonheme iron is the primary source of iron in the diet and is derived mainly from plants. Nonheme iron-absorption rates vary greatly and are negatively affected by cellulose, pectin, wheat, and soy products as well as polyphenolic compounds. Heme iron on the other hand is more favorably absorbed at 5%–35% and can be found primarily in meat products. Heme iron absorption is enhanced by the consumption of animal proteins and lowered by calcium.

There are a few factors speculated to be responsible for the increased iron needs of certain athletes including: sweat loss, gastrointestinal bleeding, hemolysis (from foot-strike impact), and heavy menstrual bleeding. During prolonged exercise or high intensity training in the heat, sweat can contribute a loss of up to 0.3 mg of iron/L of sweat. It is important to replenish iron and other minerals (i.e., sodium, potassium, zinc, magnesium) lost from sweat by including an additional 12 mg of iron to the diet during times of heavy training. Sports involving higher impacts and foot strikes such as distance running and track and field result in greater iron losses because of the increased destruction of red blood cells (hemolysis) from impact (Peeling et al. 2008).

Therefore, athletes most at risk for iron deficiencies are women, strict vegetarians, distance runners, weight-dependent, or calorically restricted athletes. The training table for these types of athletes needs to reflect this need for iron in the daily diet.

9.3.2.2 Chromium and Zinc

Chromium assists in normal carbohydrate metabolism by supporting insulin actions. Despite its perceived potential as an ergogenic aid in promoting lean body mass, it has not shown the ability to improve body composition or performance by increasing glucose uptake or glycogen synthesis. Dietary sources of chromium include cheese, seafood, nuts, asparagus, whole-grain products, and stainless-steel cookware (Table 9.7). Zinc is another important trace element that is a structural component of over 200 enzymes in the body. Zinc is responsible for nucleic acid production, protein metabolism, and energy production in the muscle. Zinc deficiency has been shown to adversely affect muscle and cardiorespiratory function during exercise (Lukaski 2001). It also plays a key role in immune function, the maintenance of membrane integrity, and the healing of injuries. The absorption of zinc is reduced when consumed with phosphorus, and it is estimated that many athletes, particularly women and vegetarians, consume below the RDA for zinc.

9.3.2.3 Selenium and Copper

Selenium is an essential trace element aiding in the defense against the harmful effects of oxidative stress from ROS (see Section 9.4). The amount of selenium in food is a direct result of concentrations in the soil, and it is readily available in the Western diet in meats, poultry, whole grains, and nuts (Table 9.7). The micromineral

TABLE 9.7
Microminerals: Trace Element RDA and Sources

Micromineral	RDA/AI Men/Women	Dietary Sources
Zinc	11 mg/8 mg	Liver, poultry, beef, dairy, whole grains, sesame, peas, almonds, spinach, and asparagus
Selenium	55 mg	Meat, poultry, liver, seafood, whole grains, and nuts
Molybdenum	45 μg	Liver, dairy, legumes, and whole grains
Manganese	2.3 mg/1.8 mg	Whole grains, nuts, seeds, leafy greens, bananas, and legumes
Iron	8 mg/18 mg	*Heme*: Meat, poultry, fish, and seafood *Nonheme*: Nuts, whole grains, beans, peas, and leafy greens
Iodine	150 μg	Iodized salt, seafood, kelp, milk, and yogurt
Fluorine	4 mg/3 mg	Drinking water, seafood, eggs, and milk
Copper	0.9 mg	Liver, meat, poultry, seafood, eggs, whole grains, nuts, avocados, broccoli, bananas, and legumes
Chromium	35 μg/25 μg	Liver, oysters, cheese, whole grains, lettuce, tomatoes, onions, asparagus, nuts, mushrooms, and stainless steel cookware

Source: Food and Nutrition Board of the Institute of Medicine. 2001. Dietary Reference Intakes for vitamin A, vitamin K, arsenic, boron, chromium, copper, iodine, iron, manganese, molybdenum, nickel, silicon, vanadium, and zinc. Washington, DC: National Academy Press.

TABLE 9.8

Micromineral Benefits and Deficiency Symptoms

Micromineral	Function/Benefits	Deficiency
Zinc	Promotes energy metabolism, protein synthesis, and tissue repair and supports immune function and antioxidant activity	Immune dysfunction, impaired healing, infections, weight loss, and impaired growth
Selenium	Antioxidant: supports glutathione peroxidase function	Impaired immune function, heart disease, and cancer
Molybdenum	Supports fat and amino-acid metabolism	Neurological dysfunction, mental, and visual disturbances
Manganese	Supports clotting factors, fat synthesis, and bone formation	Impaired growth, dermatitis, and weight loss
Iron	Supports hemoglobin synthesis and function, oxygen and electron transport, and cytochrome production and maintains immune function	Anemia, fatigue, and infections
Iodine	Constituent of thyroid hormones and maintains metabolic function	Impaired metabolic and thyroid function
Fluorine	Supports bone and tooth formation	Tooth decay and cavities
Copper	Supports iron transport, oxidative metabolism, and connective tissue, and red and white blood cell formation	Anemia, impaired immune function, arthritis, and altered glucose metabolism
Chromium	Supports insulin function	Impaired fat metabolism and glucose intolerance

copper acts as a cofactor in many important enzymes involved in the transport of iron, glucose metabolism, as well as connective tissue and bone development. It also plays an important role in the prevention of DNA oxidation and the support of catecholamine, peptide hormone, and hemoglobin synthesis. The absorption of copper may be reduced with the excessive intake of nonheme iron, zinc, and penicillin. Although rare, copper deficiency can result in drastically impaired antibody and immune function as well as inflammatory responses (Table 9.8).

9.4 ANTIOXIDANTS

Intense prolonged training and competition places stress on the body that is associated with many of the positive adaptations that result in increased performance. These adaptations include the up-regulation of endogenous antioxidant enzymes produced by the body to effectively scavenge reactive oxygen and nitrogen species generated during exercise. Oxidative stress occurs when the body's natural defenses can no longer accommodate the increased generation of reactive oxygen (ROS) and nitrogen species (RONS). The resulting damage from oxidative stress is wide ranging from inflammatory signaling to cellular membrane and DNA damage. In terms of athletic performance, this can result in delayed recovery, damage to the muscle, and impaired force production.

There are a vast number of antioxidants available in the human diet that can uniquely aid in mitigating some of the damaging effects of exercise. There are many micronutrients and compounds found in food that possess powerful antioxidative capabilities. Some of these include vitamins C and E, selenium, coenzyme Q_{10}, and phytonutrients such as carotenoids and polyphenols. As with vitamins and minerals, well-balanced nutrition rich in a variety of fruits and vegetables should provide sufficient antioxidants to the diet without the need for additional supplementation.

9.4.1 VITAMINS

Vitamin C is a strong antioxidant acting directly and indirectly through the regeneration of a-tocopherol (vitamin E). Vitamin C is released from the adrenal glands in response to free radical generating stressors such as exercise. Vitamin C assists naturally in fighting these free radicals, which contribute to cell membrane and structural protein damage, resulting in a trickle effect impacting cellular-signaling mechanisms for inflammation and various gene transcriptions. The antioxidant effects of vitamin C may be reciprocally enhanced by the additional consumption of polyphenols such as flavenoids and catechins.

Vitamin E in all of its forms is a powerful antioxidant capable of protecting free peroxyl radicals from damage to the polyunsaturated fats in cell membranes and the oxidation of lipoproteins. Consuming vitamin E in conjunction with other antioxidants such as flavonoids, vitamin C, selenium, and coenzyme Q_{10} (CoQ_{10}) can enhance its actions in maintaining cellular redox status and scavenge free radicals. Medium-chain triglycerides have also shown the ability to enhance vitamin E absorption, whereas dietary fiber can actually decrease its absorption and antioxidative properties. Much like with vitamin C, the antioxidant effects of vitamin E and selenium benefit from the combined supplementation with vitamin C.

Coenzyme Q_{10}, also referred to as ubiquinone, is a water-soluble substance that plays a pivotal role in oxidative phosphorylation, by its involvement in the electron transport chain in the mitochondria. As a powerful mitochondrial and cellular membrane antioxidant, CoQ_{10} has been speculated to improve cardiovascular function and enhance performance. No substantial evidence indicates that CoQ_{10} plays any significant ergogenic role in exercise and performance.

9.4.2 MINERALS

Selenium is a cofactor of the endogenous antioxidants glutathione peroxidase and reductase, which protect against reactive oxygen and nitrogen species. While regulating cellular redox status, selenium also affects thyroid hormone and immune functions as well. Vitamin E may have a positive synergistic effect when consumed with selenium; however, vitamin C may decrease its absorption.

9.4.3 PHYTONUTRIENTS

Phytonutrients are not considered essential nutrients because insufficient dietary intake will not result in nutritional deficiency or adverse health conditions. However, there are many benefits to their consumption because they possess a wealth of anti-oxidative capabilities that could aid in offsetting the stresses of training and potentially improving performance.

9.4.3.1   Carotenoids

The carotenoids β-carotene and lycopene, also known as A pro-vitamins, are fat-soluble pigments that cannot be synthesized by the body and must therefore be consumed in the diet. Because these substances are the pigments that give fruits and vegetables their yellow, orange, red, and green colors, foods such as carrots, dark leafy greens, red peppers, tomatoes, mangoes, and pumpkin are good sources of carotenoids in the diet. These pro-vitamins may possess antioxidative properties, which prevent DNA and cellular membrane damage by reducing lipid peroxidation by scavenging singlet oxygen and hydroperoxyl radicals.

9.4.3.2   Flavonoids

Flavonoids are a type of polyphenolic plant compound with various subtypes including flavanones (citrus fruits), flavones (fruits, vegetables), isoflavones (soybeans), and flavonols and catechins (tea, wine). Flavonoids, which have received a lot of attention for their potential to affect health and performance, include quercetin and resveratrol, which are similar in structure and function. These compounds are believed to exert additional protective effects against oxidative stress and damage from stimuli, including exercise.

Quercetin is believed to reduce low density lipoprotein oxidation and increase antioxidant enzyme capacity, anti-inflammatory transcription factors, and mitochondrial biogenesis. It also has been suggested that quercetin acts an A_1 adenosine receptor antagonist much like caffeine, contributing psychostimulatory effects such as reducing fatigue during endurance exercise. Dietary sources of quercetin include red onions, kale, broccoli, black currents, and lingoberries.

Resveratrol, which is primarily found in peanuts and the skin of grapes, is a flavonoid that has shown great promise in mitigating the negative effects of RONS on cellular membranes, muscle tissue, and inflammatory responses. Resveratrol may have the ability to alter skeletal fatty acid and glucose metabolism, increase mitochondrial biogenesis, reduce inflammation, and protect against protein and lipid peroxidation (Davis 2009).

The actions of these antioxidants are not completely understood because they are intricate, complex, and individually unique to the specific compounds exerting the effects. Therefore, it is best to strive to consume antioxidants with a diet rich in fruits and vegetables to promote overall health, recovery, and performance. However, there is not enough evidence suggesting that consuming additional antioxidant supplements could enhance performance and training adaptations. Excessive antioxidant supplementation may in fact have the reverse effect on performance by reducing the natural antioxidative enzyme adaptations to exercise training and increasing the resulting oxidative damage.

9.5   CONCLUSION

An athlete's body is as a complex machine of symbiotic components and parts all operating in unison and tuned to perfection. Each component plays a role crucial to the function of the next, as in the human body. A nutritionally dense and diverse diet can provide an athlete the vitamins and minerals required to maintain metabolic and physiologic functions essential to maximize the body's performance.

9.5.1 TRANSITIONING TEXT TO THE TRAINING TABLE

- The best way to ensure meeting the RDA for most vitamins and minerals is by selecting and consuming a well-rounded diet rich in lean meats, whole grains, and a variety of fruits and vegetables.
- If their energy intake is adequate, an athlete will not experience performance-enhancement benefits from supplementing with additional vitamins and minerals.
- In order to consistently facilitate meeting daily requirements, however, it is prudent for all adult athletes to consume a multivitamin.
- Athletes engaging in intense training may have greater demands for certain vitamins and minerals. These demands rarely exceed twice that of the RDA and can be achieved easily with the increased food consumption that generally accompanies those training cycles.
- Those at risk for vitamin and/or mineral deficiencies such as women, distance runners, and weight-controlled and vegetarian athletes should address their nutritional concerns with a registered dietician who has experience with athletic populations.
- Those with specific deficiencies can gain performance benefits from the supplementation of single or combinations of specific micronutrients.
- Dietary supplements in sports are permitted; however, the industry is poorly regulated and athletes should be advised that some products may contain banned substances.
- Athletes should use discernment when purchasing supplements and look for products with the United States Pharmacopeia (USP) certification.

REFERENCES

American College of Sports Medicine, American Dietetic Association, Dieticians of Canada. 2000. Joint position statement: Nutrition and athletic performance. *Med Sci Sports Exerc* 32: 21–30.

Bergeron, M. F. 2000. Sodium: The forgotten nutrient. *Sport Science Exchange Roundtable* 13: 1–8.

Cannell, J. J., B. Hollis, M. B. Sorenson, T. N. Taft, and J. B. Anderson. 2009. Athletic performance and vitamin D. *Med Sci Sports Exerc* 41: 1102–1110.

Davis, M. J., A. Murphy, and M. D. Carmichael. 2009. Effects of the dietary flavonoid quercetin upon performance and health. *Curr Sport Med Reports* 8(4): 206–213.

Finaud, J., G. Lac, and E. Filaire. 2006. Oxidative stress: Relationship with exercise and training. *Sports Med* 36: 327–358.

Food and Nutrition Board of the Institute of Medicine. 1997. *Dietary Reference Intakes for Calcium, Phosphorus, Magnesium, Vitamin D, and Fluoride.* Washington, D.C.: National Academies Press.

Food and Nutrition Board of the Institute of Medicine. 2000. *Dietary Reference Intakes for Thiamin, Riboflavin, Niacin, Vitamin B_6, Folate, Vitamin B_{12}, Pantothenic Acid, Biotin, and Choline.* Washington, D.C.: National Academies Press.

Food and Nutrition Board of the Institute of Medicine. 2000. *Dietary Reference Intakes for Vitamin C, Vitamin E, Selenium, and Carotenoids.* Washington, D.C.: National Academies Press.

Food and Nutrition Board of the Institute of Medicine. 2001. *Dietary Reference Intakes for Vitamin A, Vitamin K, Arsenic, Boron, Chromium, Copper, Iodine, Iron, Manganese, Molybdenum, Nickel, Silicon, Vanadium, and Zinc.* Washington, D.C.: National Academies Press.

Food and Nutrition Board of the Institute of Medicine. 2004. *Dietary Reference Intakes for Water, Potassium, Sodium, Chloride, and Sulfate.* Washington, D.C.: National Academies Press.

Food and Nutrition Board of the Institute of Medicine. 2010. *Dietary Reference Intakes for Calcium and Vitamin D.* Washington, D.C.: National Academies Press.

Hendler, S. S., and D. Rorvik. 2001. *Physician's Desk Reference for Nutritional Supplements.* Montvale, NJ: Medical Economics Company.

Lukaski, H. C. 2001. Magnesium, zinc, and chromium nutrition and athletic performance. *Can J Appl Physiol* 26(suppl): S13–S22.

Meacham, S., D. Grayscott, J. J. Chen, and C. Bergman. 2008. Review of the Dietary Reference Intake for calcium: Where do we go from here? *Critical Rev Food Sci Nutr* 48: 378–384.

Peeling, P., B. Dawson, C. Goodman, G. Landers, and D. Trinder. 2008. Athletic induced iron deficiency: New insights into the role of inflammation, cytokines and hormones. *Eur J Appl Physiol* 103: 381–391.

Volpe, S. L. 2007. Micronutrient requirements for athletes. *Clinics Sports Med* 26: 119–130.

Williams, M. H. 2004. Dietary supplements and sports performance: Introduction to vitamins. *J Int Soc Sports Nutr* 1: 1–6.

Williams, M. H. 2005. Dietary supplements and sports performance: Minerals. *J Int Soc Sports Nutr* 2: 43–49.

Woolf, K., and M. M. Manore. 2006. B-vitamins and exercise: Does exercise alter requirements? *Int J Sport Nutr Exerc Metab* 16: 453–484.

10 Fluid Needs of Athletes

Chad Kerksick

CONTENTS

10.1 FLUID, WATER, AND HYDRATION

10.1.1 INTRODUCTION

Discussions and recommendations related to water and fluids needs are an interesting paradox. The mainstream media reports and discusses daily fluid needs as well as the extent to which water is a primary constituent of the human body and its daily role in metabolism and cell function. However, a lack of appreciation from athletes themselves and coaches seems to exist regarding daily implementation of these requirements. Recently, the Institute of Medicine put forth official recommendations regarding hydration and clearly defined an adequate intake for fluid (Institute of Medicine and Food and Nutrition Board 2004). This value is based on experimentally derived intake levels that are expected to meet nutritional adequacy for essentially all members of the population.

Although most would agree regarding its importance, the ability to clearly determine a required level of water is difficult, especially in the context of this textbook, which focuses upon active exercise populations. As will be outlined, many factors (e.g., environmental and physiologic) interact, which results in daily fluid requirements of individuals. Although optimal hydration is linked with a multitude of clinical scenarios (e.g., urolithiasis, urinary tract infections, bladder cancer, constipation, heart disease, hypertension, etc.), the importance of optimal fluid and hydration during exercise remains critically important as well and will be the focus of this chapter.

Although fluid's primary role in an exercise context is thermoregulation, water functions in additional capacities. For example, water acts as a transport system for gases and various nutrients to effectively deliver substrates to their intended targets. Water plays a major part in removing wastes from our body in our feces and urine. Additionally, water provides necessary structure and form to body tissues and works to lubricate joints and provide cushioning for a number of organs and structures throughout the body.

10.1.2 PHYSIOLOGIC FLUID COMPONENTS

Total body water in an average young adult male consists of 50%–70% body mass (Sawka et al. 2005). An individual's body composition is a primary factor that influences any variability from person to person because lean body mass is approximately 73% water, whereas adipose tissue is only 10% water (Table 10.1) (Sawka et al. 2005). In this respect, total body water variability is largely accounted for by differences in body composition relative to age, gender, and aerobic fitness levels (Van Loan and Boileu 1996).

Total body water for an average 75-kg male is often reported to be around 42 L of fluid, which is comprised of two compartments: the extracellular and intracellular compartments. The intracellular compartment represents the fluid inside the cells and is often reported to comprise approximately 65% of total body water, whereas the extracellular compartment is approximately 35% of total body water (Sawka et al. 2005). Thus, approximately 27 L of body water is of an intracellular origin, and an estimated 15 L is extracellular, which is further broken down into plasma (20%; ~3–4 L) and interstitial components (80%; ~10–11 L). The interstitial compartment primarily provides cell structures with a fluid medium but also assists with lymph, saliva, eye, gland secretion, and a host of other general physiological functions. All told, typical reported values for an average 75-kg male are around 42 L of total body water, 27 L of which are intracellular and 15 L of which are extracellular, which is further divided into approximately 3–4 L of plasma and 10–11 L of interstitial fluid (Byars 2008; Sawka et al. 2005).

It is important to understand that these values are typically assumed average values, and they are not static values. Water readily traverses into and out of all cellular locations, thus making these values quite dynamic in nature. In this respect, 5%–10% of total body water is turned over on a daily basis just from non-exercise-related aspects (Raman et al. 2004). Water lost from respiration is largely offset by water produced as part of metabolism. Additionally, average urine output is 1–2 L/day, but

TABLE 10.1
Daily Water Losses and Production

Source	Loss (mL/day)	Production
Normal physiological losses and production		
Respiratory loss	−250 to −350	—
Urinary loss	−500 to −1000	—
Fecal loss	−100 to −200	—
Insensible loss	−450 to −1900	—
Metabolic production	—	+250 to +350
Total	−1300 to −3450	+250 to +350
Net loss (sedentary)	−1050 to −3100	—
Athletic losses		
Sweat losses in various sports	−455 to −3630	—
Net loss (athlete)	−1550 to −6730	—

Source: Modified from Institute of Medicine and Food and Nutrition Board. 2004. *Dietary Reference Intakes for Water, Potassium, Sodium, Chloride and Sulfate.* Washington, D.C.: National Academies Press; and Sawka, M. N., S. N. Cheuvront, and R. Carter, 3rd. 2005. Human water needs. *Nutr Rev* 63: S30–S39.

drastic up- or down-regulation can occur depending on fluid intake and sweat losses (Institute of Medicine and Food and Nutrition Board 2004; Shapiro et al. 1982).

10.1.3 Human Water Requirements

A number of factors can dictate the amount of water needed by an individual. In addition to their body mass and composition, factors such as metabolic rate, dietary consumption, clothing worn, and environmental conditions are also responsible (Institute of Medicine and Food and Nutrition Board 2004) for thermoregulatory demands placed on body. As can be seen in Table 10.2, the Institute of Medicine (Institute of Medicine and Food and Nutrition Board 2004) released suggested adequate intake values for fluid.

As an infant grows and develops into childhood, their daily water needs rise (Ballauff et al. 1988; Goellner et al. 1981). Once maturation is complete, sedentary adults are commonly reported to require a minimum of 2.5–3.3 L of daily water intake, which subsequently increases with daily physical activity. A moderately active individual is recommended to intake an average of 3.2–4.5 L of water daily, and as activity level increases further in hot (>90°F) environments, daily water needs may reach 6 L per day (Fusch et al. 1998; Leiper et al. 1996, 2001; Welch et al. 1958). Much of this fluid intake (80%), according to National Health and Nutrition Examination Survey III data, comes from beverages, whereas the remaining 20% comes from food sources (Institute of Medicine and Food and Nutrition Board

TABLE 10.2
Dietary Reference Intake Values for Total Water

Gender and Age	From Foods	From Beverages	Total Water
Males			
4–8 years	0.5	1.2	1.7
9–13 years	0.6	1.8	2.4
14–18 years	0.7	2.6	3.3
>19 years	0.7	3.0	3.7
Females			
4–8 years	0.5	1.2	1.7
9–13 years	0.5	1.6	2.1
14–18 years	0.5	1.8	2.3
>19 years	0.5	2.2	2.7

2004). Interestingly, data from this survey suggest that non-exercising individuals in all age groups (12–71 years) did a satisfactory job of maintaining water balance. Table 10.2 outlines dietary references intake values for total water from foods and beverages. In the end, the Institute of Medicine established an adequate intake for men to a value of 3.7 L/day and women 2.7 L/day, respectively. Collectively, it is important for the reader to understand that this is a guideline, and because of the extreme variability that exists in these values for different humans, especially for competitive athletes competing outside in hot/humid environments or workers/laborers performing in quite physically strenuous occupations (e.g., construction, logging, etc.), the required values will be much different. Consequently, the established adequate intake values are not intended to be interpreted as satisfactory levels in these situations and instead should be considered a minimum daily fluid intake. Regardless, maintaining some status of euhydration is important because acute and chronic body water deficits can adversely impact health and performance.

10.2 PHYSIOLOGIC CONSIDERATIONS OF HEAT STRESS AND HYDRATION

10.2.1 THERMOREGULATION AND HEAT EXHAUSTION

Exercising in the heat results in a number of changes to our physiology. The longer the exercise persists, the greater the extent of the changes. A number of factors impact how much a person sweats, how much fluid they lose, etc., and examples include the mode of exercise, sweat rate of the individual, hydration level prior to exercise, and fluid-replacement strategies to name a few.

Regardless, with the onset of exercise, the cardiac output of the heart increases to match the increased energy demand of the working muscles. Cardiac output increases as great as 400% have been reported to occur during strenuous exercise when compared with resting levels. Secondary to this massive increase in activity of the heart and other muscles is an increase in heat production. In addition, environmental radiation of the sun's rays, convection of environmental heat with the body, and potentially conduction with other competitors, the ground, or equipment can also work to further increase the temperature of the body.

Regulation of body temperature or thermoregulation is highly integrated, and the primary means by which the human body lowers its internal body temperature is through sweat production. Formation of sweat leads to rapid dissipation of heat from the body when the sweat evaporates from the skin. Over time in this environmental scenario, reductions in body water occur, and a reduction in plasma volume is a critical place where fluid is lost as the body attempts to cool itself. As more and more fluid is lost from the blood as sweat, the available volume of blood is reduced, and the heart has to work harder, resulting in a further increase in heart rate. Depending on the relative combinations of various factors such as the ambient temperature, relative humidity, level of acclimatization, hydration level, etc., the magnitude of this strain on the heart will change. The longer a person exercises, the less hydrated they are at the start of the exercise bout, or the higher their sweat rate, the more their blood volume will decrease. In fact, it has been reported that for every 1%–2% reduction in body water that occurs, heart rate can increase up to seven beats per minute. When you consider that this amount of fluid loss can easily occur during a 2-hour exercise session, sizable increases in heart rate are expected when exercising in a hot and humid environment.

Independent of obligatory losses of fluid from breathing, metabolism, wastes, etc., the primary means by which fluid is lost from the body is from sweat production. The rate at which a person sweats is a critical element when developing strategies to help sustain health and performance during hot and humid settings. Many previous reports have indicated that typical sweat rates for exercising individuals range from 0.8 to 1.4 L of sweat/hour. Many larger-framed athletes (i.e., >90 kg) will sweat at an even faster rate than this and often get up to rates of 2 L of fluid/hour. Although upper limits are not well documented, sweat rates as high as 3.7 L/hour have been reported (Armstrong 2000). In this respect, many anecdotal reports have indicated that American football lineman and other very large framed athletes (>140 kg) who wear full pads and gear when practicing in a hot/humid environment can lose over 5 L (11 pounds) of fluid in a morning or afternoon practice. Fluid losses while performing are important because it has been well documented in the literature that even minor losses of fluid (1%–2% loss of body mass as fluid) can negatively impact a person's health status and their physical and mental performance (Convertino et al. 1996; Greenleaf et al. 1983). When put into context relative to exercise, performance capacity, cognitive function, and alertness (Maughan 2003; Wilson and Morley 2003) all have been shown to decrease with a large amount of physiological strain (i.e., heart rate, tissue heat storage) experienced by the body.

To some extent, however, the type of exercise being performed dictates the extent to which performance is impacted. For example, peak force is not typically impacted at moderate to high levels of dehydration (<5% body weight loss). Therefore, strength and power athletes may not experience a noticeable decrement in physical performance, but the documented reductions in reaction time and response accuracy that have been shown to occur at low to modest levels of dehydration (2%–3% body mass loss as fluid) may influence performance. Sports (or positions) containing more of an endurance component will, however, begin to experience performance reductions. As mentioned previously, the decreases in cardiac output (secondary to the reduction in plasma volume from fluid loss as sweat) will impact performance, and in fact, sports such as long-distance cycling, soccer, and running all have documented reductions in performance. Significant reductions in VO_{2max} and endurance time to exhaustion are all impacted by dehydration and even more so when the respective exercise is being performed in a hot and humid setting. Regardless of the particular sport, the more dehydrated you become, the more it impacts performance, both physically and cognitively.

10.2.2   Preventing Hyperthermia and Dehydration

Exercising in a hot and humid environment places a tremendous amount of strain on the thermoregulatory system. The primary adaptation that results is an increase in body temperature, and in response the body will dissipate this heat through sweating and the ensuing evaporation of this water from the skin's surface. In healthy individuals, the acute and immediate rise in body temperature is often not the reason for dehydration, but rather it is the continual loss of water from the body as sweat. As body water decreases, dehydration develops, and the body's ability to cool itself begins its compromised state; importantly, many experts believe an athlete cannot recover from this compromised state once exercise has begun (Table 10.3). Many steps and strategies can be taken to help ease the physiological burden placed on the body during exercise.

10.2.2.1   Acclimatization

Although many sporting or competitive scenarios do not allow for it, acclimating your body to the temperature, humidity, and other environmental considerations is a critical factor. The physiological systems of the human body readily adapt to these changes, and as a result getting to a location several days (or weeks) ahead of schedule can make a significant difference in the amount of strain placed on the systems of the body. As initially mentioned, from a practical perspective, this is often not possible. With a regularly competitive schedule, athletes are not able to arrive several days early to allow for these changes to fully occur. To what extent

---

TABLE 10.3

Impact of Dehydration on Performance

Body Weight Loss	Exercise Environment	VO_{2max} Change	Endurance Capacity Change
−2 %	Hot	−10 %	−22 %
−4%	Hot	−27%	−48%
−5%	Mild	−7%	−12%
−5%	Mild	—	−17%

Source: Adapted from Armstrong, L. E. 2000. *Performing in Extreme Environments.* Champaign, IL: Human Kinetics.

---

an acclimation period can be provided, the body immediately senses changes in environmental cues, but it typically takes several days for a noticeable amount of physiological adaptation to occur. It is these changes that begin to occur almost immediately that will allow the body to better control its temperature and tolerate high levels of exercise intensity in this setting. As can be seen in Table 10.4, a number of physiological adaptations occur, and it is commonly accepted that after one week a great deal of adaptation has occurred, with the complete process taking an estimated 14 days (Armstrong 2000).

In this light, it is also important for coaches and athletes to train and practice during the time of the day that most closely mimics the environmental considerations to be seen during competition. Regardless of travel, training at similar times and under as similar environmental conditions as possible to what will be experienced is a key consideration. This point can be seen every year by college football or soccer teams that travel to different environments to compete or in the 2007 Chicago marathon, during which the weather was unseasonably hot and resulted in several heat-related injuries. In summary, acclimating is important not just for optimization of performance but to also optimize the various thermoregulatory control points seen when competing in these settings. Whether an athlete or team is going to compete in a hot/humid, cold/dry, or windy climate or other untoward environmental conditions, acclimation is important.

10.2.2.2   Measuring Dehydration

Currently, no universal standard exists for measuring hydration status or dehydration. Several assessment techniques are regularly employed by various research groups, and all have their advantages and disadvantages. Considering the analytical needs of many athletes and coaches, those assessment techniques that offer great practicality, ease of administration, low cost, and ease in interpretation tend to be the techniques most often recommended and employed for use in these settings. For these reasons, only three measurement techniques are discussed: 1) body-mass changes, 2) urine color, and 3) urine specific gravity.

10.2.2.2.1   Body-Mass Changes

In laboratory and field settings, changes in body mass are commonly used to assess acute changes in hydration status. The value is typically expressed as a percentage of starting body mass, of which small changes (1%–2%) have been discussed previously and are known to negatively affect physiological processes and performance (Armstrong et al. 1997; Maughan 2003; Wilson and Morley 2003). Although viewed by some as less scientific, changes in body mass are often used as the criterion upon which other techniques are compared (Armstrong 2005; Armstrong et al. 1994). For increased accuracy, body-mass changes should be measured within one hour of exercise (Shirreffs 2003), but a considerable advantage is the relative stability of body-mass changes to sufficiently assess daily fluid balance up to a period of two weeks (Leiper et al. 2001). Additionally, natural fluctuations in body mass are well documented (0.51 ± 0.20 kg) and are known to be a relatively stable measurement (intra class coefficient: 0.66 ± 0.24%) in exercising men over a three-day exercising period who replaced 100% of their sweat loss (Cheuvront et al. 2004).

TABLE 10.4
Physiological Adaptations to Heat

Days of Heat Acclimatization

Adaptation	1	2	3	4	5	6	7	8	9	10	11	12	13	14
Heart rate decrease		‹————————————›												
Expansion of plasma volume				‹————————›										
Decrease in rectal temperature														
Decreased sweat [Na⁺] and [Cl⁻]						‹——›								
Increase in sweat rate														
Decreased renal [Na⁺] and [Cl⁻]		‹———›												

Source: Adapted from Armstrong, L. E. 2000. *Performing in Extreme Environments.* Champaign, IL.: Human Kinetics.

10.2.2.2.2 Urine Color

Prolonged periods of exercise in the heat result in a marked reduction in body water that starts a cascade of physiological responses in an attempt to maintain thermo-regulatory homeostasis. Initial responses in this process include an increase in sweat as outlined throughout, resulting in a reduction in body water. In addition to fluid-replacement plans, monitoring of hydration status is important for two primary reasons. The first of these reasons is to determine the extent of further development of dehydration, and the second is to determine the overall effectiveness of already-adopted fluid-replacement strategies.

A commonly employed field approach to quickly and inexpensively determine an individual's hydration status is a visual assessment of the color of the urine being produced. Although deemed not as scientifically reliable as refractometers and other analytical devices, teaching athletes and coaches to monitor urine color as a foundational assessment of fluid status is a recommended approach because of its simplicity and practicality (Armstrong 2005). Recent texts have further advocated the use of such a scale and what the approach lacks in scientific accuracy many experts feel it makes up for in practicality, cost, and ease of assessment. As can be seen in the example in Figure 10.1, a scale of 1 to 8 is used, and alongside each number is a progressively darker shade of yellow, then orange, then brown. The more hydrated a person, the more diluted their urine, and as a result the lower the number or "clearer" their urine will appear. Vice versa, if a person is dehydrated, their body will attempt to retain as much body water as possible, leading to greater filtration of body wastes resulting in more concentrated (or darker) urine.

This scale was developed and validated as part of a three-study approach. Briefly, the first study found those individuals reporting a pale, yellow color (ranking of 1 or 2) to be within 1% of baseline euhydrated body mass (Armstrong et al. 1994). The second study compared urine color along with specific gravity, osmolality, and other hydration markers and found the changes in urine color to satisfactorily track with changes of the other markers (Armstrong et al. 1998). Finally, when women trained heavily for six weeks and completed weekly measurements of urine color and urine specific gravity, the two values tracked closely and could be used in an interchangeable fashion (Ormerod et al. 2003). Consequently, single athletes or large numbers of athletes can quickly make an assessment of their urine color. The combination of fluid-replacement strategies and monitoring urine color along with body-mass changes is one the most commonly employed and recommended approaches to maintaining optimal hydration.

10.2.2.2.3 Urinary Specific Gravity

The specific gravity of urine is a measure of the density of a urine sample when compared with water. Water has a known density of 1.000; thus any measure with a greater or lesser density will have according values (>1.000 or <1.000, respectively). Typical urine specific gravity values range from 1.013 to 1.029, whereas samples from a person in a dehydrated state often exceed 1.030 (Armstrong et al. 1994, 1998).

Advantages of urine specific gravity are that it can be measured quickly and accurately with a handheld refractometer. Such devices are portable and can be used indoors or outdoors. Mixed results exist when comparing urine specific gravity

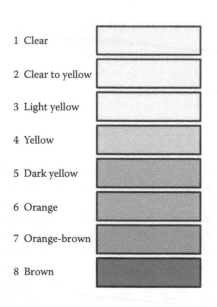

A visual-analog scale for urine color is used to provide a quick, inexpensive method to qualitatively assess fluid status.

This practice becomes more important as exercise progresses in hot and humid environments, especially for prolonged periods.

Match the color of your urine to a color on the chart. The closer the urine is to #1, the more hydrated a person. Generally speaking, a person should strive for better hydration, but values closely matched to #1, #2, or #3 are satisfactory.

If a person's urine color is dark orange, brown, or brownish-green, #6 or greater, the person is likely dehydrated, and aggressive fluid replacement strategies should be employed.

1 Clear

2 Clear to yellow

3 Light yellow

4 Yellow

5 Dark yellow

6 Orange

7 Orange-brown

8 Brown

FIGURE 10.1 Visual-analog scale for urine color. A visual-analog scale for urine color is used to provide a quick, inexpensive method to qualitatively assess fluid status. This practice becomes more important as exercise progresses in hot and humid environments, especially for prolonged periods. The closer the urine is to #1, the more hydrated a person. Generally speaking, a person should strive for better hydration, but values closely matched to #1, #2, or #3 are satisfactory. If a person's urine color is dark orange, brown, or brownish-green, #6 or greater, the person is likely dehydrated, and aggressive fluid-replacement strategies should be employed. (Adapted from Armstrong, L. E. 2000. *Performing in extreme environments.* Champaign, IL: Human Kinetics.)

measurements to urine osmolality and may not do well to track changes in body mass with acute dehydration and rehydration (Armstrong et al. 1998; Kovacs et al. 1999; Popowski et al. 2001). For example, Shirreffs and Maughan (1998) found that drinking large volumes of dilute fluids (such as water) results in copious urine production long before euhydration is achieved. For this reason, a urine sample from the first void in the morning following an overnight fast minimizes confounding influences and enhances reliability. In addition, dipsticks can be used to measure urine specific gravity; however, their use remains to be clearly accepted.

10.2.2.3 Determining Sweat Rate

An increase in heat production always occurs during exercise, especially when the exercising environment is hot and humid. Sweating is the primary mechanism the body uses to dissipate this heat, and the rate of sweat production dictates how quickly fluid loss will occur. Developing a reasonable estimate of the rate of sweat production is fairly straightforward and should be regularly used by athletes, coaches, parents, and athletic trainers to identify the sweat rate of individuals. Doing so will

TABLE 10.5
Sweat Rate Calculator

A.   Pre-exercise body mass (in pounds) = _____ pounds (1 kg = 2.2 pounds)
B.   Post-exercise body mass (in pounds) = _____ pounds (1 kg = 2.2 pounds)
C.   Body mass lost (column B – column A) = _____ pounds (1 kg = 2.2 pounds)
D.   Fluid consumed during exercise = _____ mL (30 mL = 1 fl oz)
E.   During exercise urine production = _____ mL
(Only include urine produced during exercise. If no urine was produced, this value remains zero.)
F.   Total sweat loss = _____ mL (C + D + E = F)*
*Convert everything to mL (assume 1 kg = 1000 mL)
G.   Exercise duration = _____ min
H.   Sweat rate (divide F by G) = _____ mL/min
I.   Sweat rate (L/hour) = _____ L/hour
(Divide H by 1000 and then multiply by 60)

Example:
A.   Pre-exercise body mass = 217 pounds (217/2.2 = 98.64 kg)
B.   Post-exercise body mass = 214 pounds (214/2.2 = 97.27 kg)
C.   Body mass lost from exercise = 3 pounds (3/2.2 = 1.36 kg)
D.   Fluid consumed during exercise = 32 fl oz (32 fl oz × 30 = 960 mL)
E.   During exercise urine production = 600 mL
F.   Total sweat loss = (3 pounds/2.2 = 1.36 kg = 1360 mL) = 1360 mL + 960 mL + 600 mL = 2920 mL
     of fluid lost as sweat
G.   Exercise duration = 100 minutes
H.   Sweat rate = 2920/100 = 29.2 mL/min
I.   29.2 mL/min/1000 = 0.029 L/min * 60 = 1.752 L/hour

identify those people who may be at greater risk for developing dehydration and can be used as a preliminary guide for how much environmental exposure should occur. Outlined throughout Table 10.5 is a step-by-step derivation of how an individual can determine their sweat rate. Furthermore, an example calculation is provided to assist with accurate comprehension of all calculations. For technologically motivated people, software with calculating capability can prove to be especially useful in scenarios where large numbers of people are being measured. Determining this information along with the other dehydration-assessment techniques in combination with the fluid replacement guidelines provided later in the chapter is an outstanding approach to monitor, measure, and recover from the effects of exercising in the heat and dehydration.

10.2.2.4   The Impact of Clothing

Recent advancements in fabrics of clothing worn during exercise has been a major area of development. Regardless, ideal warm-weather clothing is lightweight, loose fitting, and light colored. Dark-colored shirts, jerseys, pants, etc., are known to absorb heat and add to radiant heat gain, whereas lighter colors reflect the heat rays. Any form of clothing, no matter how technologically advanced or lightweight, retards heat exchange more than the same clothing if it is fully wet. When a shirt becomes saturated with fluid from sweat, the potential for this water to evaporate and cool the body is increased. For this reason alone, it makes very little sense to change shirts, uniforms, etc., because this will only prolong the time between sweating and evaporative cooling and in effect will increase the thermal load on the body.

Of particular concern are those sports where some form of a uniform in which helmets, pads, etc., are worn for protection because they serve as a definite barrier between the skin and the environmental air, thus reducing the potential for cooling. For example, subjects who exercised for 30 minutes in one of three conditions: 1) a full uniform, 2) shorts only, and 3) shorts and a pack equal in weight to the uniform, experienced significantly reduced rectal and skin temperatures in either condition when the full uniform was not worn (Mathews et al. 1969). In summary, lightly colored clothing that is loose fitting is preferred to facilitate evaporative cooling from sweat during exercise.

10.3 NUTRITIONAL CONSIDERATIONS TO MANAGE HYDRATION STATUS

10.3.1 GASTRIC EMPTYING

In many situations, the body's ability to empty stomach contents from the gastric region is a limiting factor regarding prevention of dehydration and performance. Many factors have been identified that impact the rate at which gastric emptying occurs, as can be seen in Table 10.6. For example, the volume of fluids ingested is one factor that has been shown to increase emptying into the intestine. When fluid is ingested on a regular basis and the volume of fluid in the stomach rises, the rate of gastric emptying from the stomach will increase (Hunt and Stubbs 1975; Mitchell and

---

TABLE 10.6
Variables That Impact the Rate of Gastric Emptying

Variables	Outcome
Volume[a]	Increasing volume promotes emptying
Energy Content[b]	Increasing energy content slows emptying
Osmolality[c]	Markedly increasing osmolality slows emptying
pH	Marked deviations from neutrality slows emptying
Exercise[d]	Hard (>70%–75% VO_{2max}) exercise slows emptying
Stress	Mental stress and anxiety slows emptying
Dehydration[e]	Slows gastric emptying; increases risk of gastrointestinal distress

[a] Hunt and Stubbs 1975; Mitchell and Voss 1990; Noakes et al. 1990.
[b] Hunt et al. 1985; Hunt and Stubbs 1975.
[c] Hunt and Pathak 1960; Hunt et al. 1985; Hunt and Stubbs 1975.
[d] Costill and Saltin 1974; Maughan et al. 1990; Rehrer et al. 1989.
[e] Rehrer et al. 1990.

Voss 1990; Noakes et al. 1990). In addition, factors such as the energy content and osmolality can be responsible for significant reductions in the rate of gastric emptying (Hunt and Pathak 1960; Hunt et al. 1985; Hunt and Stubbs 1975). Oftentimes, a highly concentrated source of fluid or food has to be broken down before it can be released and absorbed in the bloodstream. This delay in emptying in the face of increased fluid loss from sweating can negatively impact overall hydration status.

Furthermore, with more intense exercise and as dehydration develops, the rate of gastric emptying is reduced (Costill and Saltin 1974; Maughan et al. 1990; Rehrer et al. 1989, 1990). Often the combination between drastically increased rates of fluid loss caused by heavy sweating during exercise in a hot and humid environment and decreased rates of gastric emptying result in a scenario where an overall decrease in total body water is inevitable. In fact, studies have clearly shown that once dehydration develops during an exercise bout, no combination of hydration can restore hydration status to a euhydrated state no matter how severe the dehydration may be (Convertino et al. 1996). This is a humbling realization for the athlete but important to understand because it brings into clear focus the importance of managing your hydration status before the exercise bout even starts.

10.3.2 Fluid Replacement

Replacing fluids lost as a result of exercise is a critical consideration for optimal health and performance. Fluid consumption facilitates optimal maintenance of blood volume, which drives circulation, perspiration, and blood flow. Fortunately, well-published guidelines exist for these guidelines and can be found in many textbooks and review papers on the topic (Otten et al. 2006; Burke 2001; Convertino et al. 1996; Noakes 1993; Nutrient Guideslines 2000).

10.3.2.1 Before Exercise

Much of the focus for fluid replacement has centered upon fluid ingestion during the actual exercise bout, and rightfully so. Studies, however, have indicated that "pre-hydration," or ingesting fluids before the exercise bout, can serve as an effective tool to: 1) ensure the body is hydrated prior to the start of exercise and 2) help stave off the inevitable development of dehydration once the exercise bout commences. Elite soccer players hyperhydrated for one week (~4.5 L of fluid/day) in comparison with their normal hydration (~2.7 L of fluid/day) before a competition in a hot and humid environment. Greater fluid ingestion resulted in increased total body water and also increased thermoregulation throughout the exercise bout, whereas performance seemed to be unaffected (Rico-Sanz et al. 1996). As a general guideline, athletes are recommended to generously ingest fluids throughout the day. Two to three hours prior to exercise, athletes should ingest 500–600 mL (16–20 fl oz) of fluid and another 240 mL (8 fl oz) of fluid 20–30 minutes prior to exercise.

10.3.2.1.1 Glycerol Hyperhydration

In addition to increasing the ingested amount of fluids, ingestion of glycerol has been used for some time as a means to increase body water. Although body water can readily be increased by simply ingesting more fluids, a side effect of this practice is increased dieresis or urine production. Although completely acceptable in non-exercising scenarios, an increase in trips to the toilet is not possible during competitive scenarios.

Glycerol ingestion creates a favorable osmotic gradient that favors fluid retention, an amount commonly reported to be around one liter of fluid (van Rosendal et al. 2010). As a hyperhydration approach, athletes were suggested to ingest 1.2 g of glycerol/kg of body mass in 26 mL of fluid/kg of body mass over a 60-minute period, ending 30 minutes prior to exercise. Using this hyperhydration approach with either glycerol or a placebo solution, no differences in thermoregulation, performance, etc., were noticed throughout and after a 2-hour cycling ride at 66% VO_{2max}, but a significant decrease in urine volume was found (Goulet et al. 2006). However, when the glycerol hyperhydration approach was compared with a euhydrated state, the glycerol-containing conditions significantly increased total body water, prevented loss of body water, and improved performance as well as peak power output (Goulet et al. 2008). When ingested throughout an exercise bout, glycerol ingestion in lower dosages (0.125 g/kg of body mass in 5 mL of fluid/kg of body mass) can help to delay dehydration. In a post-exercise scenario, intermediate dosages (1.0 g of glycerol/kg of body mass added to each 1.5 L of fluid consumed) can accelerate restoration of plasma volume (van Rosendal et al. 2010).

10.3.2.2   During Exercise

Due to the great potential for fluid loss to occur during exercise, fluid ingestion during exercise is likely the most important factor for an athlete or coach to consider. Fortunately, guidelines for this purpose have been well-documented in position statements (Convertino et al. 1996), review papers (Noakes 1993), and other well-crafted chapters and/or books on the topic (Armstrong 2000; Byars 2008; Kleiner and Kalman 2009). A key factor for all athletes and coaches to consider is that relying upon an individual's thirst mechanism to dictate when and how much fluid is ingested is poor practice. It is well documented that the thirst mechanism is markedly delayed and that waiting to ingest fluids until the athlete is thirsty will result in a scenario where the body is already dehydrated starting from the beginning stages of exercise. Although the general guidelines that will be discussed are broad and have been developed to accommodate the hydration needs of masses of athletes, several factors discussed throughout this chapter create a situation where some level of specific and/or customizing a program may need to occur.

Generally, active individuals should strive to consume an estimated 350–500 mL (12–16 fl oz or 1–2 cups) every 15 minutes during exercise. Much research has been conducted to develop an optimal formulation of a sports drink, which provides fluid, carbohydrate, and electrolytes, all of which are lost in varying amounts as a result of exercising (especially in the heat). To date, much of the available research suggests that the optimal carbohydrate concentration is between 6% and 8% carbohydrate (6–8 g of carbohydrate for every 100 mL of fluid). As a key fuel source, carbohydrate is oxidized at a rate of 1–1.2 g of carbohydrate every minute or 60%–75 g of carbohydrate every hour of exercise.

A 6%–8% carbohydrate solution has been shown to strike the fine balance between providing enough carbohydrate to prevent deleterious reliance on muscle and liver glycogen stores, especially as exercise persists much past one hour of exercise. Similarly, this concentration also avoids providing too much carbohydrate in solution, which according to Table 10.6 would result in a decrease in gastric emptying. Lastly, a well-formulated sports drink contains sodium and other electrolytes, which can help to drive thirst and encourage more drinking while also preventing any further development of hyponatremia, which comes from drinking too much water (also called water intoxication).

For this reason and in summary, it is commonly recommended that if exercise bouts will be less than 60 minutes, ingestion of only water will suffice, but as the duration of exercise continues past one hour, the need to ingest a drink that also contains carbohydrate and sodium becomes apparent, especially if optimal performance is expected and environmental conditions are hot and humid. Finally, it should be mentioned that research is lacking to prove any level of efficacy for vitamin- or mineral-enriched waters during exercise.

10.3.2.2.1 Hyponatremia

Hyponatremia is a serious situation that often occurs as a result of misinformed individuals (although they may have great intentions). Unfortunately, each year, there are reports of athletes developing hyponatremia and very serious outcomes including seizures, coma, and death. Clinically, hyponatremia is defined as low serum sodium (<135 mmol/L) levels (Byars 2008). Hyponatremia develops during exercise as a result of an overconsumption of water as fluid (Androgue and Madias 2000). Typically, the condition develops as a person exercises for an extended period of time (>3 hours) and consumes copious amounts of water likely in a diligent attempt to stave off the development of dehydration (Gardner 2002).

As can be seen in Figure 10.2, a number of the common symptoms associated with hyponatremia are similar to dehydration, making it hard for the athlete or immediate responder to discern between the two conditions. Fortunately, hyponatremia is relatively easy to prevent. Adding sodium to a beverage or drinking a beverage that is already formulated to contain sodium is the primary consideration because relatively small amounts appear to be enough to sustain blood sodium

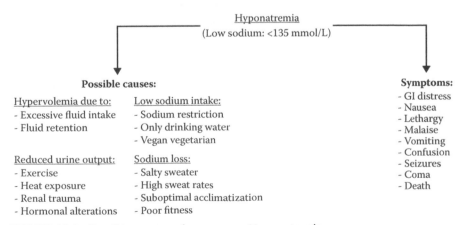

FIGURE 10.2 Possible causes and symptoms of hyponatremia.

levels. Although it is relatively easy to prevent, those individuals exercising for extended periods (>3 hours) in hot and humid environments and only ingesting water are at the greatest risk. In addition, the sodium concentration of sweat is different between individuals, and those people who are "salty sweaters" will lose sodium at rates fasterthan individuals who do not have a high concentration of sodium in their sweat and as a result will be more susceptible to developing hyponatremia. Regardless, adding salt to your drink, eating salty foods, or regularly alternating water ingestion with a sports drink are common strategies to prevent hyponatremia (Androgue and Madias 2000).

10.3.2.3   After Exercise

After exercise, prudent monitoring of body-mass changes should take place each day. As mentioned in other sections of this chapter, several techniques exist to monitor hydration, but tracking daily body-mass changes and urine color are two of the easiest and most practical measures that can be performed. An excellent, simple guideline for athletes, parents, and coaches to consider when exercising over the course of several consecutive days in a hot and humid environment is for the athlete to strive to regain all of the weight loss from the previous day before participating in practice on subsequent days. As a general guideline, athletes are encouraged to drink two cups of fluid for every pound of body mass lost as fluid after exercise.

A great debate exists as to what types of fluids are the best to consume to restore hydration status. Certainly, rehydrating with water or sports drink are excellent choices and should never be fully discounted. It is important, however, for the athlete to realize that not all of the fluid ingested has to come in beverages because many foods or snacks can be consumed that have extremely high water content. Examples of these foods include any citrus fruit, pickles, and lettuce; all of these foods are an estimated >85% water, whereas foods such as breads, cheeses, cookies, etc., are not good food sources of water.

Recently, studies have begun to elucidate the impact of adding a small amount of protein to a post-exercise carbohydrate drink and examined this combination for its ability to promote rehydration. When isocaloric amounts of carbohydrate (153 g) and a carbohydrate-protein mixture (112 g of carbohydrate + 41 g of protein) were ingested in two equal amounts after an intense glycogen-depleting bout of exercise and diet, the carbohydrate-protein combination helped to recover lost glycogen more quickly and improved time to exhaustion performance (Ivy et al. 2002).

Similarly, other studies have shown that providing one part protein to four parts carbohydrate can facilitate improved rehydration and performance, better than either water or a carbohydrate-only recovery drink (Ivy et al. 2002; Seifert et al. 2006). In fact, one of these studies reported that the carbohydrate-protein combination improved hydration by 40% over water alone and by 15% over carbohydrate alone. Although more of a recovery application, but still relevant to the scope of this chapter, studies are also available suggesting that this type of carbohydrate-protein combination may help to minimize the muscle damage seen after intense exercise and as a result may hasten recovery (Kerksick et al. 2008; Seifert et al. 2005; White et al. 2008). Finally, studies have begun to explore the impact of ingesting milk for its ability to facilitate recovery and promote rehydration. When compared with a sports drink or water, milk favorably promoted hydration after a dehydrating exercise bout that resulted in a 1.8% loss of body mass as fluid (Shirreffs et al. 2007). Results from this study suggest that milk can serve as an effective post-exercise rehydration drink.

In summary, post-exercise recovery is a critical consideration for exercising athletes. Although water- and carbohydrate-only ingestion can replenish lost fluid and muscle glycogen, adding a small amount of protein may result in more favorable recovery, minimize muscle damage, and improve performance.

10.3.2.4 Caffeinated Beverages and Dehydration

Many beverage choices include those that are caffeinated. It is often reported that caffeine will cause dehydration and as a result these beverages should be consumed in limited amounts or not at all. This consideration introduces quite a paradox when you consider that caffeine is widely known to act as an ergogenic aid during multiple sporting scenarios (Goldstein et al. 2010). When investigating its role in hydration, studies have reported no effect on urine or plasma markers of dehydration after three consecutive days of two practices per day when ingesting caffeinated Coca-Cola or its noncaffeinated version (Fiala et al. 2004). Similarly 18 males tested four beverages over a 24-hour period on changes in blood and urine markers of dehydration and clearly showed that caffeine did not invoke a dehydrating response (Grandjean et al. 2000). Although caffeine does act as a mild diuretic, closer investigations have revealed this mild effect does not result in dehydration (Millard-Stafford et al. 2007), and considering its ergogenic potential caffeine should be considered as a nutritional aid for exercise performance (Maughan and Griffin 2003).

10.4 CONCLUSIONS

Very few things exist that take on a greater level of importance for a competing athlete than maintaining required fluid levels. Repeated investigations have confirmed that fluid levels must be maintained if optimal performance is to follow. Daily water needs for humans reveal many individual factors that need be addressed on a personal level instead of using a mass-action or "cookie cutter" approach.

Daily monitoring of body-mass changes and urine color along with recording fluid ingestion are critical steps an athlete must take to effectively determine how much fluid is being lost as a part of practice and competition. Optimal daily hydration starts with regular fluid ingestion throughout the day and ingestion of foods containing high amounts of water. Prior to exercise, additional fluid should be consumed in addition to elevated ingestion during exercise to help combat the loss of fluid as sweat in the body's attempt to cool itself. Many considerations exist as to which fluids should be ingested, but the most important fluid is the one the athlete will ingest. From there, studies clearly show that providing small amounts of carbohydrate can help spare stored glycogen and increase performance, while the addition of sodium helps to minimize the development of hyponatremia. Adding one part protein to four parts carbohydrate has been shown to support hydration, promote recovery, and minimize muscle damage. Caffeinated beverages are encouraged, should not be avoided out of fear for its diuretic effects, and instead are well accepted to serve an ergogenic role.

REFERENCES

Androgue, H. J., and N. E. Madias. 2000. Hyponatremia. *New Engl J Med* 342: 1581–1589.

Armstrong, L. E. 2005. Hydration assessment techniques. *Nutr Rev* 63: S40–S54.

Armstrong, L. E. 2000. *Performing in Extreme Environments*. Champaign, IL: Human Kinetics.

Armstrong, L. E., C. M. Maresh, J. W. Castellani, M. F. Bereron, R. W. Kenefick, K. E. Lagassee, and D. Riebe. 1994. Urinary indices of hydration status. *Int J Sports Nutr* 4: 265–279.

Armstrong, L. E., C. M. Maresh, C. V. Gabaree, J. R. Hoffman, S. A. Kavouras, R. W. Kenefick, J. W. Castellani, and L. E. Ahlquist. 1997. Thermal and circulatory responses during exercise: Effects of hypohydration, dehydration, and water intake. *J Appl Physiol* 82: 2028–2035.

Armstrong, L. E., J. A. Soto, F. T. Hacker, D. J. Casa, S. A. Kavouras, and C. M. Maresh. 1998. Urinary indices during dehydration, exercise, and rehydration. *Int J Sports Nutr* 8: 345–355.

Ballauff, A., M. Kersting, and F. Manz. 1988. Do children have an adequate fluid intake? Water balance studies carried out at home. *Ann Nutr Metab* 32: 332–339.

Burke, L. M. 2001. Nutritional needs for exercise in the heat. *Comp Biochem Physiol* 128: 735–748.

Byars, A. 2008. Fluid regulation for life and human performance. In *Nutritional Supplements in Sports and Exercise*, edited by M. Greenwood, D. S. Kalman, and J. Antonio. Totawa, NJ: Humana Press.

Cheuvront, S. N., R. Carter, 3rd, S. J. Montain, and M. N. Sawka. 2004. Daily body mass variability and stability in active men undergoing exercise-heat stress. *Int J Sport Nutr Exerc Metab* 14: 532–540.

Convertino, V. A., L. E. Armstrong, E. F. Coyle, G. W. Mack, M. N. Sawka, L. C. Senay, and W. M. Sherman. 1996. ACSM position stand: Exercise and fluid replacment. *Med Sci Sports Exerc* 28: i–ix.

Costill, D. L., and B. Saltin. 1974. Factors limiting gastric emptying during rest and exercise. *J Appl Physiol* 37: 679–683.

Fiala, K. A., D. J. Casa, and M. W. Roti. 2004. Rehydration with a caffeinated beverage during the nonexercise periods of 3 consecutive days of 2-a-day practices. *Int J Sport Nutr Exerc Metab* 14: 419–429.

Fusch, C., W. Gfrorer, H. H. Dickhuth, and H. Moeller. 1998. Physical fitness influences water turnover and body water changes during trekking. *Med Sci Sports Exerc* 30: 704–708.

Gardner, J. W. 2002. Death by water intoxication. *Military Med* 5: 432–434.

Goellner, M. H., E. E. Ziegler, and S. J. Fomon. 1981. Urination during the first three years of life. *Nephron* 28: 174–178.

Goldstein, E. R., T. Ziegenfuss, D. Kalman, R. Kreider, B. Campbell, C. Wilborn, L. Taylor, D. Willoughby, J. Stout, B. S. Graves, R. Wildman, J. L. Ivy, M. Spano, A. E. Smith, and J. Antonio. 2010. International Society of Sports Nutrition position stand: Caffeine and performance. *J Int Soc Sports Nutr* 7: 5.

Goulet, E. D., R. A. Robergs, S. Labrecque, D. Royer, and I. J. Dionne. 2006. Effect of glycerol-induced hyperhydration on thermoregulatory and cardiovascular functions and endurance performance during prolonged cycling in a 25 degrees C environment. *Appl Physiol Nutr Metab* 31: 101–109.

Goulet, E. D., S. F. Rousseau, C. R. Lamboley, G. E. Plante, and I. J. Dionne. 2008. Pre-exercise hyperhydration delays dehydration and improves endurance capacity during 2 h of cycling in a temperate climate. *J Physiol Anthropol* 27: 263–271.

Grandjean, A. C., K. J. Reimers, K. E. Bannick, and M. C. Haven. 2000. The effect of caffeinated, non-caffeinated, caloric, and non-caloric beverages on hydration. *Am J Clin Nutr* 19: 591–600.

Greenleaf, J. E., P. J. Brock, L. C. Keil, and J. T. Morse. 1983. Drinking and water balance during exercise and heat acclimation. *J Appl Physiol* 54: 414–419.

Hunt, J. N., and J. D. Pathak. 1960. The osmotic effect of some simple molecules and ions on gastric emptying. *J Physiol* 154: 254–269.

Hunt, J. N., J. L. Smith, and C. L. Jiang. 1985. Effect of meal volume and energy density on the gastric emptying rate of carbohydrates. *Gastroenterology* 89: 1326–1330.

Hunt, J. N., and D. F. Stubbs. 1975. The volume and energy content of meals as determinants of gastric emptying. *J Physiol* 245: 209–225.

Institute of Medicine and Food and Nutrition Board. 2004. *Dietary Reference Intakes for Water, Potassium, Sodium, Chloride and Sulfate.* Washington, D.C.: National Academies Press.

Ivy, J. L., H. W. Goforth, Jr., B. M. Damon, T. R. Mccauley, E. C. Parsons, and T. B. Price. 2002. Early postexercise muscle glycogen recovery is enhanced with a carbohydrate-protein supplement. *J Appl Physiol* 93: 1337–1344.

Kerksick, C., T. Harvey, J. Stout, B. Campbell, C. Wilborn, R. Kreider, D. Kalman, T. Ziegenfuss, H. Lopez, J. Landis, J. L. Ivy, and J. Antonio. 2008. International Society of Sports Nutrition position stand: Nutrient timing. *J Int Soc Sports Nutr* 5: 17.

Kleiner, S. M., and D. Kalman. 2009. Hydration. In *Nutritional Concerns in Recreation, Exercise and Sport*, edited by J. A. Driskell and I. Wolinsky. Boca Raton, FL: CRC Press.

Kovacs, E. M., J. M. Senden, and F. Brouns. 1999. Urine color, osmolality and specific electrical conductance are not accurate measures of hydration status during postexercise rehydration. *J Sports Med Phys Fitness* 39: 47–53.

Leiper, J. B., A. Carnie, and R. J. Maughan. 1996. Water turnover rates in sedentary and exercising middle aged men. *Br J Sports Med* 30: 24–26.

Leiper, J. B., Y. Pitsiladis, and R. J. Maughan. 2001. Comparison of water turnover rates in men undertaking prolonged cycling exercise and sedentary men. *Int J Sports Med* 22: 181–185.

Mathews, D. K., E. L. Fox, and D. Tanzi. 1969. Physiological responses during exercise and recovery in a football uniform. *J Appl Physiol* 26: 611–615.

Maughan, R. J. 2003. Impact of mild dehydration on wellness and on exercise performance. *Eur J Clin Nutr* 57(Suppl 2): S19–S23.

Maughan, R. J., and J. Griffin. 2003. Caffeine ingestion and fluid balance: A review. *J Hum Nutr Diet* 16: 411–420.

Maughan, R. J., J. B. Leiper, and B. A. Mcgaw. 1990. Effects of exercise intensity on absorption of ingested fluids in man. *Exp Physiol* 75: 419–421.

Millard-Stafford, M. L., K. J. Cureton, J. E. Wingo, J. Trilk, G. L. Warren, and M. Buyckx. 2007. Hydration during exercise in warm, humid conditions: Effect of a caffeinated sports drink. *Int J Sport Nutr Exerc Metab* 17: 163–177.

Mitchell, J. B., and K. W. Voss. 1990. The influence of volume on gastric emptying and fluid balance during prolonged exercise. *Med Sci Sports Exerc* 23: 314–319.

Noakes, T. D. 1993. Fluid replacement during exercise. *Exerc Sport Sci Rev* 21: 297–330.

Noakes, T. D., N. J. Rehrer, and R. J. Maughan. 1990. The imporance of volume on gastric emptying and fluid balance during prolonged exercise. *Med Sci Sports Exerc* 23: 307–313.

Ormerod, J. K., T. A. Elliott, T. P. Scheett, J. L. Vanheest, L. E. Armstrong, and C. M. Maresh. 2003. Drinking behavior and perception of thirst in untrained women during 6 weeks of heat acclimation and outdoor training. *Int J Sport Nutr Exerc Metab* 13: 15–28.

Otten, J., J. Pitzi Hellwig, and L. Meyers. eds. 2006. *DRI, Dietary Reference Intakes: The Essential Guide to Nutrient Requirements.* Washington DC: The National Academics Press.

Popowski, L. A., R. A. Oppliger, G. P. Lambert, R. F. Johnson, A. Kim Johnson, and C. V. Gisolf. 2001. Blood and urinary measures of hydration status during progressive acute dehydration. *Med Sci Sports Exerc* 33: 747–753.

Raman, A., D. A. Schoeller, A. F. Subar, R. P. Troiano, A. Schatzkin, T. Harris, D. Bauer, S. A. Bingham, J. E. Everhart, A. B. Newman, and F. A. Tylavsky. 2004. Water turnover in 458 American adults 40–79 yr of age. *Am J Physiol Renal Physiol* 286: F394–F401.

Rehrer, N. J., E. J. Beckers, F. Brouns, F. Ten Hoor, and W. H. M. Saris. 1990. Effects of dehydration on gastric emptying and gastrointestinal distress while running. *Med Sci Sports Exerc* 22: 790–795.

Rehrer, N. J., E. J. Beckers, F. Brouns, F. Ten Hoor, and W. H. M. Saris. 1989. Exercise and training effects on gastric emptying of carbohdyrate beverages. *Med Sci Sports Exerc* 21: 540–549.

Rico-Sanz, J., W. R. Frontera, M. A. Rivera, A. Rivera-Brown, P. A. Mole, and C. N. Meredith. 1996. Effects of hyperhydration on total body water, temperature regulation and performance of elite young soccer players in a warm climate. *Int J Sports Med* 17: 85–91.

Sawka, M. N., S. N. Cheuvront, and R. Carter, 3rd. 2005. Human water needs. *Nutr Rev* 63: S30–S39.

Seifert, J., J. Harmon, and P. Declercq. 2006. Protein added to a sports drink improves fluid retention. *Int J Sport Nutr Exerc Metab* 16: 420–429.

Seifert, J. G., R. W. Kipp, M. Amann, and O. Gazal. 2005. Muscle damage, fluid ingestion, and energy supplementation during recreational alpine skiing. *Int J Sport Nutr Exerc Metab* 15: 528–536.

Shapiro, Y., K. B. Pandolf, and R. F. Goldman. 1982. Predicting sweat loss response to exercise, environment and clothing. *Eur J Appl Physiol Occup Physiol* 48: 83–96.

Shirreffs, S. M. 2003. Markers of hydration status. *Eur J Clin Nutr* 57(Suppl 2): S6–S9.

Shirreffs, S. M., and R. J. Maughan. 1998. Urine osmolality and conductivity as indices of hydration status in athletes in the heat. *Med Sci Sports Exerc* 30: 1598–1602.

Shirreffs, S. M., P. Watson, and R. J. Maughan. 2007. Milk as an effective post-exercise rehydration drink. *Br J Nutr* 98: 173–180.

Van Loan, M., and R. Boileu. 1996. Age, gender, and fluid balance. In *Body Fluid Balance: Exercise and Sport*, edited by E. Buskirk and S. Puhl. Boca Raton, FL: CRC Press.

van Rosendal, S. P., M. A. Osborne, R. G. Fassett, and J. S. Coombes. 2010. Guidelines for glycerol use in hyperhydration and rehydration associated with exercise. *Sports Med* 40: 113–129.

Welch, B. E., E. R. Buskirk, and P. F. Iampietro. 1958. Relation of climate and temperature to food and water intake in man. *Metabolism* 7: 141–148.

White, J. P., J. M. Wilson, K. G. Austin, B. K. Greer, N. St John, and L. B. Panton. 2008. Effect of carbohydrate-protein supplement timing on acute exercise-induced muscle damage. *J Int Soc Sports Nutr* 5: 5.

Wilson, M. M., and J. E. Morley. 2003. Impaired cognitive function and mental performance in mild dehydration. *Eur J Appl Physiol* 57(Suppl 2): S24–S29.

Section III

Other Training Table Considerations

11 Calorie Needs for Improving Body Composition

Vincent J. Dalbo and Michael D. Roberts

CONTENTS

11.1 INTRODUCTION

There are favorable body weights/body fat percentages that allow for optimal performance in sport. Table 11.1 provides information on body size and composition of elite athletes in various sports. Athletes attempting to reduce body weight should: 1) reduce weight in a healthy and efficient manner that can be maintained over time

TABLE 11.1
Body Composition of Elite Athletes in Various Sports

Sport	Gender	Position	Height (cm)	Weight (kg)	Body Fat (%)
Football	Males (Kraemer et al. 2005)[a]	Quarterback	192.0 ± 5.8	104.2 ± 2.6	14.6 ± 9.3
		Running back	180.0 ± 3.0	96.5 ± 8.1	7.3 ± 7.3
		Wide receiver	180.5 ± 3.9	85.6 ± 6.5	8.1 ± 2.8
		Tight end	194.4 ± 4.0	115.6 ± 7.2	15.1 ± 5.4
		Offensive line	193.3 ± 3.8	140.0 ± 7.5	25.1 ± 2.5
		Defensive line	191.6 ± 2.5	126.8 ± 2.4	18.5 ± 3.8
		Linebackers	186.9 ± 2.6	107.8 ± 2.9	15.7 ± 2.8
		Defensive back	179.7 ± 4.5	87.1 ± 5.6	6.3 ± 2.8
		Kicker/punter	191.4 ± 5.9	95.3 ± 0.0	11.4 ± 8.3
Basketball	Males (Ben Abdelkrim et al. 2010)[b]	Point guard	186.4 ± 5.2	78.1 ± 5.8	11.2 ± 0.7
		Shooting guard	194.0 ± 3.8	85.6 ± 5.2	8.3 ± 1.6
		Small forward	195.8 ± 3.3	87.8 ± 4.4	8.6 ± 0.7
		Power forward	202.0 ± 3.4	95.8 ± 4.3	11.6 ± 2.5
		Center	204.4 ± 4.7	97.1 ± 5.4	14.8 ± 1.9
	Females (Carbuhn et al. 2010)[c]	All positions combined	—	77.1 ± 9.4	22.7 ± 5.6
Soccer	Males (Raven et al. 1976)[d]	Forward	176.3 ± 6.5	74.5 ± 12.3	10.7 ± 2.0
		Midfield player	175.0 ± 4.1	77.3 ± 5.1	10.6 ± 3.3
		Defensive back	176.0 ± 5.7	73.6 ± 5.7	8.1 ± 3.6
		Goalkeeper	178.0 ± 3.1	86.4 ± 6.4	13.3 ± 0.1
	Females (Sedano Campo et al. 2009)[b]	All positions combined	163.0 ± 7.0	58.9 ± 9.3	23.9 ± 2.2
Baseball	Males (Coleman and Lasky 1992)[b]	Catcher	179.4 ± 2.8	90.6 ± 6.7	9.7 ± 4.0
		Infielder	182.5 ± 5.2	83.4 ± 7.3	9.3 ± 3.4
		Outfielder	182.4 ± 4.1	85.0 ± 8.0	8.4 ± 3.6
		Pitcher	186.3 ± 4.6	90.3 ± 8.0	10.4 ± 4.9
		All positions combined	—	69.5 ± 7.0	25.7 ± 5.0
Softball	Females (Carbuhn et al. 2010)[c]	All positions combined	—	69.5 ± 7.0	25.7 ± 5.0
Volleyball	Males (Calbet, et al. 1999)[c]	All positions combined	192.6 ± 6.0	87.4 ± 8.5	12.2 ± 3.4
	Females (Malousaris et al. 2008)[b]	All positions combined	179.6 ± 5.8	71.0 ± 8.2	22.7 ± 2.9

The data are reported as the means ± standard deviation.

[a] Body composition assessed using a BOD POD (air-displacement plethysmography).
[b] Body composition assessed using a skinfold equation.
[c] Body composition assessed using a DEXA (dual energy x-ray absorptiometry).
[d] Body composition assessed using a hydrostatic weighing.

and 2) maximize strength-to-weight ratio. This is especially important for weight-bearing sports such as wrestling, boxing, and mixed martial arts (MMA), where athletes should seek to compete in a weight class that optimizes their strength-to-weight ratio. This chapter will: 1) discuss how to determine body weight for a desired body fat percentage, 2) discuss how to determine caloric consumption including the calculation of resting metabolic rate (RMR) and daily energy expenditure (DEE), 3) provide dietary suggestions to promote healthy weight loss that can be maintained over time, 4) provide athletes with tests to assess their strength-to-weight ratio, and 5) provide athletes with practical take-home messages that can be applied to training table diets.

11.2 DETERMINING BODY WEIGHT FOR A GIVEN BODY FAT PERCENTAGE

After determining the optimal body fat percentage to optimize performance in your given sport and position, the next step is to determine the body weight you must achieve to obtain your target body fat percentage. The following formula can be used to determine target body weight (Howley and Franks 2007).

$$\text{Target body weight} = \text{FFM}/(1 - [\text{desired \% BF}/100])$$
$$\text{FFM (fat free mass)} = \text{body mass} - \text{fat mass}$$
$$\text{\% BF} = \text{body fat percentage}$$

To use the target body weight formula you must have an accurate estimate of percent body fat, which can be accomplished in an affordable, time-efficient manner with the use of skin fold calipers. Determination of percent body fat using 3 and 7 site skin fold equations is accurate for determining percent body fat when obtained by a qualified technician (Moon et al. 2007); however, the "average" person should be able to obtain an accurate measure of percent body fat with practice. For more information on how to obtain a measure of percent body fat and a list of population-specific skinfold equations, refer to the National Strength and Conditioning Association's Essentials of Strength and Conditioning text (Baechle and Earle 2000). For an example of how to use the target body weight equation see Topic Box 11.1.

11.3 MECHANISM FOR WEIGHT LOSS

After determination of optimal body weight, the next step is to understand the concept of energy balance. Body weight is determined by energy consumption versus energy expenditure. Weight gain occurs when energy consumption consistently exceeds energy expenditure. Energy balance (weight maintenance) occurs when energy consumption (or calories from food eaten) equals energy expenditure (or calories burned throughout the day). This chapter discusses the concept of weight loss, which occurs when energy expenditure consistently exceeds energy consumption. It is important to understand that "diets" do not have to be extreme to result in significant weight loss. Table 11.2 displays that relatively small alterations in daily energy balance over time can result in large changes in body composition over the course of a couple of months. In fact, an energy balance difference of 500 kcal/day

TOPIC BOX 11.1   DETERMINATION OF TARGET BODY WEIGHT

A 20-year-old male has a body weight of 200 pounds and was estimated to have 15% body fat. His goal is to have a body fat of 8%.

Step 1: Determine FFM

To accomplish this, you must first determine the amount of fat mass.

Fat mass = body weight × percent body fat

200 pounds × 0.15 = 30 pounds of fat mass

Then you can determine FFM

FFM = body weight − fat mass

200 pounds − 30 pounds = 170 pounds

Step 2: Enter the required variables into the target body-weight equation

Target body weight = 170/(1 − (8/100)) = 184.78 pounds

To obtain a body fat percentage of 8%, this man will have to reduce his body weight to approximately 185 pounds while maintaining skeletal muscle mass.

(3500 kcal/week) can theoretically result in a weight difference of 48 pounds over the course of a year.

11.3.1 DETERMINING CALORIC NEEDS FOR WEIGHT LOSS

Now that it has been established that weight loss occurs as a function of maintaining a negative caloric balance for an extended period of time, we need to explore

TABLE 11.2

Theoretical Weight Change of a 250-Pound Athlete in Caloric Excess or Deficit of 500 kcal/day for a Period of 1 Year

Months	Weight + 500 kcal	Weight − 500 kcal
0 (Start)	250	250
1	254	246
2	258	242
3	262	238
4	266	234
5	270	230
6	274	226
7	278	222
8	282	218
9	286	214
10	290	210
11	294	206
12	298	202

how calories are utilized by the body and how many calories should be consumed per day to stimulate weight loss. Calories are expended by the body during the process of food digestion commonly referred to as the thermic effect of food (~10% of energy expenditure), physical activity (~15–30% of energy expenditure), and the amount of energy required to sustain life known as resting energy expenditure or RMR (~60–75% of energy expenditure). Numerous formulas have been developed to estimate RMR, which is the amount of calories that are utilized independent of exercise because the majority of calories utilized for energy during the day occur in this fashion. Topic Box 11.2 provides formulas used to estimate RMR along with sample calculations.

Now that we can estimate RMR, we need to account for the amount of calories expended during physical activity, because physical activity can account for a significant portion of energy expenditure (~15–30%). Table 11.3 allows you to estimate the amount of calories you utilize during physical activity each day. See Topic Box 11.3 and Table 11.4 for an example of how to use Table 11.3 to estimate DEE.

11.3.2 WEIGHT LOSS: DIET VERSUS EXERCISE

A common misconception appears to be the belief that effective weight loss is attainable by slightly increasing physical activity such as walking. Although increasing physical activity can result in weight loss for most people, it is more practical to stimulate weight loss through a combination of diet and exercise. An important concept of weight loss is the understanding that it is much easier to achieve an energy deficit by modifying dietary habits rather than increasing physical activity, especially if the physical activity is a low-energy–expending activity such as walking. Table 11.5 demonstrates simple dietary modifications that can be implemented to reduce caloric consumption by 500 calories a day versus different forms of physical activity that would need to be performed to expend 500 calories a day. However, it is important to note that physical activity has important health implications for reducing disease risk (Paffenbarger et al. 1993), contributing to weight loss (Jeffery et al. 2003), and maintaining weight loss (Klem et al. 1997), and thus is an important component to healthy weight loss.

11.4 NUTRITIONAL GAME PLAN

11.4.1 PHASE 1: ASSESSING FOOD CONSUMPTION

Now that your caloric needs are known, the next step is to assess your daily caloric consumption. Having knowledge of your caloric consumption and nutrient profile will help you make adequate adjustments to your dietary patterns to help ensure that you stimulate weight loss in an efficient and nutritionally sound manner. A commonly used technique to assess caloric consumption is a three-day food diary. To properly perform a three-day food diary, you will track everything you eat and drink and note the correct quantities of food/drink that were consumed. See Figure 11.1 for directions on how to properly record a three-day food diary. Once you record your diet for three days, you can use the Internet to access free dietary

TOPIC BOX 11.2   FORMULAS AND SAMPLE CALCULATIONS FOR THE ESTIMATION OF RMR

Harris-Benedict (Harris and Benedict 1919)

Males: RMR = 66.47 + (13.75 × weight in kg) + (5 × height in cm)
            – (6.76 × age in years)

Example: Rob is a 27-year-old baseball player who is 6'0" tall and weighs 200 pounds. What is his RMR?
  Step 1: Solve for weight, convert pounds to kg

1 kg = 2.2046 pounds
Divide 200 pounds by 2.2046 kg = **90.72 kg**

  Step 2: Solve for height, convert feet to inches, then inches to cm

1 foot = 12 inches and 1 inch = 2.54 cm
Feet to inches: multiply 6 feet by 12 inches = 72 inches
Inches to cm: multiply 72 inches by 2.54 cm = **182.88 cm**

  Step 3: Put required information into the formula and solve

Males: RMR = 66.47 + (13.75 × 90.72 kg) + (5 × 182.88 cm) – (6.76 × 27)
            RMR = 66.47 + 1247.4 + 914.4 – 182.52
            RMR = 2045.75 kcal
            RMR = 2046 kcal

Females: RMR = 655.1 + (9.56 × weight in kg) + (1.85 × height in cm)
              – (4.68 × age in years)

Example: Amy is a 20-year-old beach-volleyball player who is 5'11" and weighs 135 pounds. What is her RMR?
  Step 1: Solve for weight, convert pounds to kg

1 kg = 2.2046 pounds
Divide 135 pounds by 2.2046 kg = **61.24 kg**

  Step 2: Solve for height, convert feet to inches, then inches to cm

1 foot = 12 inches and 1 inch = 2.54 cm
Feet to inches: multiply 5 feet by 12 inches and add 11 = 71 inches
Inches to cm: multiply 71 inches by 2.54 cm = **180.34 cm**

  Step 3: Put required information into the formula and solve

Females: RMR = 655.1 + (9.56 × weight in kg) + (1.85 × height in cm)
              – (4.68 × age in years)

$$RMR = 655.1 + 585.45 + 333.63 - 93.6$$
$$RMR = 1480.58 \text{ kcal}$$
RMR = 1481 kcal

World Health Organization (1985)
Males:

10–18 years: $(17.5 \times \text{weight in kg}) + 651$
18–30 years: $(15.3 \times \text{weight in kg}) + 679$
30–60 years: $(11.6 \times \text{weight in kg}) + 879$

Example: Rob is a 27-year-old baseball player who is 6'0" tall and weighs 200 pounds. What is his RMR?

$$RMR \ (18\text{–}30 \ yr) = (14.7 \times \text{weight in kg}) + 496$$
$$RMR = (14.7 \times 90.72) + 496$$
$$RMR = 1829.58 \text{ kcal}$$
RMR = 1830 kcal

Females:

10–18 years: $(12.2 \times \text{weight in kg}) + 746$
18–30 years: $(14.7 \times \text{weight in kg}) + 496$
30–60 years: $(8.7 \times \text{weight in kg}) + 829$

Example: Amy is a 20-year-old beach-volleyball player who is 5'11" and weighs 135 pounds. What is her RMR?

$$RMR \ (18\text{–}30 \ yr) = (14.7 \times \text{weight in kg}) + 496$$
$$RMR = (14.7 \times 61.24) + 496$$
$$RMR = 1396.23 \text{ kcal}$$
RMR = 1396 kcal

Note the relatively small difference in estimated RMR between equations: for males: Harris-Benedict versus World Health Organization (2045.75 kcal versus 1829.58 kcal); and for females: Harris-Benedict versus World Health Organization (1480.58 kcal versus 1396.23 kcal). However, from this example you can see that the equation from the World Health Organization provides a more conservative estimate of RMR than then Harris-Benedict equation, and research has suggested that the Harris-Benedict equation overestimates RMR (Burke and Deakin 2000).

assessment programs. The following web sites have provided free nutritional assessment programs and are user friendly: http://nutritiondata.self.com/ and http://www.mypyramidtracker.gov/.

Protein, carbohydrate, and fat are referred to as macronutrients, all of which have been discussed in previous chapters. The suggested macronutrient breakdown is

TABLE 11.3
Estimates of Caloric Expenditure during Various Activities of Daily Living

Activity	kcal/per pound/min
Aerobics	
Moderate	0.065
Vigorous	0.095
Baseball	0.031
Basketball	
Recreation	0.038
Competition	0.065
Cycling	
5.5 mph	0.033
10.0 mph	0.050
13.0 mph	0.071
Dance	
Moderate	0.030
Vigorous	0.055
Golf	0.030
Jogging	
6.0 min/mile	0.114
7.0 min/mile	0.102
8.5 min/mile	0.090
11.0 min/mile	0.070
Judo	0.086
Racquetball	0.065
Soccer	0.059
Stairmaster	
Moderate	0.070
Vigorous	0.090
Swimming	
25 yards/min	0.040
50 yards/min	0.070
Tennis	
Recreation	0.045
Competition	0.064
Walking (4.5 mph)	0.045
Weightlifting	0.050
Wrestling	0.085

Source: Adapted from Hoeger, W. K., and S. A. Hoeger. 2009. *Lifetime Physical Fitness and Wellness: A Personalized Program*, 10th Ed. Belmont, CA: Wadsworth Cengage Learning.

TOPIC BOX 11.3 EXAMPLE FOR ESTIMATING DEE

In the previous example to calculate RMR, we used Rob, who is a 27-year-old baseball player that is 6'0" tall and weighs 200 pounds. Rob's RMR using the equation from the World Health Organization was estimated to be 1830 kcal/day. Table 11.4 lists Rob's daily physical activity and demonstrates how to estimate DEE utilizing caloric energy expenditure values from Table 11.3.

TABLE 11.4
Estimated Total Daily Energy Expenditure Based upon Physical Activity Level

Time	Physical Activity	Duration (min)	Energy Expended (kcal)
RMR from World Health Organization equation			1830
9:00 a.m.	Walk the dog (4.5 mph)	15	135
12:30 to 2:00 p.m.	Play baseball	90	93
4:00 to 5:00 p.m.	Weightlifting	60	150
Calories used not factoring in food intake		165 min (2 h 45 min)	2208
Calories used factoring in food intake; this is the value above multiplied by 0.1 and then re-added to the value above			**2429**

Please note that this calculation takes the thermic effect of food into account (~10% of DEE).

TABLE 11.5
Weight Management: Diet versus Exercise

Food/Drink	Serving Size	kcal	Amount per 500 kcal	Mode of Exercise	kcal/pound/min[a]	Minutes to Expend 500 kcal[b]
Soda	1 cup, 8 oz	120	4.2 cups	Walking 4.5 mph	0.045	56
Orange juice	1 cup, 8 oz	134	3.7 cups	Jogging 7.0 mph	0.102	25
Chocolate milk shake	1 cup, 8 oz	264	1.9 cups	Cycling 10 mph	0.050	50
Frosted Flakes	1 cup, 39 g	143	3.5 cups	Swimming 25 yd/min	0.040	63
Brownie	1 square, 56 g	227	2.2 squares	Weightlifting	0.050	50

[a] Caloric values were obtained from Table 11.3.
[b] Caloric expenditure is based on an individual weighting 200 pounds.

Date: _____

Instructions:

1) Record everything that you eat for three weekdays:

   Two weekdays and one weekend day

2) Precisely record the food item (brand if applicable), preparation method, and TOTAL quantity consumed

3) Break down mixed dishes or recipes by listing their component parts

4) For dairy and meat products, indicate fat level (low fat, extra lean, 2% etc.)

DAY 1

FOOD ITEM	PREPARATION METHOD (e.g. baked, fried, grilled, etc.)	QUANTITY							
		g	mL	cups	Tbsp or tsp.	oz.	Pieces	Sm, Med, Lg	Other
MEAL 1:									
MEAL 2:									
MEAL 3:									
MEAL 4:									
SNACKS:									

FIGURE 11.1   Sample food log and instructions for recording dietary habits.

TABLE 11.6
Caloric and Physiological Relevance of Each Macronutrient

	Protein	Carbohydrate	Fat
Calories (per gram)	4	4	9
Physiological relevance (Hoeger and Hoeger 2007)	– Used to build and repair tissue – Form parts of antibody, hormone, and enzyme molecules – Help maintain normal balance of body fluids	– Energy source for brain – Maintain cells – Generate heat	– Component of cells – Aids in absorption of fat soluble vitamins – Needed for production of steroids

Note there are 7 calories/g of alcohol.

10–35% protein, 45–65% carbohydrate, and 20–35% fat (Williams 2010). During weight loss you reduce the total amount of calories consumed, and during this process it is typically suggested to reduce the percentage of calories consumed from carbohydrate and increase percentage calories consumed from protein in an attempt to maintain skeletal muscle mass (Williams 2010). It is important to note that each macronutrient has a specific caloric content associated with it, and each serves different yet vital processes in the body (Table 11.6).

11.4.1.1 Protein

Protein is required to build and repair tissue, including skeletal muscle. Protein is composed of amino acids. There are 20 amino acids, of which 9 are considered essential amino acids, meaning they are not produced by the body or are produced by the body but in very low quantities so that more of the amino acid is needed from external food sources. Proteins can be separated into complete and incomplete proteins. Complete proteins contain each of the essential amino acids, whereas incomplete proteins lack one or more of the essential amino acids (refer to Table 11.7). Animal proteins form complete proteins, whereas grains, legumes, and nuts serve as incomplete proteins. It is important to note that certain incomplete proteins (such as rice and beans) can be consumed in conjunction with one another to make a complete protein; these are called complementary proteins.

11.4.1.2 Carbohydrate

Carbohydrate serves many important functions such as providing the body with an immediate energy source and aiding in recovery from exercise (Ivy and Portman 2004). Carbohydrates can be classified as low or high glycemic index (GI). When carbohydrates are consumed, there is a resulting increase in blood glucose concentrations. In healthy individuals, blood glucose concentrations range between 80 and 100 mg/dL (Williams 2010). The glycemic index is a measure of the effects of carbohydrate consumption on blood glucose concentrations. Low GI carbohydrates are classified as having a GI rating of ≤55. Low GI carbohydrates are digested at a slower rate than high GI carbohydrates and result in a slow stable rise in blood glucose concentrations. High

TABLE 11.7

List of Essential and Nonessential Amino Acids

Nonessential	Essential
Alanine	Isoleucine
Arginine	Histidine
Asparagine	Leucine
Aspartic acid	Lysine
Cysteine	Methionine
Glutamic acid	Phenylalanine
Glycine	Threonine
Ornithine	Tryptophan
Proline	Valine
Selenocysteine	
Serine	
Tyrosine	

GI carbohydrates are classified as having a GI rating of ≥70. High GI carbohydrates are digested quickly and result in a rapid increase in blood glucose concentrations.

Table 11.8 displays the glycemic index of commonly consumed foods and is adapted from the work of Foster-Powell et al. (2002). As a general rule of thumb, particularly for weight loss, you should limit the consumption of high–glycemic-index carbohydrates to avoid insulin spikes throughout the day. Insulin is secreted from the pancreas to reduce blood glucose concentrations. When there is excess glucose in the

TABLE 11.8

Classification of Various Low–, Medium–, and High–Glycemic-Index Carbohydrates

Food Type	Low GI (≤55)	Medium GI (56–69)	High GI (≥70)
Peanut	14		
Grapefruit	25		
Apple	38		
Strawberry	40		
Pineapple		59	
Table sugar (sucrose)		64	
White bread			70
Wheat bread			71
Watermelon			72
Russet potatoes			85

Source: Adapted from Foster-Powell, K., S. H. Holt, and J. C. Brand-Miller. 2002. International table of glycemic index and glycemic load values: 2002. *Am J Clin Nutr* 76: 5–56.

blood, glucose can be used for energy in other tissues, converted to glycogen to be stored in the liver and skeletal muscle, excreted in the form of urine by the kidneys, or stored as fat (Williams 2010). Thus, if an athlete consumes an overabundance of high glycemic and/or total carbohydrates, it may be more difficult to lose body fat, because this food source can be readily converted into and stored as fat.

11.4.1.3 Fat

Fat serves important functions in the body and is an essential nutrient; however, you need to monitor the types of fat you consume. Specifically, saturated fat should be limited to <7% of energy consumption, trans fat to <1% of energy consumption, and cholesterol to less than <300 mg/day (Lichtenstein et al. 2006). However, fat is not evil even when attempting to lose weight. From a physiological standpoint, all of the body's tissues require fat for fuel and cellular integrity. Dietary fat also aids the absorption of fat-soluble vitamins (A, E, D, and K) and is needed for the production of steroids (Hoeger and Hoeger 2007). Furthermore, there are essential fatty acids including omega-3 fatty acids, higher consumption of which has been associated with decreased risk of coronary heart disease and coronary heart disease deaths (Hu et al. 2002). Therefore, it would be counterproductive for an athlete to severely reduce fat intakes with the notion that weight loss would be accelerated.

11.4.2 Phase 2: General Recommendations for Healthy Weight Loss

The rate of healthy weight loss has been suggested to be no more than 2.2 pounds/week (Burke and Deakin 2000). This may not seem like much, but in order to lose 2 pounds of fat in a week, you must achieve a weekly caloric deficit of 7000 calories or a daily caloric deficit of 1000 calories (3500 calories is the energy stored in 1 pound of fat). There are circumstances in which it may be feasible to lose more than 2 pounds in week in a healthy manner, particularly in obese populations, but for athletic, healthy populations, 2 pounds/week should be considered the benchmark for "healthy" weight loss. When restricting calories, you want to be certain you are receiving all of the required vitamins and minerals, and therefore a balanced diet is key during the period of caloric restriction.

In terms of the macronutrient profile, it is difficult to make exact recommendations, because nutritional needs will vary for each individual depending on numerous factors including gender, amount of daily physical activity, exercise type, exercise intensity, exercise duration, and protein quality (Lemon 2000). General benchmarks to shoot for are 30–35% of calories from protein, 40–45% of calories from carbohydrate, and 30–35% of calories from fat (Farnsworth et al. 2003). When customizing your diet you need to keep the following in mind:

1. Ensure you are consuming a minimum of 1.8 g of protein/kg of body weight (Lemon 2000). The protein requirement is particularly important if you are engaging in daily physical activity.
2. Pay attention to the GI of the carbohydrates consumed, because research has found high-protein, low-GI index carbohydrate diets to be highly effective at optimizing body fat loss (McMillan-Price et al. 2006).

TOPIC BOX 11.4   SAMPLE WEIGHT-LOSS PROGRAM WITH THE AIM OF LOSING 1 POUND/WEEK.

Rob is used as the sample participant, and he weighs ~91 kg. Keeping in mind that 3500 kcal is equal to 1 pound, Rob must obtain a caloric deficit of 3500 kcal/week (500 kcal/day) to achieve his weight loss goal of 1 pound/week. In Table 11.4, we estimated Rob's DEE to be 2429 kcal. Given this information, to lose 1 pound of weight/week, Rob must limit his daily caloric consumption to 1929 kcal. See Table 11.10 for Rob's ideal macronutrient profile.

---

3. Ensure the fat consumed is low in saturated and trans fats. Topic Box 11.4 and Table 11.9 display the macronutrient profile designed for weight loss of 1 pound per week in Rob, the baseball player.

11.5   TIPS TO PROMOTE WEIGHT LOSS

11.5.1   REMOVE DRINKS OTHER THAN WATER AND MILK FROM YOUR DIET

Added sweeteners contribute approximately 318 kcal/day to the average American diet (Nielsen et al. 2002), equivalent to 33.2 pounds/year. More importantly, sweet corn-based syrups compose nearly half of the caloric sweeteners consumed by Americans (Vuilleumier 1993). Specifically, the consumption of high-fructose corn syrup (HFCS) has increased over 1000% from 1970 to 1990 and represents over 40% of caloric sweeteners added to food and drinks and is the only caloric sweetener in soft drinks in the United States (Bray et al. 2004). A conservative estimate of HFCS consumption for Americans is 132 kcal/day (Bray et al. 2004), equating to 13.8 pounds/year. However, the effects of HFCS are worse than just added calories. For instance, *in vitro* (studies conducted in a controlled environment such as a test tube) investigations have found that fructose does not stimulate insulin secretion. This is important, because when you consume glucose (sugar), blood glucose concentrations increase, and insulin is secreted to maintain blood glucose concentrations in an acceptable range. Insulin has been suggested to directly reduce food intake and to stimulate the release of leptin (Saad et al. 1998). Leptin is a protein that when released signals the body to stop eating (Bray et al. 2004). When consuming sugar in the form of fructose, less insulin is secreted from the pancreas, and thus

---

TABLE 11.9
Ideal Macronutrient Profile for Rob

Macronutrient	Ratio of Each Macronutrient (%)	kcal	g	g/kg of body weight
Protein	35	675	169	1.86
Carbohydrate	45	868	217	2.38
Fat	20	386	43	0.47

TABLE 11.10
Elimination of Drinks and Resulting Weight Loss

Beverage	Calories/cup (8 oz)	Calories/year (8 oz/day)	Weight Loss in a Year (lbs)
Cranberry juice	137	50,005	14.2
Apple juice	114	41,610	11.9
Orange juice	110	40,150	11.5
Beer	96	35,040	10.0
Coke	93	33,945	9.7
Kool-Aid	60	10,950	3.1

less leptin will be secreted, leading to increased feelings of hunger in addition to the useless calories in HFCS.

Table 11.10 provides a visual display of the caloric content of various drinks and the amount of weight that can be lost per year with the elimination of a single serving of each drink per day over the course of a year. If seeking to lose body fat, a key first step is to examine how many calories you consume per day in the form of drinks. Milk is a high-quality protein and contains calcium, a nutrient that is deficient in the diet of American children (Fleming and Heimbach 1994), and should not be eliminated from the diet. However, a switch from whole milk (3.5% fat) to skim milk (0% fat) can theoretically result in the loss of over 6 pounds of body fat over the course of the year, assuming that one serving of milk is consumed daily. Skim milk also greatly reduces the amount of saturated fat consumed over the course of the year, which may promote cardiovascular health (Table 11.11).

11.5.2 MONITOR YOUR CARBOHYDRATE CONSUMPTION

Over the years, fat has garnered much of the attention regarding the obesity epidemic and thus weight gain; however, empty calories primarily in the form of carbohydrates and HFCS appear to be more damaging in terms of weight control. Carbohydrates serve numerous biological functions, but you need to be conscience of the types and amount of carbohydrates being consumed. Keep in mind that this discussion is limited to the extent of carbohydrate consumption in athletic populations, and excessive carbohydrate intakes contributes to several disorders, with type 2 diabetes being the primary result.

We have already discussed the practicality of eliminating liquid calories, but you should also be aware of the GI of carbohydrates consumed. We spoke previously about the ideal diet for weight loss to be composed primarily of protein (30–35% of calories) and low-GI carbohydrates (40–45% of calories); however, there is a place for high-GI carbohydrates. In order to optimize performance and promote recovery, high–GI-index carbohydrates should be consumed with protein prior to and during exercise. A general recommendation for nutrient consumption surrounding resistance exercise can be segmented into three phases: preparation (prior to exercise), exercise, and recovery (post-exercise). Prior to exercise, 20–26 g of high-GI carbohydrates should be consumed with 5–6 g of protein. During exercise, 40–50 g

TABLE 11.11

Comparison of Whole versus Skim Milk

	Single Serving (244 g)		Yearly Comparison (244 g/day)		
	Whole Milk (3.5% Fat)	Skim Milk (0% Fat)	Whole Milk (3.5% Fat)	Skim Milk (0% Fat)	Whole versus Skim Milk
Calories	146	86	53,290	31,390	+21,900[a]
Protein (g)	8	8	2920	2920	0
Carbohydrate (g)	13	12	4745	4380	+365
Fat (g)	8	0	2920	0	+2920
Saturated fat (g)	5	0	1825	0	+1825

[a] Note that the caloric difference between whole and skim milk equates to a caloric difference associated with a weight loss of 6.3 pounds over the course of the year.

of high–GI-index carbohydrates should be consumed with 13–15 g of protein. Following exercise, another 2–4 g of high-GI carbohydrate should be consumed with 14 g of protein (Ivy and Portman 2004). From examining Table 11.9, we can see that Rob can consume 217 g of carbohydrate/day. Even if Rob consumes the upper limit of high-GI carbohydrates surrounding training (78 g), the majority of his carbohydrates (64%) should be in the form of low-GI carbohydrates. Because a majority of consumed carbohydrate should be in the form of fruit, Table 11.12 lists the caloric content, fiber content, and GI of various fruits. For weight loss, the ideal fruits will be high in fiber and low in calories and have a low GI.

11.5.3 INCREASE FIBER CONSUMPTION

The average American has been reported to consume ~12 g of fiber daily, which is below the recommendation of 26–30 g suggested for adults (Slavin 2005). Fiber serves numerous health-promoting purposes such as decreasing the risk for cardiovascular disease, cancer, diverticulitis, hemorrhoids, gallbladder disease, and obesity (Hoeger and Hoeger 2007). Furthermore, fiber can also aid weight loss by increasing feelings of fullness while adding minimal calories to the diet (Hoeger and Hoeger 2007).

Fiber intake can be increased by consuming whole grains, high fiber cereals, legumes, fruits, and vegetables (Hoeger and Hoeger 2007). Fiber can be classified as soluble fiber and insoluble fiber. Soluble fiber dissolves in water and can bind to fat, improving cholesterol and blood glucose levels (Hoeger and Hoeger 2007). Insoluble fiber does not dissolve easily in water and cannot be digested, which reduces the amount of time stool remains in the digestive system.

When selecting breads and cereals to incorporate in the diet, it is important to pay attention to the fiber and carbohydrate content of the food item. A general suggestion is to purchase cereals that provide 5 g or more of dietary fiber and protein while having no more than 40 g of carbohydrate. An example of a good cereal would

TABLE 11.12
Carbohydrate, Glycemic Index, and Fiber Contents of Various Fruits

Type of Fruit	kcal/100 g	Fiber/100 g	Glycemic Index
Apple	52	2	40
Banana	89	3	47
Blackberry	43	5	—
Blueberry	57	2	—
Cantaloupe	34	1	65
Cherry	63	2	22
Grape	67	1	43
Grapefruit	42	2	25
Kiwi	61	3	58
Mango	55	2	51
Nectarine	44	2	—
Orange	46	2	40
Peach	39	1	28
Pear	58	3	33
Pineapple	50	1	66
Plum	46	1	24
Pomegranate	83	4	—
Raisins	299	4	64
Raspberry	52	6	—
Strawberry	32	2	40
Tangerine	53	2	—
Watermelon	30	0	72

be Kashi Go Lean Crunch, which contains 200 kcal, 9 g of protein, 4.5 g of fat, 0 g of saturated fat, 36 g of carbohydrate, and 8 g of fiber (4 g of soluble fiber and 4 g of insoluble fiber). You want to find breads that have similar qualities: high fiber (~5 g), moderate protein (≥5 g), whole grains, and minimal carbohydrates (≤40 g).

11.5.4 Do Not Waste Calories in the Form of Protein

It should be noted that if you were to overconsume any of the macronutrients while attempting to lose body fat, protein would be the best choice because protein provides the greatest thermic effect of food (protein: 20–30%, carbohydrate: 5–10%, fat: 0–3%) (Tappy 1996). Furthermore, isocaloric diets higher in protein have been found to result in better maintenance of lean weight compared with lower-protein diets (Farnsworth et al. 2003; Layman et al. 2003; Mettler et al. 2010). However, in weight-bearing sports where an ounce can make the difference between being able to compete and disqualification, every calorie counts.

In this regard it should be noted that protein/meal should be limited to 25–30 g of protein because this amount has been found to maximally stimulate muscle protein synthesis (a process in muscle tissue that leads to increases in muscle building and strength over time) (Paddon-Jones and Rasmussen 2009). The consumption of 25–30 g of protein/meal has been suggested based on several significant findings. The lower limit of 25 g is suggested based on the finding that a typical 20-g serving of most animal or plant-based proteins contains approximately 5–8 g of essential amino acids, which are primarily responsible for skeletal-muscle protein synthesis (Volpi et al. 2003). The upper limit recommendation of protein (30 g/serving) is based on the results of an investigation in which healthy younger and older adults did not experience a greater anabolic response from 90 g of protein compared with 30 g of protein, suggesting that the consumption of 30 g of protein in a single meal may elicit an optimal anabolic response in regard to muscle protein synthesis (Symons et al. 2007).

11.6   AGENTS THAT MAY SUPPORT WEIGHT LOSS

11.6.1   Weight-Loss Agents: Orlistat, Caffeine, and Ephedrine

Although diet and exercise should be the primary components to any weight loss program, there are supplements that can increase the rate of weight loss such as orlistat, caffeine, and ephedrine. Orlistat is an interesting compound because it has been found to lower serum cholesterol, reduce blood pressure, and aid in the control of diabetes (Burke and Deakin 2000). Although the efficacy of orlistat has not been examined in athletic populations, the physiological effects of the compound on fat absorption should promote weight loss in athletic populations. Orlistat inhibits the activity of pancreatic and gastric lipases, which are involved in triglyceride hydrolysis (Finer et al. 2000), which is essential for the absorption of fat (Hauptman et al. 1992). Specifically, a 120-mg dose consumed three times daily (breakfast, lunch, and dinner) can reduce dietary fat absorption by up to 35% (Zhi et al. 1994). However, orlistat is not a miracle compound. Because orlistat reduces fat absorption, the fat that is not absorbed is passed through the digestive system and excreted in bowel movements. As a result you need to be on a low-fat diet when consuming orlistat, or diarrhea and fat or oil loss through the stool may result (Burke and Deakin 2000). Do note, however, that taking orlistat on a low-fat diet may compromise the amount of fat available for the body to use for important physiological processes, so it is not a preferable practice for athletes striving to maintain nutritional adequacy during periods of weight loss. Finally, orlistat will not interfere with carbohydrate or protein absorption (Burke and Deakin 2000), so it is possible for weight gain to occur if a proper diet is not consumed.

Caffeine and ephedrine are stimulants that have been scientifically proven to promote weight loss. Caffeine can promote weight loss by causing an increase in circulating epinephrine (a fat-burning hormone) (Bangsbo et al. 1992) and free fatty acids (Dalbo et al. 2008a; Powers and Dodd 1985). Like caffeine, ephedrine also promotes weight loss by increasing circulating levels of epinephrine (Astrup et al. 1986). Specifically, 50 mg of ephedrine has been found to increase 24-hour energy expenditure by 3.6% (Shannon et al. 1999). Another investigation reported the 3-month consumption of 60 mg a day of ephedrine increased metabolic rate by 10% (Astrup et al. 1986). Interestingly, caffeine and ephedrine have a synergist effect, meaning they work better for weight loss when consumed together rather than consuming one or the other. A scientifically proven dosage of these compounds includes 20 mg of ephedrine and 200 mg of caffeine (Bell et al. 2000), because this combination will effectively increase metabolic rate and the amount of energy utilized in the form of fat. To further increase the fat-burning capabilities of caffeine and ephedrine, you can add 80 mg of aspirin (Daly et al. 1993). However, it is important to note that ephedrine and caffeine can cause a rise in systolic blood pressure and heart rate. Therefore, it is important that athletes with pre-existing cardiovascular conditions (i.e., high blood pressure, arrhythmias, etc.) consult a physician prior to using these compounds as weight-loss aids.

It should be stressed that the optimal doses of ephedrine and caffeine are 20 and 200 mg, respectively. Increasing these doses will not effectively enhance caloric expenditure but can have more pronounced negative effects on heart rate and blood pressure (Bell et al. 2000). It is not advised to consume caffeine or ephedrine prior to vigorous exercise particularly in heat because of the influence of each on heart rate and systolic blood pressure. The use of caffeine and ephedrine have also been linked to heart palpitations (Shekelle et al. 2003).

11.6.2 MUSCLE MAINTENANCE AGENTS: LEUCINE AND CREATINE

Leucine is an amino acid that potentially has numerous health-promoting benefits and may provide benefit in a standard diet and a diet to promote weight loss. Several investigations have found the consumption of leucine (an amino acid found in high concentrations in milk and animal proteins) with mixed-nutrient meals to improve protein synthesis (Rieu et al. 2006; Layman 2002). Moreover, the consumption of leucine, protein, and carbohydrate were found to increase whole-body net protein balance (a rough indication of muscle building) to a significantly greater degree than protein and carbohydrate alone (Koopman et al. 2005). Based on the available research, it appears that the optimal time to consume leucine is with each meal at a total dose of 16 g (leucine from meal plus leucine in form of supplement if needed) (Koopman et al. 2005; Zhang et al. 2007).

Creatine has been found in numerous investigations to increase skeletal-muscle strength and hypertrophy (Dalbo et al. 2009). However, creatine may also reduce skeletal-muscle breakdown associated with caloric restriction because 20 g of creatine consumed with a diet of 18 kcal/kg of body mass resulted in less loss of lean mass compared with a placebo (Rockwell et al. 2001). It should also be noted that creatine promotes a state of hyperhydration because creatine supplementation has been found to increase total body water (Volek et al. 2001; Weiss and Powers 2006; Ziegenfuss et al. 1998), intracellular water (Weiss and Powers 2006; Ziegenfuss et al. 1998), and extracellular water (Weiss and Powers 2006) and has also been found to reduce heart rate (Easton et al. 2007), body temperature (Easton et al. 2007), and ratings of perceived exertion (Easton et al. 2007) following exercise compared with a placebo. As a result, creatine supplementation may also function to reduce the risk of heat illness during exercise, particularly when exercising in hot and or humid climates (Dalbo et al. 2008b). Athletes in weight-bearing sports must realize that creatine results in an increase in body weight, primarily in the form of water, so they must consider this effect of creatine surrounding competition.

11.7   SPECIAL CONSIDERATIONS FOR WEIGHT-BEARING ATHLETES

Athletes in weight-bearing sports have different considerations in terms of body weight than athletes in non-weight-bearing sports. For example, a wide receiver in football may try to obtain 8% body fat in an attempt to optimize his performance, but this receiver will not be concerned with his body weight in the days immediately prior to competition. However, a collegiate wrestler or an MMA fighter may have to make a weight of 185 pounds prior to competition, and although it does not matter what his body composition is during the weigh-in, it will be beneficial for the athlete to have as much lean mass as possible during the competition. As a result, in many instances these athletes will reduce body weight in the form of water weight, via dehydration prior to weigh-ins. For most athletes in weight-bearing sports (there are some exceptions such as many heavyweight competitors), maintaining a body fat percentage of no more than 8% is suggested because this is a sustainable level of body composition, particularly in-season.

When losing body weight in the form of water, be aware that decrements occur as the result of impaired cardiovascular, thermoregulatory, central nervous system, and metabolic functioning (Cheuvront et al. 2003; Judelson et al. 2007), resulting in decreased aerobic performance (Cheuvront et al. 2003), muscle strength (Judelson et al. 2007), and muscle endurance (Judelson et al. 2007) when dehydration exceeds 2.0% of body weight (Cheuvront et al. 2003; Judelson et al. 2007) (Topic Box 11.5). As a result, athletes dropping body weight through the loss of water should attempt to rehydrate as quickly as possible prior to competition. When rehydrating, it is a good idea for the beverage to contain electrolytes and carbohydrate; with that in mind, Gatorade is a good beverage for the use of rehydration.

There are sports, such as wrestling, where many athletes intentionally dehydrate themselves to "make" weight, and unfortunately this practice can sometimes have dire consequences. In November and December of 1997, three collegiate wrestlers died of dehydration-related deaths. In each case, the wrestler restricted his consumption of food and water while engaging in vigorous exercise wearing vapor-impermeable suits under clothing in hot environments to promote weight loss, primarily in the form of water. One of the wrestlers went into cardiorespiratory arrest and had a body temperature of 108°F, while another wrestler underwent rhabdomyolysis, which is the rapid breakdown of skeletal muscle resulting in the release of products into the bloodstream that can result in acute kidney failure and in this case death (Centers for Disease Control 1998).

It is unfortunate that in many instances high-school children receive information about training and nutrition from high school coaches who often give poor advice regarding lifting technique, hydration, and nutrition strategies. The government needs to take a stand and require coaches and gym teachers to obtain certificates from a recognized organization such as the American College of Sports Medicine or National Strength and Conditioning Association before being able to coach/teach

TOPIC BOX 11.5   THE BIRTH OF GATORADE
AND THE DANGERS OF DEHYDRATION

The birth of the most popular sports drink in the world, Gatorade, began in 1965. Dwayne Douglas, an assistant football coach at the University of Florida and a former NFL player, questioned Dr. Robert Cade, then director of the University of Florida College of Medicine's renal and electrolyte division, about why players would lose so much weight over the course of a game but never had the need to urinate. Dr. Cade quickly came to the conclusion that players were sweating so much they did not have any fluids left to urinate, which also influenced the body's electrolyte balance.

To develop a solution to the problem, Dr. Cade approached then football coach Ray Graves about using football players as test subjects, to determine the physiological effects of football training on the body. Coach Graves agreed to let Dr. Cade use freshman football players as test subjects. The results obtained from the test subjects were "jaw-dropping": the players blood volume was low (a sign of dehydration), their blood sugar was low (which hinders performance), and their electrolytes were out of balance (which also hinders performance). As a result Dr. Cade and his research team knew that players had to be given water to promote hydration, salt to restore electrolytes, and sugar to maintain blood sugar. The first formula of Gatorade tasted so bad that the scientists could not drink it, so Dr. Cade's wife suggested adding lemon juice to the drink to make it more palatable (Kays and Phillips-Han 2003).

The first on-field test of the effects of Gatorade was in 1965 in a scrimmage between the Gators B team versus the freshman. The Gators B team was drinking water while the freshman team was drinking Gatorade. The B team went into the half with a 13-0 lead over the freshman, but in the second half, the tide turned as the freshman scored two or three touchdowns in the third quarter and five or six more in the fourth quarter! Coach Graves was so impressed, he asked Dr. Cade to make enough Gatorade for the varsity team's game against Louisiana State University the following day. Needless to say, Florida beat the heavily favored Louisiana State University in 102°F temperatures, which led to Gatorade becoming a staple of recreational and professional teams worldwide (Kays and Phillips-Han 2003).

Besides enhancing performance, Gatorade also improved safety. Over a period of 2 days in 1966, 24 players were brought to the Shands Hospital emergency room with heat-related illnesses. As a result, coach Graves asked Dr. Cade to supply the football team with enough Gatorade to keep all players supplied during practice and games. Over the next 5 years, only one player was hospitalized due to a heat-related illness, and he reportedly had not consumed Gatorade (Kays and Phillips-Han 2003).

children. Currently there is no accountability, and the children end up paying the price after receiving misguided information.

11.7.1 Tests to Assess Strength-to-Weight Ratio

Numerous investigations have demonstrated that during the process of weight loss, the body loses fat mass and muscle mass (Farnsworth et al. 2003; Layman et al. 2003). In an athletic population, decreases in muscle mass will directly result in decreases in strength and thus potentially inhibit performance. As previously noted, increasing protein consumption (Layman et al. 2003; Mettler et al. 2010; Farnsworth et al. 2003) and the use of creatine at a dose of 20 g a day (Rockwell et al. 2001) can reduce the amount of muscle lost while in caloric deficit. The addition of these nutrients is important from a training-table prospective. As a result, it is important to track changes in your strength-to-weight ratio during the process of weight loss. You can assess your strength-to-weight ratio by performing a one repetition maximum bench press test for upper-body strength and a one repetition maximum squat test for lower-body strength. To assess your strength-to-weight ratio for bench press and squat, take the amount you lift in pounds and divide that weight by your weight in pounds. Vertical jump can be used to access another important component of sport, power. To assess vertical jump, stand next to a wall with your dominant hand closest to wall. Reach up as high as possible with your dominant hand while keeping your nondominant hand down and feet flat on the floor and mark the wall at the highest point you can reach. Then bend your knees and jump as high possible, marking the wall at the highest point you reach. The equation below can be used to calculate peak power (Harman et al. 1991):

$$\text{Peak power (W)} = (61.9 \times \text{jump height (cm)}) + (36 \times \text{body mass (kg)}) + 1822$$

11.8 TRAINING TABLE

This chapter described the concept of caloric control for weight loss and provided nutritional recommendations for healthy weight loss for athletes of various sports. Simple suggestions you should keep in mind while at the training table are the following:

- Remember your caloric goal (amount of kcal/day you can consume)
- Track your macronutrient consumption. General recommendations are as follows:
    - Protein: 10–35% of kcal
    - Carbohydrate: 45–65% kcal
    - Fat: 20–35% of kcal
- Think of calories as you think of money: you do not want to waste them. You can maximize your calories by:
    - Not consuming calories in the form of drinks (other than milk)
    - Eating more fiber
    - Not wasting protein (limit protein to 25–30 g/meal)

- Eat for performance. Remember not all carbohydrates and proteins are equal.
- High–glycemic-index carbohydrates should be consumed immediately prior to and during exercise to promote performance and recovery. Low–glycemic-index carbohydrates should be consumed during recovery (following exercise).
- Complete proteins contain all essential amino acids, whereas incomplete proteins lack some essential amino acids.
- Dehydration is a component of many weight-bearing sports. Take precaution not to let the practice of dehydration hurt your performance or, more importantly, your health.
- Maintain a low body fat percentage (~8%).
- Remember a 2% loss of water starts to hinder performance. If you are losing more than 2% of your body weight in water prior to competition, lose more body fat or compete at a higher weight.
- You have the knowledge to lose weight. It is up to you to decide if you want to achieve your desired body composition.

11.9   CONCLUSIONS

There are numerous factors that must be considered when making nutritional adjustments in an attempt to modify body composition to allow for optimal athletic performance. The most important factor to keep in mind is to lose weight in a healthy manner. Weight loss of 2 pounds per week does not sound like much in terms of total body weight, but in terms of calories you much achieve a caloric deficit of ~7000 kcal/week or 1000 kcal/day. Protein must also be on your mind because protein is required to build and repair muscle following training, is needed for growth in younger athletes, results in the greatest thermic effect of food, and helps to minimize the rate of skeletal-muscle loss during periods of caloric deficit. Fruits and vegetables also need to be incorporated into the diet to provide the body with vitamins, minerals, and fiber, which will help reduce the feeling of hunger.

Supplements such as orlistat, caffeine, and ephedrine can be added to your nutritional game plan to promote weight loss, although caution should be exercised when using weight-loss agents because of the potentially negative aforementioned health effects. It is also a good idea to supplement the diet with leucine and creatine to help reduce the loss of muscle during caloric restriction, although creatine results in water retention, which may limit its practicality for use among athletes in weight-bearing sports. Finally, during weight loss, it is a good idea to keep track of your strength-to-weight ratio. If your strength-to-weight ratio is dropping, you may need to make modifications to your diet or exercise program to maintain more skeletal-muscle mass.

REFERENCES

Astrup, A., J. Madsen, J. J. Holst, and N. J. Christensen. 1986. The effect of chronic ephedrine treatment on substrate utilization, the sympathoadrenal activity, and energy expenditure during glucose-induced thermogenesis in man. *Metabolism* 35: 260–265.

Baechle, T. R., and R. W. Earle. 2000. *Essentials of Strength Training and Conditioning*, 2nd Ed. Champaign, IL: Human Kinetics.

Bangsbo, J., K. Jacobsen, N. Nordberg, N. J. Christensen, and T. Graham. 1992. Acute and habitual caffeine ingestion and metabolic responses to steady-state exercise. *J Appl Physiol* 72: 1297–1303.

Bell, D. G., I. Jacobs, T. M. McLellan, and J. Zamecnik. 2000. Reducing the dose of combined caffeine and ephedrine preserves the ergogenic effect. *Aviat Space Environ Med* 71: 415–419.

Ben Abdelkrim, N., A. Chaouachi, K. Chamari, M. Chtara, and C. Castagna. 2010. Positional role and competitive-level differences in elite-level men's basketball players. *J Strength Cond Res* 24: 1346–1355.

Bray, G. A., S. J. Nielsen, and B. M. Popkin. 2004. Consumption of high-fructose corn syrup in beverages may play a role in the epidemic of obesity. *Am J Clin Nutr* 79: 537–543.

Burke, L , and V. Deakin. 2000. *Clinical Sports Nutrition*, 2nd Ed. Roseville, CA: McGraw-Hill Company.

Calbet, J. A., P. Diaz Herrera, and L. P. Rodriguez. 1999. High bone mineral density in male elite professional volleyball players. *Osteoporos Int* 10: 468–474.

Carbuhn, A. F., T. E. Fernandez, A. F. Bragg, J. S. Green, and S. F. Crouse. 2010. Sport and training influence bone and body composition in women collegiate athletes. *J Strength Cond Res* 24: 1710–1707.

Centers for Disease Control. 1998. Hyperthermia and dehydration-related deaths associated with intentional rapid weight loss in three collegiate wrestlers—North Carolina, Wisconsin, and Michigan, November-December 1997. *Morbidity and Mortality Weekly Report* 47: 105–108.

Cheuvront, S. N., R. Carter, 3rd, and M. N. Sawka. 2003. Fluid balance and endurance exercise performance. *Curr Sports Med Rep* 2: 202–208.

Coleman, E. A., and L. M. Lasky. 1992. Assessing running speed and body composition in professional baseball players. *J Appl Sport Sci Res* 6: 207–213.

Dalbo, V. J., M. D. Roberts, C. M. Lockwood, P. S. Tucker, R. B. Kreider, and C. M. Kerksick. 2009. The effects of age on skeletal muscle and the phosphocreatine energy system: Can creatine supplementation help older adults? *Dyn Med* 8: 6.

Dalbo, V. J., M. D. Roberts, J. R. Stout, and C. M. Kerksick. 2008a. Acute effects of ingesting a commercial thermogenic drink on changes in energy expenditure and markers of lipolysis. *J Int Soc Sports Nutr* 5: 6.

Dalbo, V. J., M. D. Roberts, J. R. Stout, and C. M. Kerksick. 2008b. Putting to rest the myth of creatine supplementation leading to muscle cramps and dehydration. *Br J Sports Med* 42: 567–573.

Daly, P. A., D. R. Krieger, A. G. Dulloo, J. B. Young, and L. Landsberg. 1993. Ephedrine, caffeine and aspirin: Safety and efficacy for treatment of human obesity. *Int J Obes Relat Metab Disord* 17(Suppl 1): S73–S78.

Easton, C., S. Turner, and Y. P. Pitsiladis. 2007. Creatine and glycerol hyperhydration in trained subjects before exercise in the heat. *Int J Sport Nutr Exerc Metab* 17: 70–91.

Farnsworth, E., N. D. Luscombe, M. Noakes, G. Wittert, E. Argyiou, and P. M. Clifton. 2003. Effect of a high-protein, energy-restricted diet on body composition, glycemic control, and lipid concentrations in overweight and obese hyperinsulinemic men and women. *Am J Clin Nutr* 78: 31–39.

Finer, N., W. P. James, P. G. Kopelman, M. E. Lean, and G. Williams. 2000. One-year treatment of obesity: A randomized, double-blind, placebo-controlled, multicentre study of orlistat, a gastrointestinal lipase inhibitor. *Int J Obes Relat Metab Disord* 24: 306–313.

Fleming, K. H., and J. T. Heimbach. 1994. Consumption of calcium in the U.S.: Food sources and intake levels. *J Nutr* 124(8 Suppl): 1426S–1430S.

Foster-Powell, K., S. H. Holt, and J. C. Brand-Miller. 2002. International table of glycemic index and glycemic load values: 2002. *Am J Clin Nutr* 76: 5–56.

Harman, E. A., M. T. Rosenstein, P. N. Frykman, R. M. Rosenstein, and W. J. Kraemer. 1991. Estimation of human power output from vertical jump. *J Appl Sport Sci Res* 5: 116–120.

Harris, J. A., and F. G. Benedict. 1919. *A biometric study of basal metabolism in man.* Philadelphia, PA: J. B. Lippincott Company.

Hauptman, J. B., F. S. Jeunet, and D. Hartmann. 1992. Initial studies in humans with the novel gastrointestinal lipase inhibitor Ro 18-0647 (tetrahydrolipstatin). *Am J Clin Nutr* 55(1 Suppl): 309S–313S.

Hoeger, W. K., and S. A. Hoeger. 2007. *Lifetime Physical Fitness and Wellbeing*, 9th Ed. Belmont, CA: Cengage Brooks Cole.

Hoeger, W. K., and S. A. Hoeger. 2009. *Lifetime Physical Fitness and Wellness: A Personalized Program*, 10th Ed. Belmont, CA: Wadsworth Cengage Learning.

Howley, E. T., and B. D. Franks. 2007. *Health Fitness Instructor's Handbook*, 5th Ed. Champaign, IL: Human Kinetics.

Hu, F. B., L. Bronner, W. C. Willett, M. J. Stampfer, K. M. Rexrode, C. M. Albert, D. Hunter, and J. E. Manson. 2002. Fish and omega-3 fatty acid intake and risk of coronary heart disease in women. *JAMA* 287: 1815–1821.

Ivy, J, and R. Portman. 2004. *Nutrient timining: The future of sports nutrition.* North Bergen, NJ: Basic Health Publications, Inc.

Jeffery, R. W., R. R. Wing, N. E. Sherwood, and D. F. Tate. 2003. Physical activity and weight loss: Does prescribing higher physical activity goals improve outcome? *Am J Clin Nutr* 78: 684–689.

Judelson, D. A., C. M. Maresh, J. M. Anderson, L. E. Armstrong, D. J. Casa, W. J. Kraemer, and J. S. Volek. 2007. Hydration and muscular performance: Does fluid balance affect strength, power and high-intensity endurance? *Sports Med* 37: 907–921.

Kays, J., and A. Phillips-Han. 2003. Gatorade: The idea that launched an industry. *Explore Magazine.* 8. Retrieved from http://www.research.ufl.edu/explore/v08n1/gatorade.html

Klem, M. L., R. R. Wing, L. Simkin-Silverman, and L. H. Kuller. 1997. The psychological consequences of weight gain prevention in healthy, premenopausal women. *Int J Eat Disord* 21: 167–174.

Koopman, R., A. J. Wagenmakers, R. J. Manders, A. H. Zorenc, J. M. Senden, M. Gorselink, H. A. Keizer, and L. J. van Loon. 2005. Combined ingestion of protein and free leucine with carbohydrate increases postexercise muscle protein synthesis in vivo in male subjects. *Am J Physiol Endocrinol Metab* 288: E645–E653.

Kraemer, W. J., J. C. Torine, R. Silvestre, D. N. French, N. A. Ratamess, B. A. Spiering, D. L. Hatfield, J. L. Vingren, and J. S. Volek. 2005. Body size and composition of National Football League players. *J Strength Cond Res* 19: 485–489.

Layman, D. K. 2002. Role of leucine in protein metabolism during exercise and recovery. *Can J Appl Physiol* 27: 646–663.

Layman, D. K., R. A. Boileau, D. J. Erickson, J. E. Painter, H. Shiue, C. Sather, and D. D. Christou. 2003. A reduced ratio of dietary carbohydrate to protein improves body composition and blood lipid profiles during weight loss in adult women. *J Nutr* 133: 411–417.

Lemon, P. W. 2000. Beyond the zone: Protein needs of active individuals. *J Am Coll Nutr* 19(5 Suppl): 513S–521S.

Lichtenstein, A. H., L. J. Appel, M. Brands, M. Carnethon, S. Daniels, H. A. Franch, B. Franklin, P. Kris-Etherton, W. S. Harris, B. Howard, N. Karanja, M. Lefevre, L. Rudel, F. Sacks, L. Van Horn, M. Winston, and J. Wylie-Rosett. 2006. Diet and lifestyle recommendations revision 2006: A scientific statement from the American Heart Association Nutrition Committee. *Circulation* 114: 82–96.

Malousaris, G. G., N. K. Bergeles, K. G. Barzouka, I. A. Bayios, G. P. Nassis, and M. D. Koskolou. 2008. Somatotype, size and body composition of competitive female volleyball players. *J Sci Med Sport* 11: 337–344.

McMillan-Price, J., P. Petocz, F. Atkinson, K. O'Neill, S. Samman, K. Steinbeck, I. Caterson, and J. Brand-Miller. 2006. Comparison of 4 diets of varying glycemic load on weight loss and cardiovascular risk reduction in overweight and obese young adults: A randomized controlled trial. *Arch Intern Med* 166: 1466–1475.

Mettler, S., N. Mitchell, and K. D. Tipton. 2010. Increased protein intake reduces lean body mass loss during weight loss in athletes. *Med Sci Sports Exerc* 42: 326–337.

Moon, J. R., H. R. Hull, S. E. Tobkin, M. Teramoto, M. Karabulut, M. D. Roberts, E. D. Ryan, S. J. Kim, V. J. Dalbo, A. A. Walter, A. T. Smith, J. T. Cramer, and J. R. Stout. 2007. Percent body fat estimations in college women using field and laboratory methods: A three-compartment model approach. *J Int Soc Sports Nutr* 4: 16.

Nielsen, S. J., A. M. Siega-Riz, and B. M. Popkin. 2002. Trends in energy intake in U.S. between 1977 and 1996: Similar shifts seen across age groups. *Obes Res* 10: 370–378.

Paddon-Jones, D., and B. B. Rasmussen. 2009. Dietary protein recommendations and the prevention of sarcopenia. *Curr Opin Clin Nutr Metab Care* 12: 86–90.

Paffenbarger, R. S., Jr., R. T. Hyde, A. L. Wing, I. M. Lee, D. L. Jung, and J. B. Kampert. 1993. The association of changes in physical-activity level and other lifestyle characteristics with mortality among men. *N Engl J Med* 328: 538–545.

Powers, S. K., and S. Dodd. 1985. Caffeine and endurance performance. *Sports Med* 2: 165–174.

Raven, P. B., L. R. Gettman, M. L. Pollock, and K. H. Cooper. 1976. A physiological evaluation of professional soccer players. *Br J Sports Med* 10: 209–216.

Rieu, I., M. Balage, C. Sornet, C. Giraudet, E. Pujos, J. Grizard, L. Mosoni, and D. Dardevet. 2006. Leucine supplementation improves muscle protein synthesis in elderly men independently of hyperaminoacidaemia. *J Physiol* 575: 305–315.

Rockwell, J. A., J. W. Rankin, and B. Toderico. 2001. Creatine supplementation affects muscle creatine during energy restriction. *Med Sci Sports Exerc* 33: 61–68.

Saad, M. F., A. Khan, A. Sharma, R. Michael, M. G. Riad-Gabriel, R. Boyadjian, S. D. Jinagouda, G. M. Steil, and V. Kamdar. 1998. Physiological insulinemia acutely modulates plasma leptin. *Diabetes* 47: 544–549.

Sedano Campo, S., R. Vaeyens, R. M. Philippaerts, J. C. Redondo, A. M. de Benito, and G. Cuadrado. 2009. Effects of lower-limb plyometric training on body composition, explosive strength, and kicking speed in female soccer players. *J Strength Cond Res* 23: 1714–1722.

Shannon, J. R., K. Gottesdiener, J. Jordan, K. Chen, S. Flattery, P. J. Larson, M. R. Candelore, B. Gertz, D. Robertson, and M. Sun. 1999. Acute effect of ephedrine on 24-h energy balance. *Clin Sci (Lond)* 96: 483–491.

Shekelle, P., M. L. Hardy, S. C. Morton, M. Maglione, M. Suttorp, E. Roth, L. Jungvig, W. A. Mojica, J. Gagne, S. Rhodes, and E. McKinnon. 2003. Ephedra and ephedrine for weight loss and athletic performance enhancement: Clinical efficacy and side effects. *Evid Rep Technol Assess (Summ)* 76: 1–4.

Slavin, J. L. 2005. Dietary fiber and body weight. *Nutrition* 21: 411–418.

Symons, T. B., S. E. Schutzler, T. L. Cocke, D. L. Chinkes, R. R. Wolfe, and D. Paddon-Jones. 2007. Aging does not impair the anabolic response to a protein-rich meal. *Am J Clin Nutr* 86: 451–456.

Tappy, L. 1996. Thermic effect of food and sympathetic nervous system activity in humans. *Reprod Nutr Dev* 36: 391–397.

Volek, J. S., S. A. Mazzetti, W. B. Farquhar, B. R. Barnes, A. L. Gomez, and W. J. Kraemer. 2001. Physiological responses to short-term exercise in the heat after creatine loading. *Med Sci Sports Exerc* 33: 1101–1108.

Volpi, E., H. Kobayashi, M. Sheffield-Moore, B. Mittendorfer, and R. R. Wolfe. 2003. Essential amino acids are primarily responsible for the amino acid stimulation of muscle protein anabolism in healthy elderly adults. *Am J Clin Nutr* 78: 250–258.

Vuilleumier, S. 1993. Worldwide production of high-fructose syrup and crystalline fructose. *Am J Clin Nutr* 58(5 Suppl): 733S–736S.

Weiss, B. A., and M. E. Powers. 2006. Creatine supplementation does not impair the thermoregulatory response during a bout of exercise in the heat. *J Sports Med Phys Fitness* 46: 555–563.

Williams, M. H. 2010. *Nutrition for health, fitness, & sport*, 9th Ed. New York: McGraw-Hill.

World Health Organization. 1985. *Energy and protein requirments*, Technical Report Series 724. Geneva, Switzerland: World Health Organization.

Zhang, Y., K. Guo, R. E. LeBlanc, D. Loh, G. J. Schwartz, and Y. H. Yu. 2007. Increasing dietary leucine intake reduces diet-induced obesity and improves glucose and cholesterol metabolism in mice via multimechanisms. *Diabetes* 56: 1647–1654.

Zhi, J., A. T. Melia, R. Guerciolini, J. Chung, J. Kinberg, J. B. Hauptman, and I. H. Patel. 1994. Retrospective population-based analysis of the dose-response (fecal fat excretion) relationship of orlistat in normal and obese volunteers. *Clin Pharmacol Ther* 56: 82–85.

Ziegenfuss, T. N., L. M. Lowery, and P. W. Lemon. 1998. Acute fluid volume changes in men during three days of creatine supplementation. *J Exerc Physiol Online* 1: 3.

12 Calorie Needs for Inducing Muscle Hypertrophy

Michael D. Roberts

CONTENTS

12.1 INTRODUCTION

Recent research has indicated that many athletes practice poor nutritional habits that are not conducive to optimizing muscle mass and/or athletic performance. Such examples reported in the scientific literature include the following:

- A sampled group of South American female strength/power athletes ingested an inadequate amount of carbohydrates to support their physical activity levels (de Sousa et al. 2008).
- A sampled cohort of North American athletes consumed substantially less calories compared to the recommendations for physically active persons (Lun et al. 2009).
- A surveyed cohort of Brazilian tennis players possessed a caloric intake that was 10% lower than daily energy expenditure in one-third of the athletes (Juzwiak et al. 2008).

Contrary to the above-mentioned data, however, it is commonly preached that athletes should ingest more dietary calories on a daily basis in order to match increased energy-expenditure levels incurred during rigorous training. If an athlete is in a chronic calorically depleted state, severe physiological repercussions can ensue including: 1) muscle and liver glycogen stores can be exhausted, which lowers performance capabilities through impaired energy production, and 2) muscle mass can

225

be catabolized (i.e., broken down for energy), which further depresses force and/or power production capabilities.

An example illustrating these concepts comes from the research of Reynolds et al. (1999), who demonstrated that mountain climbers undertaking a 21-day expedition developed severe lethargy and lost 6.1 pounds of body mass because they had consumed 2920 calories/day while expending 5390 calories/day. The aforementioned research proves that an athlete must be aware of his/her physical activity levels as well as his/her calorie intake levels in order to sustain an optimal body weight and energy levels. Therefore, this chapter will thoroughly discuss the following topics including: 1) the difference between energy intake and energy expenditure, 2) how athletes can eat to build muscle and optimize performance, and 3) a practical take-home messages that athletes can apply to their training-table habits.

12.2 CONCEPTS OF ENERGY BALANCE

Simply stated, energy balance is the summation of energy consumed through food-stuffs (typically expressed as dietary calories, kilocalories, or kilojoules; will be written as calories herein) versus total daily energy expenditure; for textual consistency, dietary energy will be expressed as calories. Total daily energy expenditure is comprised of three components including:

1. Resting energy expenditure (or REE): the energy needed to maintain organ function not taking into account physical activity. This value is best thought of as the number of calories used per day if an individual were to lay motionless.
2. Energy expenditure during exercise: the energy needed to sustain physical activity. This value is best thought of as the number of calories used (or "burned") during stints of physical activity.
3. Energy expenditure of eating (or the thermic effect of food): the energy needed to digest and reassimilate (i.e., "burn" or store glucose, fat, and protein) ingested foodstuff.

Figure 12.1 estimates how much each of the aforementioned components contributes to an individual's daily energy expenditure.

As mentioned previously, it is instrumental that an athlete is aware of his/her physical activity levels as well as calorie intake levels in order to sustain an appropriate energy balance. If an athlete is in a negative energy balance, then this person metabolizes or "burns" more calories than he/she is eating. Conversely, if an athlete is in a positive energy balance, then this person consumes an extraneous amount of food energy; if this pattern of overeating ensues over chronic periods, then positive "energy" or calories will be converted into and stored as extra body fat. Therefore, in order to achieve an optimal energy balance, an athlete must be aware of his/her: 1) REE, 2) physical activity levels, 3) thermic effect of food value (which is approximately 10% of REE + physical activity levels, and 4) calorie intake. In order to calculate REE, the Harris-Benedict equation is commonly used (Harris and Benedict 1919).

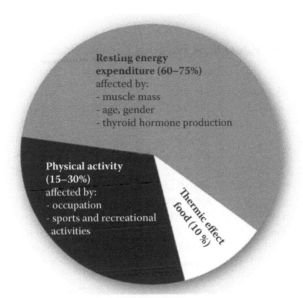

FIGURE 12.1   Components of energy expenditure. (Adapted from McArdle, W. D., F. I. Katch, and V. L. Katch. 2001. *Exercise physiology: Energy, nutrition, and human performance.* 5th Ed. Philadelphia, PA: Lippincott Williams & Wilkins.)

For men,

$$REE = 66.5 + (13.75 \times \text{weight in kg}) + (5.003 \times \text{height in cm})$$
$$- (6.775 \times \text{age in years})$$

For women,

$$REE = 655.1 + (9.563 \times \text{weight in kg}) + (1.850 \times \text{height in cm})$$
$$- (4.676 \times \text{age in years})$$

For example metabolic calculations, we will continually refer to John Doe throughout the chapter; John Doe is a 25-year-old, 5'10" (177.8-cm) male athlete weighing 200 pounds (90.7 kg). According to the Harris-Benedict equation above, John's REE is calculated here:

$$REE = 66.5 + (13.75 \times \textbf{90.7 kg}) + (5.003 \times \textbf{177.8 cm}) - (6.775 \times \textbf{25 years old})$$
$$= 66.5 + 1247.1 + 889.5 - 169.4$$
$$= 2033.7, \text{ which will be estimated as } {\sim}2040 \text{ calories/day}$$

Hence, 2040 calories/day is the energy that John needs to consume from his diet in order to match his metabolic needs in a resting state. Assuming John performs more rigorous activities throughout the day, then his caloric demands increase. If John consumes below this number for prolonged periods (i.e., days to weeks), then he will be able to fuel the metabolic costs of living from energy that is stored as body fat. However, if his calorie intake is depressed for months, then he will inevitably catabolize skeletal-muscle fuel stores and inevitably muscle mass for energy, which will

TABLE 12.1

Energy Expenditure Values (kcal/hour) for Various Physical Activities

Physical Activity	100 Pounds	150 Pounds	200 Pounds	250 Pounds
Weightlifting (moderate intensity)	140 (2.33)	210 (3.50)	290 (4.83)	360 (6.00)
Weightlifting (high intensity)	280 (4.67)	430 (7.17)	570 (9.5)	710 (11.8)
Walking, 2 mph	160 (2.67)	240 (4.00)	312 (5.20)	380 (6.33)
Walking, 3 mph	210 (3.50)	320 (5.33)	416 (6.93)	500 (8.33)
Walking, 4.5 mph	295 (4.92)	440 (7.33)	572 (9.53)	690 (11.5)
Running, 5.5 mph	440 (7.33)	660 (11.00)	962 (16.03)	1080 (18.00)
Running, 7 mph	610 (10.17)	920 (15.33)	1230 (20.50)	1540 (25.67)
Running, 10 mph	850 (14.20)	1280 (21.33)	1664 (27.73)	2010 (33.5)
Swimming, 25 yards/min	185 (3.08)	275 (4.58)	358 (5.97)	440 (7.33)
Swimming, 50 yards/min	325 (5.42)	500 (8.33)	650 (10.83)	825 (13.75)
Bicycling, 6 mph	160 (2.67)	240 (4.00)	312 (5.20)	380 (6.33)
Bicycling, 12 mph	270 (4.50)	410 (6.83)	534 (8.90)	650 (10.83)

The values in parentheses indicate the number of calories used per minute.

Source: Adapted from Haskell W. L., I. M. Lee, R.R. Pate, K. E. Powell, S. N. Blair, B. A. Franklin, C. A. Macera, G. W. Heath, P. D. Thompson, A. Bauman; American College of Sports Medicine; Heart Association. Physical activity and public health: Updated recommendation for adults from the American College of Sports Medicine and the American Heart Association. *Circulation.* Aug. 28, 2007, 116(9):1081–1093.

compromise his athletic capabilities. Furthermore, being in a chronically calorically depleted state will substantially depress resting energy expenditure and compromise John's ability to burn calories; this may lead to an increased propensity for body fat accumulation once John brings up his calories to predepletion levels.

Next, athletes must accurately account for energy expended during physical activity on a daily basis. Table 12.1 provides energy expenditures for various physical activities. Thus, in the case of John Doe, if he were to provide us with a daily log of various activities (see an example in Table 12.2), then he would be able to derive his total daily energy expenditure.

Based upon the aforementioned calculations, John Doe should consume approximately 2960 calories/day in order to sustain his current body weight given his physical activity level. Without these meticulous calculations, assuming the precise caloric needs of John Doe would become more challenging and could lead to less optimal energy-balance states. Hence, it is advised that an athlete calculates his/her average daily energy expenditure as performed prior to designing an eating regimen in order to effectively optimize his/her energy balance and potentially build muscle as discussed in the next section.

12.3   EATING TO BUILD MUSCLE: INTRODUCTORY CONCEPTS

Prior to discussing how to eat in order to build muscle, it is necessary to discuss the current macronutrient recommendations for athletes. In 2009, the American College

TABLE 12.2

Estimated Total Daily Energy Expenditure Based upon Physical Activity Level

Time	Physical activity	Duration (min)	Calories Expended (Estimated from Table 12.1)
REE (based upon Harris-Benedict calculation)			2,040
8:00 AM	Walk from car to office (3 mph)	5	35
9:00 AM -5:00 PM	Walk around office (3 mph)	30	208
5:00 PM	Walk from office to car (3 mph)	5	35
6:00 PM	Bicycling (6 mph)	20	156
6:20 PM	Resistance training (moderate intensity)	45	217
Calories used not factoring in food intake 105 min			2,691
Calories used factoring in food intake. This is the value above multiplied by 0.1 and then added again to the value above.			2,960

These values are based upon a 200-pound (90.7-kg), 5'10" (177.8-cm), 25-year-old male. Furthermore, the thermic effect of food must be accounted for; this value being ~10% of (REE + physical activity).

of Sports Medicine, American Dietetic Association, and the Dieticians of Canada released a joint position stand stating that athletes should fulfill the following macronutrient requirements (Rodriguez et al. 2009):

- 6–10 g/kg of body weight (2.7–4.5 g/pound) of carbohydrates/day. This amount depends upon total daily energy expenditure.
- 1.2–1.7 g/kg of body weight (0.5–0.8 g/pound) of protein per day. It has been reported that athletes wishing to build muscle typically consume more than 2 g/kg/day (Lambert et al. 2004).
- Fat intake should range from 20 to 35% of total caloric intake. This is approximately 1.0–1.5 g/kg (0.5–0.7 g/pound) of fat/day.
- Following exercise, athletes should replace lost fluids, electrolytes, and glycogen by taking in 1.0–1.5 g/kg (0.5–0.7 g/pound) of a carbohydrate-laden beverage.
- Consuming protein rich in amino acids (i.e., whey or casein isolate or hydrolysates) following exercise will facilitate muscle recovery and accelerate post-exercise muscle hypertrophy. Although quantity recommendations have not been made, researchers have determined that approximately 20 g of whey/casein protein sources increases muscle-building mechanisms following exercise (Tipton et al. 2004)

The Atwater Conversion System is also another important concept to grasp prior to planning dietary regimens. American chemist Wilbur Atwater determined the gross energy in various food sources by studying the heat generated while combusting these foodstuffs. Atwater took these experiments a step further and derived the amount of energy lost from these foodstuffs through fecal and urine energy analysis.

To summarize, Atwater determined that carbohydrates and proteins contained 4 calories of available energy, whereas fat contained 9 calories of available energy. Thus, consuming a cinnamon roll containing 29 g of fat, 80 g of carbohydrates, and 9 g of protein would yield the following caloric value:

Caloric value = 29 g of fat (×9 calories/g) + 80 g of carbohydrates (×4 calories/g)
+ 9 g of protein (×4 calories/g)
= 261 calories from fat + 320 calories from carbohydrates
+ 36 calories from protein
= 617 calories

Using the example from the previous section of John Doe, who weighs 200 pounds (90.6 kg), the aforementioned guidelines dictate that he should consume: 1) 544–906 g of carbohydrates/day, 2) 109–154 g of protein/day, and 3) 91–136 g of fat/day. Extrapolating these macronutrient quantities to caloric values using the Atwater Conversion System indicates that John Doe should be ingesting between 3422 calories (544 g of carbohydrates, 109 g of protein, and 91 g of fat) and 5464 kcal (906 g of carbohydrates, 154 g of protein, and 136 g of fat) per day. However, these recommendations are highly indicative of daily physical activity patterns. If John Doe were to merely expend 2960 calories/day as calculated above and he were to ingest 3422–5464 calories/day, then he would be consuming up to 460–2504 excessive calories/day, thus putting him in an extraneously positive energy balance, which would lead to a gain body fat. Therefore, individuals like John Doe (i.e., "weekend warriors" or recreational athletes) should base their macronutrient intakes on caloric percentages using a 25-50-25 scheme (i.e., 25% of ingested calories from protein, 50% from carbohydrates, and 25% from fat) presented here:

- As mentioned, John Doe needs 2960 calories/day to maintain his body weight
- Protein needs: 25% of ingested calories = 0.25 × 2960 calories or 740 calories from protein, which is 185 g of protein (= 740 kcal ÷ 4 calories/g of protein)
- Carbohydrate needs: 50% of ingested calories = 0.50 × 2960 calories or 1480 calories from carbohydrates, which is 370 g of carbohydrates (= 1480 calories ÷ 4 calories/g of carbohydrate)
- Fat needs: 25% of ingested calories = 0.25 × 2960 calories or 740 calories from fat, which is 82 g of fat (= 1480 calories ÷ 9 calories/g of fat)

Although the 25-50-25 scheme goes against the conventional 15% protein, 55% carbohydrate, 30% fat scheme proposed by the United States Department of Agriculture (USDA), recent research contends that athletes (and perhaps the general population) need more protein to support the recovery and muscle-building processes that accompany the rigors of training. For instance, Bilsborough and Mann state (2006):

A suggested maximum protein intake based on bodily needs, weight control evidence, and avoiding protein toxicity would be approximately of 25% of energy requirements at approximately 2 to 2.5 g per kg [on a daily basis] corresponding to 176 g protein per day for an 80 kg individual on a 12,000 kJ/d (2873 kcal/d) diet. This is well below the theoretical maximum safe intake range for an 80 kg person (up to 365 g/d).

Furthermore, athletes that do not consume food sources rich in bioavailable essential amino acids (i.e., strict vegans who do not consume meat and dairy products) are advised to consume 2.0+ g of protein/kg of body weight (0.91 g/pound) on a daily basis to ensure that enough essential amino acids are ingested (McArdle et al. 2001). In this regard, a similar sports-nutrition article claims that milk-based foods contain 10% (milk isolate, casein) to 12% (whey) leucine content, meat and egg-based products contain approximately 8–9% leucine, and plant-based products such as wheat protein contain less than 8% leucine; this, the authors contend, make the latter foods "not optimal" for stimulation of skeletal muscle growth (Kim et al. 2009). Thus, it is integral that athletes consume an adequate amount and the proper sources of protein to optimize bodily protein needs. This is a topic that will be further discussed in subsequent sections.

12.4   EATING TO BUILD MUSCLE: WHAT THE SCIENCE SAYS

Enriching the diet with more calories and/or higher quality protein sources has been found to increase strength and muscle mass in resistance-trained individuals. Illustrating this point, data from our laboratory (Roberts et al. 2007) illustrated that college-aged resistance-trained males increasing their calorie intake by 580 calories through two supplemental high-protein beverages (45 g of protein, 24 g of carbohydrate, and 1 g of fat) daily experienced the following after a 50-day intervention: 1) a 2.4-pound (1.1 kg) increase in muscle mass, 2) an 18–25-pound (8–11 kg) increase in bench press strength, 3) an 50–55-pound (23–25 kg) increase in leg press strength, and 4) an increase in the amount of muscle contractile proteins as evidenced through muscle biopsy analyses.

Similarly, Singh et al. (1999) demonstrated that supplementing older men and women who resistance trained on a regular basis and consumed less than the recommended dietary allowance for energy intake with a 360-calorie beverage (i.e., 15 g of soy protein, 54 g of carbohydrates, and 9 g of fat) achieved the following outcomes following a 10-week study: 1) strength levels increased nearly two times in those who resistance trained and supplemented compared with those who trained without the supplemental beverage (i.e., a 250% increase versus a 100% increase, respectively), 2) muscle biopsy analysis revealed that those who supplemented exhibited a 10% increase in muscle cell size, indicating that these individuals experienced greater muscle protein synthesis throughout the course of the study, and 3) statistical analysis revealed that changes in strength and muscle cell size were prominently caused by the increase in calorie intake.

Interestingly, other data exist demonstrating that increasing the intake of higher-quality protein sources or protein sources that contain more highly digestible essential amino acids, which the body cannot make, increases muscle mass in the absence of increasing calorie intake. For instance, our laboratory (Kerksick et al. 2006) has demonstrated that resistance-trained males ingesting a supplemental protein beverage containing 40 g of whey protein and 8 g of casein protein exhibited a 4.2-pound (1.9 kg) increase in muscle mass following a 12-week study. As mentioned, what is interesting is that this increase in muscle mass occurred in the absence of an increase in calorie intake, demonstrating that an athlete's macronutrient profile may be just as crucial in optimizing body composition in comparison with his/her energy balance. Taking all of this data into consideration, it is integral that athletes aspiring to increase muscle mass consume more calories as well as higher-quality protein sources. Other sections in this chapter will outline explicit calorie and macronutrient intakes to achieve these goals.

So the inevitable question remains: how many extra calories are needed to build muscle mass without increasing body fat mass? Although this question is seemingly broad and is difficult to answer on an interindividual basis, it is known that individuals carrying more muscle mass metabolize more and thus need to ingest more calories on a daily basis. For instance, our laboratory (Roberts et al. 2008) has determined that for each pound (0.45 kg) of lean tissue mass, college-aged males metabolize approximately 408 extra calories/day, whereas females metabolize 153 extra calories/day (Figure 12.2). However, our data are limited for interpretation because age, physical activity patterns, and interindividual genetic differences were

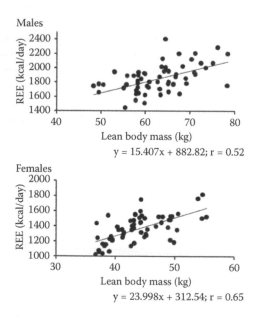

FIGURE 12.2   Relationships between lean body mass and REE in college-aged males and females. For each pound (0.45 kg) of lean tissue mass, college-aged males metabolize approximately 408 extra calories/day. Likewise, for each pound (0.45 kg) of lean tissue mass, females metabolize 153 extra calories/day. These data illustrate the need for more calories for individuals that strive to maintain or gain muscle mass. (Adapted from Roberts, M. D., V. J. Dalbo, S. E. Hassell, J. R. Stout, and C. M. Kerksick. 2008. *J Int Soc Sports Nutr* 5: 19.)

not taken into account prior to these calculations. A more conservative estimation from scientist Robert Wolfe suggest that each additional pound of muscle mass metabolizes an extra 5 or 6 calories when accounted for in resting-energy expenditure estimations (Wolfe 2006). Hence, if John Doe were to increase his muscle mass by 10 pounds after a year of extensive training, then according to Wolfe's estimations, he would raise his REE by 50 kcal (or calories)/day. Nonetheless, these data illustrate the need for more calories for individuals that strive to maintain or gain muscle mass.

According to other scientific estimations (i.e., that muscle tissue is approximately 70% water, 22% protein, and 8% fat), approximately 2500 calories above metabolic needs incurred via total daily energy expenditure are required to synthesize 1 pound (0.45 kg) of muscle in athletes that resistance train. Although the mechanisms behind muscle growth are beyond the realm of this chapter, extra energy needs are integral to muscle growth because adding more protein (i.e., myofibrils, cytoskeletal, cytosolic, etc.) to pre-existing muscle tissue requires skeletal muscle to be in a positive state of muscle protein balance, this being a state that requires an abundance of dietary protein as well as energy that is derived from foodstuff. Specifically, it has been estimated that 4 moles of ATP (or 28 dietary calories) are needed to integrate 1 mole of protein into skeletal muscle structures (Wolfe 2006). Skeletal muscle tissue inherently has a protein turnover rate, meaning that proteins within skeletal muscle are continually broken down and rebuilt or synthesized (Elliot et al. 2006).

In general, consuming an abundance of calories (i.e., more than is burned) will ensure that muscle protein balance is relatively stable. Without modifying dietary habits, resistance exercise tends to accelerate protein turnover rate and even slightly favors muscle protein synthesis. When athletes weight train and consume extraneous protein-laden meals, muscle protein synthesis rates far exceed muscle protein breakdown rates, leading to the eventual increase in muscle mass (Elliot et al. 2006). Based upon these concepts, the National Strength and Conditioning Association advises athletes wishing to gain muscle mass to strive for a 1–2-pound (0.45–0.90 kg) increase in body mass/week, which increases caloric needs to 350–700 kcal/day above what the athlete metabolizes (Baechle and Earle 2000). A template dietary intake pattern is provided at the conclusion of the chapter illustrating how athletes can strive to achieve these intakes.

Beyond consuming more calories, scientists have determined that increasing eating frequency, especially following exercise, is important for building muscle mass. For instance, researchers Rene Koopman et al. (2005) demonstrated that administering macronutrients to participants every 30 minutes following resistance training up to 6 hours optimally stimulated muscle protein synthesis; note that participants on average ingested either: 1) 22.2 g of carbohydrates, 14.4 g of whey hydrolysate, and 7 g of leucine, 2) 22.2 g of carbohydrates and 14.4 g of whey hydrolysate, or 3) 22.2 g of carbohydrates every 30 minutes for 6 hours. Moreover, ingesting a carbohydrate/protein/leucine-laden beverage following an exercise stimulus achieved the greatest muscle-building effects following exercise compared with isocaloric carbohydrate/protein or carbohydrate beverages. Although it is impractical to eat or consume nutritional supplements every 30 minutes following each workout, the aforementioned data suggest that post-exercise muscle-building mechanisms are extremely responsive to macronutrients following training, with quickly digestible protein/carbohydrate sources spiked with leucine being the most optimal macronutrient mixture. Therefore, it is recommended that athletes consume a post-exercise protein/carbohydrate beverage as well as numerous rapidly digestible protein-laden meals following training sessions. Table 12.3 provides slowly versus rapidly digestible protein sources as a reference for athletes.

Finally, researchers have recently determined that nutrient timing is an integral aspect of building muscle. Illustrating this concept, Cribb and Hayes (2006) performed a 10-week study demonstrating that participants ingesting ~30 g of whey protein, ~30 g carbohydrate, and ~5 g of creatine monohydrate immediately prior to and immediately after resistance exercise experienced a greater increase in strength and muscle mass compared with a separate group that consumed this drink in the morning and evening. Specifically, the pre-/post-exercise group gained 6.2 pounds (2.8 kg) of muscle mass compared to 3.3 pounds (1.5 kg) in the latter group. Further, the pre-/post-exercise group gained 45.0 pounds (20.4 kg) of lower-body strength compared to 35.5 pounds (16.1 kg) in the latter group.

When examining muscle biopsies from these subjects, the pre-/post-exercise group gained significantly more contractile protein and had a substantially greater increase in other molecular characteristics (i.e., muscle fiber area, more creatine, more muscle glycogen, etc.). The authors also emphasize the importance of

---

TABLE 12.3
Estimated Absorption Rates of Various Protein Sources

Protein Source	Absorption Rate (g/hour)
Egg protein (raw)	1.3
Pea flour	2.4
Egg protein, cooked	2.8
Milk protein	3.5
Soy isolate	3.9
Casein isolate	6.1
Free amino acids	7.0–7.5
Whey protein isolate	8.0–10.0

Note that researchers have indicated that it is advantageous to consume rapidly digestible protein sources immediately following exercise. Likewise, it is advantageous to consume protein-laden meals (10+ g) frequently (i.e., 3+ times) following an exercise bout in order to maximally stimulate muscle-building mechanisms.

Source: Adapted from Bilsborough, S., and N. Mann. 2006. A review of issues of dietary protein intake in humans. *Int J Sport Nutr Exerc Metab* 16: 129–152.

---

consuming a protein/carbohydrate-laden beverage surrounding (i.e., immediately before and after) exercise because acute research settings have shown this practice to provide a rapid influx into exercised skeletal muscle of essential amino acids, which can be used for muscle rebuilding processes. Likewise, the International Society of Sports Nutrition has released position statements on protein and exercise (Campbell et al. 2007) and nutrient timing (Kerksick et al. 2008), respectively, stating that:

> While it is possible for physically active individuals to obtain their daily protein requirements through a varied, regular diet, supplemental protein in various forms are a practical way of ensuring adequate and quality protein intake for athletes

and,

> Ingesting carbohydrate alone or in combination with protein during resistance exercise increases muscle glycogen, offsets muscle damage, and facilitates greater training adaptations after either acute or prolonged periods of supplementation with resistance training.

Hence, although it has been deemed unnecessary for athletes to consume supplemental protein beverages versus whole meals, this scientific literature provides sound evidence that this sort of supplementation scheme is beneficial for building muscle mass.

12.5   TRANSITIONING FROM TEXT TO TRAINING TABLE

In summary, it is integral that athletes grasp the concepts of energy intake versus energy expenditure in order to ensure that they are achieving optimal energy balance. Calculations are provided in this chapter, and athletes are advised to perform these tabulations prior to adjusting their diet with the intent of increasing muscle mass. For athletes wishing to accrue muscle mass, it is important to consume slightly more energy than what is being expended. In this regard, these athletes should strive to consume 350–700 extra calories/day than what is being metabolized, and weight gain should not exceed 2 pounds (0.91 kg)/week.

Finally, whereas this point was not emphasized in this chapter, it is integral that athletes consume a well-balanced diet that also contains various fruit and vegetable sources in order to ensure that they obtain adequate micronutrients (i.e., vitamins and minerals), as well as fiber, on a daily basis. In this regard, it is recommended that athletes follow USDA guidelines and consume 2–4 servings of fruit and 3–5 servings of vegetable sources per day. When increasing calorie intake, these servings can be increased to enhance energy intake while adequately ensuring that micronutrient intakes are appropriate. Table 12.4, which contains muscle-building foods, can be used by athletes for food selection purposes in conjunction with Figure 12.3 in training-table environments. The following sections as well as Figure 12.3 further summarize integral take-home messages.

TABLE 12.4
Common Foods Found at Training-Table Settings

Food (Serving Size)	Protein (g)	Carbohydrates (g)	Fat (g)	Calories
Common protein sources				
Lean ground beef, 4–7% fat (3 oz)	18	0	~3	~120
Ground beef, 20% fat (3 oz)	15	0	18	210
Sirloin steak, fat trimmed (3 oz)	26	0	5	156
Chicken: white meat, no skin (3 oz)	18	0	0	93
Chicken: dark meat, no skin (3 oz)	24	0	9	174
Turkey: white meat (3 oz)	24	0	0	114
Fish: salmon (3 oz)	18	0	12	174
Fish: halibut, tilapia, cod (3 oz)	18	0	2	93
Fish: tuna, canned in water (3 oz)	21	0	0	96
Eggs: whole (1 medium)	6	0	5	71
Eggs: whites only (1 large)	4	0	0	16
Skim milk (1 cup or 8 fl oz)	8	12	0	83
Tofu (3 oz)	6	3	3	51
Cheese: made from whole milk (1 oz)	6	0	9	105
Yogurt: low fat (1 cup or 8 oz)	13	17	4	154
Cottage cheese: low fat (1 cup or 8 oz)	28	2	6	163
Ham: sliced, lean (3 oz)	15	0	3	90
Pork loin: lean meat only (3 oz)	15	0	6	132
Common starches				
Pasta: spaghetti, macaroni, etc. (1 cup, cooked)	8	43	1	220
White/wheat bread or rolls (1 roll, 1 oz)	2	13	2	76
Baked potato: plain (medium)	4	46	0	200
Sweet potato: plain (large)	4	37	0	162
White rice (1 cup)	4	45	0	205
Brown rice (1 cup)	5	45	2	216
Bagel: plain (regular size)	11	56	2	290
Beans: red, black, pinto (1 cup)	16	40	0	220
Oatmeal (1 cup, cooked)	6	29	3	160
Low-fat granola: bar or cereal (1 oz)	2	23	2	109
Corn (1 cup)	4	46	1	184
Common fruits and vegetables				
Apple, medium size	0	25	0	95
Orange, medium size	1	17	0	69
Banana, medium size	1	27	0	105
Grapes (1 cup, 30 grapes)	1	27	0	104
Berries: blueberries, cranberries, blackberries, strawberries, etc. (1 cup)	1	13–21	0	53–84
Tomatoes (1 cup, chopped)	2	5	0	25
Root vegetables: carrots, beets, turnips (1 cup)	1	12	0	52
Cruciferous vegetables: greens, broccoli, cauliflower, cabbage, etc. (1 cup cooked)	2–3	6–7	0	30–40

TABLE 12.4 (CONTINUED)
Common Foods Found at Training-Table Settings

Food (Serving Size)	Protein (g)	Carbohydrates (g)	Fat (g)	Calories
Common fat sources				
Butter (1 oz)	1	0	15	140
Whole milk (1 cup or 8 fl oz)	8	13	8	146
2% milk (1 cup or 8 fl oz)	8	12	5	120
Peanuts (1 oz)	5	7	14	166
Almonds (1 oz)	4	6	17	177
Peanut butter: commercial, sweetened (1 oz)	7	6	14	165
Cream cheese (1 oz)	2	1	10	96
Creamy salad dressing: ranch, bleu cheese, Italian (1 oz)	0	2	14	136
Avocado (1/2 of fruit without seed)	1.5	6	10.5	114

For measurement conceptualizations:
- 3 oz = size of a deck of playing cards or a Dixie cup
- 1 oz = 2 tablespoons, except for rolls or bread, which is porous
- 8 oz or 8 fl oz = approximately three small Dixie cups

Source: http://www.nutritiondata.com.

12.5.1 RECREATIONAL ATHLETES

- For weight maintenance, recreational athletes should calculate daily energy expenditure as presented in Table 12.2 and base their macronutrient intakes on the 25-50-25 scheme as previously discussed. Although research has deemed it unnecessary for well-fed athletes to consume nutritional supplements, some research has indicated that that athletes should consume a post-exercise supplemental beverage (~240 calories) containing 30 g of whey protein isolate and 30 g of carbohydrate immediately following weight-training sessions for optimal muscle recovery.
- To steadily increase muscle mass, recreational athletes should calculate daily energy expenditure as presented in Table 12.2, add 350–700 calories/day to this figure, and base their macronutrient intakes on the 25-50-25 scheme as previously discussed. Increases in caloric intake can be achieved by eating more at mealtime and increasing eating frequency. Importantly, recent research has indicated that individuals wishing to optimize muscle mass should consume a pre- and post-exercise supplemental beverage (~240 calories) containing 30 g of whey protein isolate, 30 g of carbohydrate, and 5 g of creatine monohydrate immediately prior to and immediately following a weight-training session (Cribb and Hayes 2006). If weight gain exceeds 2 pounds/week, then it is advised the athlete re-evaluate his/her diet and reduce caloric intake.

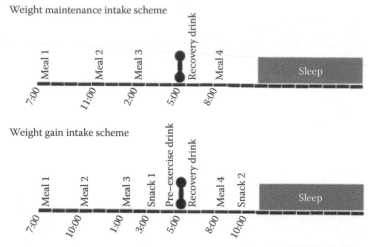

Bodyweight	100 lb	150 lb	200 lb	250 lb
Meals 1–4				
Kcal	300–400	500–600	700–800	900–950
PRO (g)	19–25	31–38	44–50	56–59
CHO (g)	38–50	62–76	88–100	112–118
FAT (g)	8–11	13–18	19–22	25–27
*Snacks 1–2				
Kcal	200+	200+	200+	200+
PRO (g)	13+	13+	13+	13+
CHO (g)	25+	25+	25+	25+
FAT (g)	6+	6+	6+	6+
*†Pre-exercise drink				
Kcal	240	240	240	240
PRO (g)	30	30	30	30
CHO (g)	30	30	30	30
FAT (g)	<1	<1	<1	<1
†Recovery drink				
Kcal	240	240	240	240
PRO (g)	30	30	30	30
CHO (g)	30	20	30	30
FAT (g)	<1	<1	<1	<1
Weight maintenance				
Kcal/day	1440–1840	2240–2640	3040–3460	3840–4040
PRO (g/day)	106–130	154–182	206–230	254–266
CHO (g/day)	152–230	278–334	982–430	478–502
FAT (g/day)	32–44	52–72	76–88	100–108
Weight gain				
Kcal/day	2080–2480	2880–3280	3680–4100	4480–4680
PRO (g/day)	162–186	210–238	262–286	310–322
CHO (g/day)	232–266	358–414	462–510	558–582
FAT (g/day)	44–56	64–84	88–100	112–120

FIGURE 12.3 Typical dietary schemes for weight maintenance or weight gain for recreational or competitive strength-training athletes. Weight maintenance values include meals 1–4 and a post-exercise recovery shake, whereas weight gain includes meals 1–4, snacks 1 and 2, and pre- and post-exercise shakes. Note that value ranges account for variations in physical activity patterns. *These meals should be eaten during weight-gaining phases. †These beverages should contain 5 g of creatine monohydrate in order to optimize gains in muscle mass.

12.5.2 COMPETITIVE STRENGTH ATHLETES

- For weight maintenance, strength athletes should consume 6–10 g/kg of body weight (2.7–4.5 g/pound) of carbohydrates/day. This amount depends upon total daily energy expenditure. Consume at least 1.2–1.7 g/kg of body weight (0.5–0.8 g/pound) of protein/day; it has been reported that athletes wishing to build muscle typically consume more than 2 g/kg/day. Consume approximately 1.0–1.5 g/kg (0.5–0.7 g/pound) of fat/day. For optimal muscle recovery, it is advised that athletes consume a post-exercise supplemental beverage (~240 calories) containing 30 g of whey protein isolate and 30 g of carbohydrate immediately prior to and immediately following a weight-training session.
- For weight gain, strength athletes should consume 6–10 g/kg of body weight (2.7–4.5 g/pound) of carbohydrates/day; this amount depends upon total daily energy expenditure. Consume 1.2–1.7 g/kg of body weight (0.5–0.8 g/pound) of protein/day; it has been reported that athletes wishing to build muscle typically consume more than 2 g/kg/day. Consume approximately 1.0–1.5 g/kg (0.5–0.7 g/pound) of fat/day. Increases in caloric intake should be 350–700 kcal above what is expended, and this can be achieved by eating more at mealtime and/or increasing eating frequency. Importantly, recent research has indicated that individuals wishing to optimize muscle mass should consume a pre- and post-exercise supplemental beverage (~240 calories) containing 30 g of whey protein isolate, 30 g of carbohydrate, and 5 g of creatine monohydrate immediately prior to and immediately following a weight-training session (Cribb and Hayes 2006). If weight gain exceeds 2 pounds/week, then it is advised that the athlete re-evaluate his/her diet and reduce caloric intake.

Finally, this chapter will conclude with a sample menu that athletes can mimic when wishing to add muscle mass. Using the John Doe example as done throughout this chapter, if John wished to increase muscle mass then he would have to consume up to 700 calories/day greater than his total daily energy expenditure, which is equivalent to 3660 calories/day (i.e., 2960 calories to maintain weight + 700 extra calories). The meal plan in Table 12.5 for John Doe was adapted from Figure 12.2.

The following items are additional online sources for athletes further highlighting the physiological and nutritional concepts discussed in this chapter:

- http://www.nutritionadata.com: Athletes can find general nutrition information on a wide variety of foods and analysis tools that allow users to determine how various foods affect their health.
- http://www.mypyramid.gov: This website designed by the USDA offers personalized eating plans and other interactive applications that assists athletes to assess their current intakes and plan diets.
- http://www.gssiweb.com: This website designed by the Gatorade Sports Science Institute assists athletes in optimizing health and performance by presenting research-based sports-nutrition information.

TABLE 12.5

Sample Meal Plan for Athletes Striving for Weight Gain

Meal	Protein (g)	Carbohydrates (g)	Fat (g)	Calories
Meal 1 (7:00 AM)				
Four large eggs, scrambled	24	0	20	284
Two pieces toast	4	26	4	152
Butter (1/2 tbsp)	0.5	0	7.5	70
One banana	1	27	0	105
Subtotal	*29.5*	*53*	*31.5*	*611*
Meal 2 (10:00 AM)				
Two pieces wheat bread	4	26	4	152
Ham, sliced, lean (3 oz)	15	0	3	90
One apple	0	25	0	95
Almonds (1 oz)	4	6	17	177
Subtotal	*27*	*63*	*41*	*691*
Meal 3 (1:00 PM)				
Chicken breast (6 oz)	36	0	0	186
Black beans (1 cup)	16	40	0	220
Chopped strawberries (2 cups)	2	~30	0	128
Subtotal	*54*	*70*	*0*	*534*
Snack 1 (3:00 PM)				
Low-fat granola (3 oz)	6	69	6	327
One apple	0	25	0	95
Subtotal	*6*	*94*	*6*	*422*
Pre-exercise beverage (before exercise) *with optional 3 g of creatine monohydrate*	30	30	0	240
Post-exercise beverage (after exercise) *with optional 3 g of creatine monohydrate*	30	30	0	240
Meal 4 (8:00 PM)				
Sirloin steak (6 oz)	52	0	10	312
Green beans (1 cup)	3	7	0	40
Corn (2 cups)	8	92	2	368
Subtotal	*63*	*99*	*12*	*720*
Snack 2 (10:00 PM)				
Cottage cheese (1/2 cup)	14	1	3	81.5
Chopped pineapple (1 oz)	1	22	0	82
Subtotal	*15*	*23*	*3*	*163.5*
Totals	254.5	462	93.5	3621.5

REFERENCES

Baechle, T. R., and R. W. Earle, eds. 2000. *Essentials of Strength and Conditioning*, 2nd Ed. Champaign, IL: Human Kinetics.

Bilsborough, S., and N. Mann. 2006. A review of issues of dietary protein intake in humans. *Int J Sport Nutr Exerc Metab* 16: 129–152.

Campbell, B., R. B. Kreider, T. Ziegenfuss, P. La Bounty, M. Roberts, D. Burke, J. Landis, H. Lopez, and J. Antonio. 2007. International Society of Sports Nutrition position stand: Protein and exercise. *J Int Soc Sports Nutr* 4: 8.

Cribb, P. J., and A. Hayes. 2006. Effects of supplement timing and resistance exercise on skeletal muscle hypertrophy. *Med Sci Sports Exerc* 38: 1918–1925.

de Sousa, E. F., T. H. Da Costa, J. A. Nogueira, and L. J. Vivaldi. 2008. Assessment of nutrient and water intake among adolescents from sports federations in the Federal District, Brazil. *Br J Nutr* 99: 1275–1283.

Elliot, T. A., M. G. Cree, A. P. Sanford, R. R. Wolfe, and K. D. Tipton. 2006. Milk ingestion stimulates net muscle protein synthesis following resistance exercise. *Med Sci Sports Exerc* 38: 667–674.

Harris, J., and F. Benedict. 1919. *A Biometric Study of Basal Metabolism in Man*. Washington, D.C.: Carnegie Institute of Washington.

Haskell W. L., I. M. Lee, R.R. Pate, K. E. Powell, S. N. Blair, B. A. Franklin, C. A. Macera, G. W. Heath, P. D. Thompson, A. Bauman; American College of Sports Medicine; Heart Association. Physical activity and public health: Updated recommendation for adults from the American College of Sports Medicine and the American Heart Association. *Circulation*. 2007 Aug 28;116(9):1081–1093.

Juzwiak, C. R., O. M. Amancio, M. S. Vitalle, M. M. Pinheiro, and V. L. Szejnfeld. 2008. Body composition and nutritional profile of male adolescent tennis players. *J Sports Sci* 26: 1209–1217.

Kerksick, C., T. Harvey, J. Stout, B. Campbell, C. Wilborn, R. Kreider, D. Kalman, T. Ziegenfuss, H. Lopez, J. Landis, J. L. Ivy, and J. Antonio. 2008. International Society of Sports Nutrition position stand: Nutrient timing, *J Int Soc Sports Nutr* 5: 17.

Kerksick, C. M., C. J. Rasmussen, S. L. Lancaster, B. Magu, P. Smith, C. Melton, M. Greenwood, A. L. Almada, C. P. Earnest, and R. B. Kreider. 2006. The effects of protein and amino acid supplementation on performance and training adaptations during ten weeks of resistance training. *J Strength Cond Res* 20: 643–653.

Kim, J. S., J. M. Wilson, and S. R. Lee. 2009. Dietary implications on mechanisms of sarcopenia: Roles of protein, amino acids and antioxidants. *J Nutr Biochem* 21: 1–13.

Koopman, R., A. J. Wagenmakers, R. J. Manders, A. H. Zorenc, J. M. Senden, M. Gorselink, H. A. Keizer, and L. J. van Loon. 2005. Combined ingestion of protein and free leucine with carbohydrate increases postexercise muscle protein synthesis in vivo in male subjects. *Am J Physiol Endocrinol Metab* 288: E645–E653.

Lambert, C. P., L. L. Frank, and W. J. Evans. 2004. Macronutrient considerations for the sport of bodybuilding. *Sports Med* 34: 317–327.

Lun, V., K. A. Erdman, and R. A. Reimer. 2009. Evaluation of nutritional intake in Canadian high-performance athletes. *Clin J Sport Med* 19: 405–411.

McArdle, W. D., F. I. Katch, and V. L. Katch. 2001. *Exercise Physiology: Energy, Nutrition, and Human Performance*. 5th Ed. Philadelphia, PA: Lippincott Williams & Wilkins.

Reynolds, R. D., J. A. Lickteig, P. A. Deuster, M. P. Howard, J. M. Conway, A. Pietersma, J. deStoppelaar, and P. Deurenberg. 1999. Energy metabolism increases and regional body fat decreases while regional muscle mass is spared in humans climbing Mt. Everest. *J Nutr* 129: 1307–1314.

Roberts, M. D., V. J. Dalbo, S. E. Hassell, J. R. Stout, and C. M. Kerksick. 2008. Efficacy and safety of a popular thermogenic drink after 28 days of ingestion. *J Int Soc Sports Nutr* 5: 19.

Roberts, M. D., M. Iosia, C. M. Kerksick, L. W. Taylor, B. Campbell, C. D. Wilborn, T. Harvey, M. Cooke, C. Rasmussen, M. Greenwood, R. Wilson, J. Jitomir, D. Willoughby, and R. B. Kreider. 2007. Effects of arachidonic acid supplementation on training adaptations in resistance-trained males. *J Int Soc Sports Nutr* 4: 21.

Rodriguez, N. R., N. M. Di Marco, and S. Langley. 2009. American College of Sports Medicine position stand: Nutrition and athletic performance. *Med Sci Sports Exerc* 41: 709–731.

Singh, M. A., W. Ding, T. J. Manfredi, G. S. Solares, E. F. O'Neill, K. M. Clements, N. D. Ryan, J. J. Kehayias, R. A. Fielding, and W. J. Evans. 1999. Insulin-like growth factor I in skeletal muscle after weight-lifting exercise in frail elders. *Am J Physiol* 277: E135–E143.

Tipton, K. D., T. A. Elliott, M. G. Cree, S. E. Wolf, A. P. Sanford, and R. R. Wolfe. 2004. Ingestion of casein and whey proteins result in muscle anabolism after resistance exercise. *Med Sci Sports Exerc* 36: 2073–2081.

Wolfe, R. R. 2006. The underappreciated role of muscle in health and disease. *Am J Clin Nutr* 84: 475–482.

13 Nutrient Timing for Optimal Adaptation and Recovery

Brian D. Shelmadine, Paul M. La Bounty, and Kara A. Sample

CONTENTS

13.1 INTRODUCTION: WHAT IS NUTRIENT TIMING?

For years, it has been generally acknowledged that both what and how much an athlete eats can affect exercise performance. However, the time the athlete eats relative to when the workout occurs can also affect the extent of the physiological adaptations. In order to run faster, jump farther, and simply improve athletic performance, the athlete needs to optimize adaptation and enhance recovery. How is this accomplished? This chapter is intended to explain exactly that: to teach what to eat, when to eat, and how much to eat so that adaptation and recovery can be optimized.

Specifically, the purpose of this chapter is to provide scientific strategies on how to time the ingestion of meals and snacks in relation to a bout of exercise to more effectively replenish glycogen, increase protein synthesis, and blunt protein degradation. However, this chapter will spend little time on the various physiological mechanisms that pertain to adaptation or recovery. That information can be found in other chapters in this book. The principles in this chapter can be applied to different types of training such as running, cycling, swimming, rowing, or weight lifting.

The following pages address the consumption of carbohydrate, fat, and protein prior to exercise, during exercise, and after exercise relative to recovery and adaptation of skeletal muscle from training. Although the majority of recent research has involved examining the effect of singular macronutrients or the combination of those nutrients in supplemental form, the concept of the "training table" implies the consumption of whole foods. As such, relevant research concerning the consumption of whole foods and actual meals will be emphasized when that information is available. One such example is the consumption of milk or chocolate milk instead of a commercial protein powder post-exercise to improve recovery and adaptation. However, the use of whole foods and meals during training is an area in need of more research. Thus, it is still a necessity to review articles using macronutrients in supplemental form. In keeping with the concept of the training table, though, examples of meals and snacks that can be found in any grocery store and/or dining hall will be provided.

Before delving into the nuances of nutrient timing, it needs to be briefly stated that proper adaptation and recovery will not occur without adequate caloric consumption. In other words, if an athlete does not meet the number of calories expended during the day, which includes enough for basal metabolic function as well as that expended during activity, then proper adaptation will not occur. Subsequently, performance will not be optimized. With that said, a review of current recommendations for macronutrient intake is prudent. The American Dietetic Association (ADA) states that carbohydrate intake should range from 2.7 to 4.5 g/lb (6 to 10 g/kg) of body weight, protein intake should range from 0.5 to 0.8 g/lb (1.2 to 1.7 g/kg) body weight, and fat intake should range from 20 to 35% of total daily intake (Rodriguez et al. 2009). The ADA also recommends that nutrients should be consumed prior to exercise, during exercise, and after exercise.

Because the purpose of this chapter is to focus on timing macronutrient intake to optimize adaptation and recovery, the idea of nutrient intake or meal timing to optimize athletic performance for a single bout of exercise will not be emphasized. Where appropriate this topic will be addressed, but only to point out how increasing the performance or work output during one bout can be parlayed into long-term results. Instead, this chapter will speak to increasing athletic performance over time by ensuring glycogen repletion and by maximizing a net positive protein balance, which is associated more with changes in protein synthesis than protein breakdown (Biolo et al. 1997; Tipton et al. 1999), for it is actually the cumulative effect of training, adaptation, and recovery from training that leads to improved performance. Proper nutrition aids in that adaptation and recovery. This includes consuming adequate amounts of calories and can be improved with nutrient timing.

13.2 NUTRIENT TIMING PRIOR TO EXERCISE

13.2.1 CARBOHYDRATE

13.2.1.1 Loading

Approximately 45 years ago, it was first demonstrated that skeletal muscle glycogen levels are a good predictor of an individual's ability to perform prolonged, strenuous exercise (Bergstrom et al. 1967). Ever since that time, scientists and athletes alike have sought effective ways to maximally increase muscle glycogen levels. Carbohydrate loading, also known as glycogen supercompensation, is the process of ingesting relatively high amounts of carbohydrate, often in conjunction with a tapering exercise program, several days prior to an athletic event or bout of exercise. The goal of carbohydrate loading is to increase skeletal muscle glycogen content and ultimately enhance exercise performance, specifically endurance-based performance (Arnall et al. 2007).

Several studies have demonstrated that increased baseline muscle glycogen levels can increase aerobic-exercise performance lasting longer than 90 minutes (Galbo et al. 1979; Lamb et al. 1991; Rauch et al. 1995). In fact, it has been reported in an extensive review of carbohydrate-loading studies that glycogen supercompensation may postpone fatigue by as much as 20% in endurance events lasting longer than 90 minutes (Hawley et al. 1997). Additionally, it has been reported that glycogen supercompensation may improve performance by 2–3% in endurance events in which a predetermined distance is covered as fast as possible (Hawley et al. 1997). On the other hand, carbohydrate loading may not play a significant role in exercise lasting less than 90 minutes (Hawley et al. 1997; Madsen et al. 1990; Sherman et al. 1981). Currently, there are varying methods of carbohydrate loading that have shown to be effective (Bergstrom et al. 1967; Sherman et al. 1981). These models, which will be discussed, differ by the amount and duration of the carbohydrate consumption, as well as the intensity and volume of exercise being performed during the protocol (Sedlock 2008).

Some of the earliest work investigating the effects of carbohydrate loading was performed by Bergstrom et al. (1967) and is now commonly referred to as the "classic" model of carbohydrate loading (Jeukendrup et al. 2005; Sedlock 2008). This protocol involves performing a glycogen-depleting bout of exercise followed by three days of consuming a high-fat and -protein diet. On the fourth day, an individual performs a second exhausting bout of exercise and follows it up with three days of eating a high-carbohydrate diet (Bergstrom et al. 1967). This protocol resulted in significantly increased skeletal muscle glycogen levels (Bergstrom et al. 1967). However, there are potential areas for concern using these methods, such as the disruption of the athlete's normal training cycle (i.e., altering their "normal" training and eating regimen the week before an event), which could affect mental outlook, as well as possible gastrointestinal distress and increased risk of injury (Jeukendrup et al. 2005; Lamb et al. 1991; Sedlock 2008).

In 1981, Sherman et al. compared the effects of six days of carbohydrate (CHO) loading on a subsequent 20.9-km (~13-mile) run in trained runners. The subjects consumed either a high-CHO (70% of total calories), moderate-CHO (50% of total calories), or low-CHO (15% of total calories) diet for the first three days and then were assigned one of the other two diets for the remaining three days (i.e., trial A, low/high; trial B, moderate/high; and trial C, moderate/moderate). In addition to following the dietary intervention, the participants also performed a five-day depletion/taper exercise regimen (90, 40, 40, 20, and 20 minutes of running at 73% VO_{2max} for days 1–5, respectively). The athletes rested on day six and performed the performance run on the day seven. The authors reported that trials A and B led to the largest increases in resting muscle glycogen and actual glycogen utilization during the performance run (Sherman et al. 1981). However, no significant differences in either run times or post-performance glycogen levels between the trials were reported (Sherman et al. 1981). As a result of this study, it was demonstrated that a more "moderate" approach to carbohydrate loading could produce comparable results to the more "classic" model and with less potential problems. In other words, the athlete does not have to perform an exhaustive/depleting bout of exercise, and they could still perform some exercise on most days during the protocol (which may aid in mental preparedness). Lastly, the athlete would also not have to subject himself to ingesting low levels of carbohydrate and its potential deleterious effects.

Since the moderate approach to carbohydrate loading was introduced, scientists have continued to discover methods that enhance muscle glycogen levels while utilizing even shorter protocols. In 2000, scientists reported that trained cyclists significantly increased their muscle glycogen by simply ingesting 9 g of carbohydrate/kg of body weight for three days while maintaining normal exercise including a tapering period (Burke et al. 2000). Subsequent research demonstrated that consuming ~10 g of high-glycemic carbohydrates/kg of body mass for even one day while remaining inactive led to maximal glycogen stores in types I, IIa, and IIb muscle fibers (Bussau et al. 2002). These findings are very important and practical because this would allow an athlete to carbohydrate load with very minimal disruption to their normal dietary and training regimen (Bussau et al. 2002). Thus, as a general rule based on existing research, it is suggested by Jeukendrup et al. (2005) that experienced endurance athletes should consume ~10 g/kg of body weight at least 1 day before competition and should attempt to substantially reduce glycogen stores 1–4 days prior to competition.

Although it is not common, an athlete may be subjected to an event being cancelled or possibly postponed for a couple of days. In these cases, it was originally unknown how long an individual would remain in a glycogen-supercompensated state or if they needed to "start over" again. To address this concern, researchers had trained cyclists perform an exhaustive, glycogen-depleting bout of exercise and then consume a very–high-carbohydrate diet (85% carbohydrate, 8% protein, and 7% fat) for 3 days. For the next 3 days the participants consumed a moderate-carbohydrate diet (i.e., 60%), while limiting physical activity. It was demonstrated that muscle glycogen content following glycogen supercompensation remained higher than normal for up to 5 days (Arnall et al. 2007), thus having a sustained response that could benefit an athlete if a scenario developed in which their performance was delayed from the anticipated start time.

13.2.1.2 Pre-exercise

Pre-exercise carbohydrate consumption is partially undertaken to maximize hepatic and skeletal muscle glycogen levels (Coyle et al. 1986; Hargreaves 2001) because endogenous glycogen stores may only last between 1.5 and 3 hours when exercising between 65 and 85% VO_{2max} (Tarnopolsky et al. 2005). The level of muscle glycogen depletion is dependent upon exercise intensity and duration (Millard-Stafford et al. 2008), but glycogen levels can be restored with a pre-exercise meal containing 140–330 g of carbohydrate 2–4 hours before the exercise bout (Coyle et al. 1985, 1986). Additional value may be gained by ingesting carbohydrate in relatively close proximity (<60 minutes) to the exercise bout (Hargreaves 2001; Tokmakidis and Karamanolis 2008). This serves to increase levels of circulating glucose from exogenous sources for fuel utilization. Without adequate circulating levels of glucose and adequate glycogen stores, the level of training and subsequent adaptations from that training may be compromised.

13.2.1.2.1 Endurance Exercise

There has been continued debate as to whether low- or high-glycemic index carbohydrates should be consumed because carbohydrate ingestion prior to exercise has been shown to result in hypoglycemia also referred to as "rebound hypoglycemia" (Foster et al. 1979; Kuipers et al. 1999). In attempts to avoid this potentially deleterious effect, the ingestion of specific kinds of carbohydrates have been advocated. Strong evidence exists for the use of low-glycemic foods less than an hour before exercise because it frequently results in lower immediate glucose and insulin responses than high-glycemic foods but greater levels of blood glucose and free fatty acids after the exercise bout (DeMarco et al. 1999; Thomas et al. 1991, 1994). High-glycemic foods <1-hour prior to exercise result in high blood glucose responses immediately prior to exercise (DeMarco et al. 1999; Febbraio et al. 2000; Sparks et al. 1998), but within the first 20 minutes of endurance exercise lower blood glucose responses have been reported compared to low-glycemic foods or control (DeMarco et al. 1999; Febbraio et al. 2000; Sparks et al. 1998).

As for performance, in some studies low-glycemic foods increased time to exhaustion (DeMarco et al. 1999; Thomas et al. 1991) and better time-trial performance (Moore et al. 2010), whereas in others there were no differences in performance despite differences in glucose and insulin responses (Febbraio et al. 2000; Febbraio and Stewart 1996; Sparks et al. 1998). It should be noted that the use of high-glycemic foods did not hinder performance. In fact, more recently the use of glucose, which is high on the glycemic index, just 15 minutes prior to exercise bouts resulted in 12.8% longer times to exhaustion when compared with placebo despite having a peak glucose response as exercise was initiated (Tokmakidis and Karamanolis 2008). One study compared medium-glycemic foods to controls that ingested water alone. Carbohydrate utilization was increased, and glycerol and free fatty acids were decreased, but performance time was not different compared with controls (Kirwan et al. 2001a). However, other evidence has compared medium- and high-glycemic foods to control and found improved time to exhaustion, maintenance of euglycemia, and increased carbohydrate oxidation for medium glycemic foods (Kirwan et al. 2001b).

Just as the use of low-glycemic foods <1 hour before exercise resulted in higher levels of glucose after exercise (DeMarco et al. 1999; Thomas et al. 1991), the use of low-glycemic foods >1 hour before exercise, when compared with high-glycemic foods, resulted in higher levels of available glucose during exercise and supported the idea that low-glycemic foods decrease glycogen utilization (Wee et al. 1999; Wong et al. 2008; Wu and Williams 2006). However, only two studies showed improvement in performance (Wong et al. 2008; Wu and Williams 2006).

Additionally, contrasting results have been reported suggesting that high-glycemic foods result in optimal glycogen stores (Bussau et al. 2002; Goforth et al. 2003). It should be noted that these studies were conducted to examine different carbohydrate loading protocols; thus, they are not necessarily applicable in this instance because it is not a common practice to carbohydrate load every few days during training. However, there is a training regimen that is reported to improve adaptations and performance from training in a glycogen-depleting state during base conditioning. The athlete then trains in the presence of increased glycogen stores as training intensity increases and the competitive season begins. This practice is showing promise, but needs more research before it is recommended. As such, the practice of attaining proper glycogen repletion before the next training session is encouraged to ensure optimal adaptation and recovery for endurance exercise. As the previous paragraphs indicate, this can be accomplished with varying types of carbohydrates. The key point is to consume adequate amounts of those carbohydrates. As long as the exercise session is started with full glycogen stores and adequate circulating levels of glucose, the athlete should be able to train harder or longer for that particular session. In time, given adequate glycogen repletion and recovery, prolonged training under these conditions should result in improved performance.

13.2.1.2.2   Strength/Power Exercise

Although carbohydrate supplementation prior to endurance exercise has been extensively studied, there is currently much less research available on carbohydrate supplementation alone prior to resistance training. However, as with endurance exercise, muscle glycogen content is important for strength and power performance. For example, performing resistance-training sessions after completing two glycogen-depleting protocols trials in either a low-carbohydrate or a high-carbohydrate fed state resulted in low and normal glycogen levels, respectively (Creer et al. 2005). This research supported previous findings that resistance exercise can decrease muscle glycogen content (Tesch and Berg 1998). Additionally, resistance training in a glycogen-depleted state did not appear to increase Akt activation, whereas exercising with normal levels of glycogen did (Creer et al. 2005). Thus, the literature suggests that exercising in the absence of adequate glycogen levels may blunt the effect of resistance-training bouts.

The previous articles point to the importance of proper glycogen content prior to one exercise bout, but they do not provide evidence of the effect of carbohydrate consumption alone prior to resistance training after that training has been maintained for any substantial amount of time. For this evidence, it may actually be helpful to look at studies using carbohydrate as a placebo prior to resistance-training programs. For example, recreationally active men resistance trained for 28 days and ingested either 28 g of a creatine- and amino acid-containing supplement or a carbohydrate placebo of maltodextrin 30 minutes prior to each training session or first thing in the morning on days they did not train (Shelmadine et al. 2009). In both groups, total body mass, fat-free mass, bench-press strength, and leg-press strength increased, whereas fat mass remained unchanged. Additionally, there were not significant differences in total calories or macronutrient consumption between the groups (Shelmadine et al. 2009). This study did not use a true control group (i.e., a group that did not ingest any supplement), but the data suggest that carbohydrate ingested prior to resistance training aided in physiological adaptations evidenced in the increase in total body mass and fat-free mass, without a concomitant increase in fat mass.

13.2.2 Fat Consumption

13.2.2.1 Endurance Exercise

Although it is less common today, the idea of ingesting fat, either in the form of long-chain triacylglycerols (i.e. triglycerides) (Satabin et al. 1987) or medium-chain triacylglycerols (Decombaz et al. 1983; Horowitz et al. 2000; Ivy et al. 1980; Massicotte et al. 1992) has been employed to improve endurance performance and training. As with carbohydrate ingestion before exercise, the idea was to provide an energy source for use in hopes of sparing glycogen stores. Because of differences in absorption, long-chain triacylglycerols were typically ingested 1–4 hours before exercise, whereas medium-chain triacylgcerols were ingested ~1 hour before exercise; both were purported to improve endurance capacity and reduce muscle glycogen breakdown (Jeukendrup and Aldred 2004). However, long-chain triacylglycerols in the absence of heparin did not get metabolized to the extent previously found (Satabin et al. 1987). Furthermore, medium-chain triacylglycerols were found to be oxidized during endurance exercise (Decombaz et al. 1983; Massicotte et al. 1992; Satabin et al. 1987), but this had no effect on carbohydrate utilization (Ivy et al. 1980), did not increase free fatty acids (Horowitz et al. 2000), and did not have an effect on muscle glycogen breakdown (Decombaz et al. 1983; Horowitz et al. 2000). Taken together, research does not suggest that the ingestion of lipids improves performance.

Adding further evidence against the use of lipids, researchers had athletes perform glycogen-depleting exercise and then consume either a high-carbohydrate, low-fat diet for several days or a high-carbohydrate, higher-fat diet (Zehnder et al. 2006). After a few days of the same glycogen-depleting exercise, a 20-km cycling time trial were performed. Although the higher-fat diet resulted in larger intramuscular lipid stores, glycogen depletion was similar for both groups during exercise, and there were no differences in time-trial performances (Zehnder et al. 2006). Based on the evidence presented above, the ingestion of lipids would not have ergogenic effects if ingested in a "loading" manner over several days or in an acute manner.

13.2.3 PROTEIN CONSUMPTION

The optimal amount of protein intake for highly active individuals involved in endurance and strength exercise is debatable. However, the importance of protein is not. It is suggested that endurance athletes need between 1.2 and 1.4 g/kg/day, with ultraendurance athletes needing slightly higher amounts like that recommended for strength-trained athletes (1.2–1.7 g/kg) (Rodriguez et al. 2009).

13.2.3.1 Strength/Power Exercise

Resistance training alone has been shown to increase protein synthesis (Biolo et al. 1995; MacDougall et al. 1995; Tipton and Wolfe 1998), but the intake of protein in proximity to exercise may improve the anabolic response to resistance training (Levenhagen et al. 2001; Tipton et al. 2001, 2007). It has been reported that non-resistance-trained individuals showed enhanced stimulation of muscle anabolism when resistance exercise followed ingestion of 16 g of intact protein (whey protein) and 3.4 g of leucine (Tipton et al. 2009). Although this study used a combination of intact protein and leucine, the results support previous research indicating that pre-exercise consumption of either free essential amino acids (EAA) or intact whole protein (whey) results in an anabolic environment following a resistance-training session (Tipton et al. 2001, 2007). Ingestion of 20 g of intact protein (whey protein) prior to resistance exercise resulted in an increase in amino-acid uptake into the skeletal muscle of untrained individuals (Tipton et al. 2007). Consumption of EAA also resulted in an anabolic environment in recreationally active individuals (Tipton et al. 2001).

Although these studies were excellent studies, a closer look at the results and explanation of the results is needed before firm conclusions can be drawn. In both studies, the ingestion of an amino-acid source before resistance training was compared with ingestion of the same source after resistance training. It appears that the anabolic response to EAA ingested prior to exercise is greater than the anabolic response to ingesting EAA post-exercise (Tipton et al. 2001), whereas the anabolic response to ingestion of intact protein prior to exercise was similar to the anabolic response when the same protein was ingested one hour following resistance training (Tipton et al. 2007).

Distinctions and limitations made by the authors will aid in optimizing adaptations and recovery using the training table. First, muscle protein accretion does appear to be stimulated by ingestion of intact protein, but the timing of ingestion is not as important because it may be relative to the timing of EAA supplementation alone (Tipton et al. 2007). The authors suggest that the differences in results may be due to a couple key points:

1. EAA supplementation may result in increased amino-acid delivery to the muscle because it does not need to be broken down (Tipton et al. 2001, 2007).
2. The 6 g of EAA used in that study was accompanied by 35 g of carbohydrate solution (Tipton et al. 2001), which may have resulted in a greater insulin response than whey protein alone.

The authors do point out, however, that insulin response was similar in both studies (Tipton et al. 2007).

So, what can be drawn from these two studies that can apply to the training table? First, ingestion of an intact protein source prior to resistance training can result in an anabolic environment. Second, ingestion of free amino acid supplements is not necessary for an anabolic environment to occur. Third, the time frame of protein ingestion prior to exercise may be further divided into hours before exercise, minutes before exercise, and minutes after exercise. In the research where the amino-acid source was delivered immediately before exercise, the EAA resulted in greater amino-acid uptake into active skeletal muscle (Tipton et al. 2001, 2007). However, as the authors pointed out, ingestion of intact protein further in advance may also provide greater availability of free amino acid by allowing time for the intact protein to be digested (Tipton et al. 2007).

Moreover, if ingesting protein hours before the exercise session *and* minutes before the exercise session then the composition, or type, of intact protein may make a difference in amino acid availability because different proteins have different amino-acid profiles and are digested slightly differently. For example, whey protein contains a greater percentage of branched-chain amino acids, namely leucine, than all other natural protein sources (Pasin and Miller 2000), and under resting conditions whey protein will result in a faster increase in circulating amino acids than casein because of differences in digestive properties (Boirie et al. 1997; Dangin et al. 2001). Consequently, it may be more advantageous to eat a meal higher in casein hours before the exercise session and then eat a small meal containing more whey protein <1 hour prior to exercise.

Evidence for this approach can be found in a recent study on the timed ingestion of a casein-based supplement during a resistance-training program (Burk et al. 2009). Physically active but untrained young men took part in two eight-week resistance-training programs while ingesting a casein-based supplement at 10 a.m. and 3:50 p.m. or at 10 a.m. and 10:30 p.m. (Burk et al. 2009). All of the workouts took place at 4 p.m. Ingestion of the casein-based supplement at 10 a.m. and 10:30 p.m. resulted in a significant increase in fat-free mass and a significant decrease in percent body fat, whereas this was not observed in the group that ingested the casein-based supplement immediately before the training session (Burk et al. 2009). In essence, because of the slow digestive properties of casein, it would not be as advantageous to eat a meal high in casein in close proximity to a resistance-training bout as it would to ingest a meal lower in casein and higher in other natural protein sources.

13.2.4 MACRONUTRIENT COMBINATIONS

Unless the athlete is taking individual macronutrient supplements to achieve the required levels of nutrients, it is likely that the pre-exercise meal will be a combination of the macronutrients such as that found in whole foods. The pre-exercise meal or snack should be relatively high in carbohydrates, contain moderate amounts of protein, and be low in fat and fiber to facilitate gastric emptying (Rodriguez et al. 2009). Additionally, it has been emphasized that the pre-exercise meal should contain foods that are well-tolerated by the athlete and should be dependent on the intensity and duration of the workout (Kerksick et al. 2008; Rodriguez et al. 2009). It is suggested that athletes experiment with new foods during training and not prior to a competition (Rodriguez et al. 2009). This will hopefully avoid gastrointestinal distress during competition.

Interestingly, a study examining the effects of pre-exercise meals on metabolism and performance during cycling suggested that there was little difference in sprint or 50-km time-trial performance between diets high in fat, high in protein, and high in carbohydrate (Rowlands and Hopkins 2002). This indicates that when considering performance, the composition of the pre-exercise meal may not be as important as previously thought, as long as glycogen repletion is ensured and there is an adequate amount of glucose circulating in the blood during exercise. These results support the findings of a similar study using high- and low-glycemic meals (Burke et al. 1998) and either a high-carbohydrate or an isoenergetic-fat meal (Paul et al. 2003) prior to cycling bouts where there were no differences between performance variables.

However, before drawing practical conclusions from these studies, a few things need to be examined. First, neither of the studies presented in the preceding paragraph presented any difference in performance measures (Burke et al. 1998; Rowlands and Hopkins 2002). Second, carbohydrates were consumed during the ride, which ensured adequate levels of circulating glucose. These points indicate that as long as carbohydrate is consumed during exercise and as long as the pre-exercise diet provides enough calories for ensuing exercise bouts >1 hour, given adequate glycogen stores, effort during that bout will not be affected. Practically speaking, this is an important point. In today's sporting world, it is rare that athletes will not have access to some source of carbohydrate or sports drink containing carbohydrate. Unless this is not the case, the pre-exercise meal can be highly variable between athletes. Hargreaves (2001) makes the point that if the only form of carbohydrate received around the workout to increase glucose availability during exercise is pre-exercise ingested carbohydrates, the athlete may want to ingest as much carbohydrate as possible without causing gastrointestinal distress. Depending on when the meal is consumed, the meal could be a high- or low-glycemic meal.

13.2.5 PRE-EXERCISE MEALS AND SNACKS

The following paragraphs provide practical advice for pre-exercise nutrition and are divided into what to eat 3–4 hours before exercise and what to eat <1 hour before exercise. The ADA recommends the pre-exercise meal take place between three and four hours before the exercise session and provide 200–300 g of carbohydrate, with no emphasis on the glycemic index of the carbohydrate and a recommendation of only a moderate amount of protein (Rodriguez et al. 2009), whereas the position stand of the International Society of Sport Nutrition (ISSN) on nutrient timing suggests that a meal should provide 1–2 g of carbohydrate and 0.15–0.25 g of protein/kg of body mass (Kerksick et al. 2008). For practical purposes, two theoretical athletes will be used to give examples of how to apply these recommendations: one of 55 kg and one of 70 kg.

13.2.5.1 What to Eat Hours before Exercise

Table 13.1 provides the pre-exercise macronutrient quantities for carbohydrate and protein and the range of calories for the pre-exercise meal that should be consumed between three and four hours before the workout. These ranges are those suggested by the ISSN. Figure 13.1 provides a sample meal plan, as well as the amount of each food that should be consumed, how many grams of carbohydrate and protein of each food, and the amount of kcal each food provides. Figure 13.1 is an example of a breakfast meal for those that may exercise in the morning, and Figure 13.2 provides the same information as Figure 13.1, but the example is of a meal for those that may workout in the afternoon or early evening.

13.2.5.2 What to Eat Less than an Hour before Exercise

As can be seen in Table 13.1, the recommended upper level of pre-exercise quantities of carbohydrate easily falls in the range provided by the ADA. However, the lower end of the range in Table 13.1 does not meet the lower range of that provided by the ADA. The ADA does not provide hard recommendations on nutrient intake <1 hour before exercise; thus, the difference in the ISSN and ADA quantities 3–4 hours before exercise can be made up in the hour before exercise, provided the athlete in question is not adversely affected by transient hypoglycemia, which can occur with carbohydrate ingestion immediately prior to an exercise session. Table 13.2 provides the pre-exercise macronutrient quantities for carbohydrate and protein and the range of calories for the pre-exercise snack that should be consumed <1 hour before the workout. Figure 13.3 provides sample snack plans, as well as the amount of each food that should be consumed, the grams of carbohydrate and protein of each food, and the amount of kcal each food provides.

TABLE 13.1
Pre-exercise Meal (3–4 Hours Prior to Exercise)

	Carbohydrate	Protein	Calories
Guidelines	1–2 g/kg	0.15–0.25 g/kg	600–900
For a 55-kg individual	55–110 g	8.25–13.75 g	600–700
For a 70-kg individual	70–140 g	10.5–17.5 g	700–900

55 kg individual				
ITEM	QUANTITY	CHO (g)	Pro (g)	Kcal
Oatmeal (*plain prepared w/ water*)	1 cup	17	4	97
English muffin* (*toasted & topped w/ 1 T. butter*)	2 oz	26	4	236
Jam	1 Tbsp	14	0	56
Banana	1 medium	27	1	109
100% Fruit juice	8 oz	27	2	110
Substitute 1 slice of whole wheat toast for English muffin if desired.	**TOTALS**	**111**	**11**	**608**
70 kg individual				
ITEM	QUANTITY	CHO (g)	Pro (g)	Kcal
Oatmeal (*plain prepared w/ water*)	1.5 cups	26	6	146
English muffin* (*toasted & topped w/ 1 T. butter*)	2 oz	26	4	236
Jam	1 Tbsp	14	0	56
Banana	1 medium	27	1	109
100% Fruit juice	12 oz	41	3	165
Substitute 1 slice of whole wheat toast for English muffin if desired.	**TOTALS**	**134**	**14**	**712**

FIGURE 13.1 Example pre-exercise breakfast meal (3–4 hours prior to exercise) for 55-kg and 70-kg individuals.

55 kg individual				
ITEM	QUANTITY	CHO (g)	Pro (g)	Kcal
Angel hair pasta (*tossed w/ 1 t. olive oil & 1 t. lemon juice**)	1 cup	40	7	237
Breadstick	2 (.35 oz)	14	2	82
Mixed fruit cup	2 cups	40	0	180
Zucchini (*sauteed in 1 t. olive oil & topped w/ 1 T. grated parmesan cheese*)	1 cup	8	5	138
Substitute 1/2 cup marinara sauce for olive oil and lemon juice if desired.	**TOTALS**	**102**	**14**	**637**
70 kg individual				
ITEM	QUANTITY	CHO (g)	Pro (g)	Kcal
Angel hair pasta (*tossed w/ 2 t. olive oil & 2 t. lemon juice**)	1.5 cups	60	11	356
Breadstick	2 (.35 oz)	14	2	82
Mixed fruit cup	2 cups	40	0	180
Zucchini (*sauteed in 1 t. olive oil & topped w/ 1 T. grated parmesan cheese*)	1 cup	8	5	138
Substitute 1 cup marinara sauce for olive oil and lemon juice if desired.	**TOTALS**	**122**	**18**	**756**

FIGURE 13.2 Example pre-exercise lunch or dinner meal (3–4 hours prior to exercise) for 55-kg and 70-kg individuals.

13.3 NUTRIENT TIMING DURING EXERCISE

13.3.1 CARBOHYDRATE CONSUMPTION

13.3.1.1 Endurance Exercise

Near the end of the previous section, two studies were covered indicating that carbohydrate consumption during exercise may trump the contents of the pre-exercise meal as long as adequate calories were consumed and glycogen stores are adequate (Burke et al. 1998; Rowlands and Hopkins 2002). It has been reported that the ingestion of carbohydrate during exercise allows athletes to train longer and harder (Hawley et al. 2006). Regardless of mechanism, the quantity and type of carbohydrate used to achieve these effects may be of interest.

Research within the past decade indicates that a mixture of glucose and fructose produces 20–50% greater rates of exogenous carbohydrate oxidation rates later in

TABLE 13.2

Pre-exercise Snack (<1 Hour Prior to Exercise)

	Carbohydrate	Protein	Calories
Guidelines	0.7–0.9 g/kg	0.2 g/kg	200–350
For a 55-kg individual	40–50 g	10–12 g	200–250
For a 70-kg individual	50–60 g	12–15 g	250–350

55 kg individual				
ITEM	QUANTITY	CHO (g)	Pro (g)	Kcal
Pita bread (6.5")	1/2 each	17	3	85
Hummus*	1/4 cup	10	5	100
Grapes	1 cup	16	1	62
*Substitute 8 oz (1%) milk for hummus if desired.	TOTALS	43	9	247
70 kg individual				
ITEM	QUANTITY	CHO (g)	Pro (g)	Kcal
Pita bread (6.5")	1/2 each	17	3	85
Hummus*	1/3 cup	15	8	150
Grapes	1.5 cup	24	2	93
*Substitute 12 oz (1%) milk for hummus if desired.	TOTALS	56	13	328

FIGURE 13.3 Example pre-exercise snack (<1 hour before exercise) for 55-kg and 70-kg individuals.

the exercise bout than glucose only (Jentjens et al. 2004a, 2004b; Jeukendrup et al. 2006; Wallis et al. 2005), as well as an improvement in endurance performance (Currell and Jeukendrup 2008). However, the quantity of carbohydrate ingested has been rather high, ranging from 1.5 to 2.5 g/min (Jentjens et al. 2004a, 2004b; Jeukendrup et al. 2006; Wallis et al. 2005) and has used large fluid volumes that are not close to the volume reportedly ingested during actual sporting events (Lambert et al. 2008; Pfeiffer et al. 2009, 2010a, 2010b). These concentrations of carbohydrate (>10% carbohydrate solution, >100 g of carbohydrate/h, and 0.8–1 L of fluid/h) are greater than most sports drinks, which are between 4 and 8% (Pfeiffer et al. 2010a). Thus, gels or solids may be an alternative means to provide carbohydrate during exercise.

Recently, two studies by the same research group were conducted comparing the oxidation of carbohydrates in liquids versus gels and solids during bouts of cycling (Pfeiffer et al. 2010a, 2010b). The study comparing gels to liquids used sources that both provided a 2:1 ratio of glucose to fructose at a rate of 1.8 g/min while ingesting equivalent volumes of fluid 0.867 L/h (Pfeiffer et al. 2010a). The oxidation rate of the exogenous carbohydrates was not different between the gel and the liquid, nor was oxidation efficiency. However, when a 2:1 glucose-to-fructose ratio providing 1.55 g/min was provided in bar form compared to liquid, exogenous carbohydrate oxidation was lower compared to the drink (Pfeiffer et al. 2010b). However, the peak oxidation rate of exogenous carbohydrates was high for both groups indicating that consumption of carbohydrates in solid form is an effective source of carbohydrate during exercise. It should be pointed out, though, that the ADA suggests that for events lasting

>1 hour, the athlete only needs to consume 30–60 g/h (0.5–1 g/min) to maintain blood glucose levels (Rodriguez et al. 2009). Further support for the use of alternative forms of carbohydrate sources such as gels and solids is found in a study that found sports beans (jelly beans), a sports drink, and a sports gel each to be equally effective at maintaining blood glucose levels during 80 minutes of exercise as well as improving performance in a subsequent 10-km time trial (Campbell et al. 2008).

An example of a food that can be found in the grocery store or at the training table used in research involves the use of honey as a carbohydrate source. Fifteen grams of honey, dextrose, or placebo plus 250 ml of water was ingested every 16 km of a 64-km event to assess the relationship between ingestion of these carbohydrates and time-trial performance (Earnest et al. 2004). During the final 16 km of the 64-km time trial, the ingestion of dextrose and honey allowed the riders to complete this section faster than placebo (Earnest et al. 2004). Additionally, the ingestion of dextrose and honey allowed for a significant increase in power output over the last 16 km. Taken from a practical standpoint, the athletes were able to work harder toward the end of the exercise bout than they were if they would have only consumed water. Again, coupled with proper post-exercise nutrition to ensure glycogen repletion and protein balance, being able to train harder should result in enhanced performance over the duration of months and years through chronic training.

One final point should be made. Thus far, research presented in this chapter regarding the effects of carbohydrate in proximity to endurance exercise has mostly involved cycling as a model. However, it is worth noting that similar results have been found when using events where the running pattern is not one of a long continuous duration but involves intermittent bouts of running at varying intensities such as soccer (Patterson and Gray 2007). When a carbohydrate gel was consumed with water before exercise and every 15 minutes during the exercise bout, blood glucose levels remained elevated compared with an artificially sweetened placebo. During a subsequent run to exhaustion, there was a significant increase in the time when the carbohydrate gel was ingested. Additionally, carbohydrate consumption during a soccer match was shown to attenuate the loss of muscle glycogen (Leatt and Jacobs 1989).

13.3.1.2 Strength/Power Exercise

Carbohydrate consumption prior to and during resistance training can help reduce the loss of muscle glycogen documented with resistance exercise (Haff et al. 2000). This has been observed in highly–resistance-trained men that consumed either carbohydrate or placebo while performing isokinetic knee flexion/extension and isotonic squats (Haff et al. 2000). The quantity of carbohydrate consumed 10 minutes before the exercise bout was 1.0 g/kg of body mass, whereas the carbohydrate consumed every 10 minutes during the training session provided 0.3 g/kg of body mass (Haff et al. 2000).

Although there were no differences between isokinetic performances between the groups, there was a significant attenuation of muscle glycogen from the isotonic squat protocol in the carbohydrate group. Furthermore, when resistance-trained men ingest glucose before and during isotonic leg-extension exercise, blood glucose levels are elevated, and improvement in performance during several bouts of resistance exercise was shown (Lambert et al. 1991). All of the participants consumed the same meal after a 10-hour fast and then 4 hours later. Before exercise, they ingested either a placebo or a glucose solution. Participants performed as many sets of 10 repetitions as they could until fatigue and ingested a placebo or glucose solution after every fifth set (Lambert et al. 1991). The carbohydrate group had significantly elevated blood glucose levels after the seventh set and after their final set, as well as performed three more sets on average when consuming carbohydrate.

As with the ingestion of carbohydrate during endurance exercise, ingesting carbohydrate during resistance training may allow athletes to train at higher intensities for longer periods of time. This is due to the increase in circulating glucose levels and subsequent reduction in the loss of glycogen. As such, it stands to reason that when an athlete can work harder for longer periods of time there is a greater chance that performance will improve in the long term.

13.3.2   FAT CONSUMPTION

13.3.2.1   Endurance Exercise

The idea of consuming sources of fat during exercise is similar to that of consuming carbohydrate during exercise. The hypothesis is that this will cause increased oxidation of the ingested fat with a concomitant decrease in reliance on glycogen. Thus, researchers have sought to gain a performance advantage via ingestion of medium-chain triacylglycerols, but studies to date have not generally found a performance benefit or glycogen sparing effect. In a great review on the topic, Jeukendrup and Aldred (2004) found that although the ingestion of medium-chain triacylglycerols at 10- or 15-minute intervals during exercise did result in an increase in oxidation of the medium-chain triacylglycerols (Jeukendrup et al. 1995, 1996b), it did not improve metabolism (Goedecke et al. 1999; Jeukendrup et al. 1995, 1996b), did not have any effect on glycogen (Jeukendrup et al. 1996a, 1998), and did not improve performance (Goedecke et al. 1999; Jeukendrup et al. 1998; Vistisen et al. 2003). However, one study has found improved time-trial performance and reduced glycogen oxidation (Van Zyl et al. 1996), but the results from this study have not been replicated. In fact, larger quantities of fat like that ingested in the trial that did find improvement in performance and a reduction of glycogen oxidation (86 g) (Van Zyl et al. 1996) have since been associated with gastrointestinal distress during exercise (Jeukendrup et al. 1998).

13.3.3   MACRONUTRIENT COMBINATIONS

13.3.3.1   Endurance Exercise

Because the addition of protein to a carbohydrate drink had been purported to increase plasma insulin responses following longer-duration aerobic exercise, it was hypothesized that a carbohydrate-protein supplement would prove beneficial during variable-intensity exercise by sparing muscle and liver glycogen (Ivy et al. 2003). When trained male cyclists ingested either a placebo, carbohydrate supplement (7.75%), or carbohydrate-protein supplement (7.75% carbohydrate, 1.94% protein) while exercising at varying intensities and then performing a subsequent ride to exhaustion at 85% VO_{2max}, it was found that blood glucose and insulin levels were elevated in both the carbohydrate and carbohydrate-protein groups compared with placebo alone. The carbohydrate-protein supplement resulted in significantly longer times to exhaustion than carbohydrate and placebo, leading the authors to conclude that the addition of protein to carbohydrate supplements enhanced aerobic endurance performance (Ivy et al. 2003).

Similar findings have been observed when carbohydrate supplements were compared with carbohydrate-protein supplements consumed during time to exhaustion events (Saunders et al. 2004, 2007). The addition of protein to carbohydrate supplements also resulted in reduced muscle damage after exhaustive exercise as indicated by creatine phosphokinase levels (Saunders et al. 2004, 2007). However, it was difficult to ascertain whether the results of these studies were due to any particular mechanism through which the amino acids could act or were merely due to the increased energy supply provided by the addition of protein to the carbohydrate drink because the carbohydrate and carbohydrate-protein supplements were not isoenergetic. The amount of carbohydrate delivered in these studies was also less than that recommended by some to be ingested during exercise (>1 g/min) (Jeukendrup 2004). However, the amounts provided (0.5–0.75 g/min) are within the dosage recommended by the ADA (Rodriguez et al. 2009).

Additionally perplexing to the scientific community was the applicability of a time-to-exhaustion bout to improved performance, because it does not mimic real life competition. Thus, ensuing research into the area sought to elucidate whether a carbohydrate-protein supplement improved performance in a time trial (Osterberg et al. 2008; van Essen and Gibala 2006). Under time-trial conditions, there were no added benefits to drinking a carbohydrate-protein supplement compared with carbohydrate alone. The carbohydrate group had faster average times than the carbohydrate-protein group and placebo (Osterberg et al. 2008) and showed no difference in time-trial performance between groups (van Essen and Gibala 2006).

Further research on the topic did not support the assertion that adding protein improved performance when the supplements were isocaloric (Romano-Ely et al. 2006; Valentine et al. 2008). Again, timed rides to exhaustion were used, leaving only one known study comparing isocaloric carbohydrate supplements to carbohydrate-protein supplements during a time trial (Toone and Betts 2010). When 12 highly trained cyclists and triathletes consumed either a carbohydrate-protein drink or an isocaloric-carbohydrate drink during a 45-minute ride of variable intensity, followed by a 6-km time trial, the carbohydrate-protein solution resulted in significantly slower times than the carbohydrate alone (Toone and Betts 2010).

Although research has mainly examined the effects of the combination of carbohydrate and protein on performance variables, a few points can be made that relate to adaptation and recovery. Combined results add further support for the consumption of macronutrients during exercise to either prolong the time to fatigue or improve performance. Additionally, when carbohydrate is of equal caloric content to a carbohydrate-protein supplement, there is no added benefit to performance. However, the carbohydrate-protein supplements do appear to confer a protective benefit against muscle damage. Compared with carbohydrate alone, carbohydrate-protein drinks, with and without anti-oxidants, resulted in less muscle damage as indicated by creatine phosphokinase (Ivy et al. 2003; Romano-Ely et al. 2006; Valentine et al. 2008), lactate dehydrogenase (Romano-Ely et al. 2006), and serum myoglobin (Valentine et al. 2008) levels. This could lead to quicker recovery between exercise bouts, thus resulting in the ability to train harder over time.

An alternative to consuming a commercially available sports drink that contains a carbohydrate-protein mixture would be to consume milk during endurance exercise. Milk consumed during prolonged endurance exercise resulted in greater growth-hormone levels following exercise (Miller et al. 2002) as well as a reduction in whole body protein breakdown with a concomitant increase in protein oxidation (Miller et al. 2007) compared with carbohydrate alone. During a timed ride to exhaustion at a set intensity, ingesting milk did not result in greater performance than a carbohydrate-electrolyte solution, but it was greater than water alone (Lee et al. 2008). Although consuming milk during exercise may not necessarily be palatable to some, it is may be a viable option for others. Consuming milk during exercise may confer a protective benefit against muscle damage in a similar fashion as a commercially available carbohydrate-protein sports drink. Because milk can be easily obtained at any grocery store or cafeteria, it could be more cost effective than purchasing a carbohydrate-protein mixture at the local nutrition store.

13.3.3.2 Strength/Power Exercise

When carbohydrate alone or in combination with EAA has been ingested before and during a single bout of resistance exercise, the serum cortisol response following the bout was blunted, as was protein degradation (Bird et al. 2006a and c). Additionally, the insulin response was stimulated from ingesting either carbohydrate or carbohydrate-EAA. Together, these results indicate an improved anabolic environment for the strength and power athlete. When a similar protocol was followed during 12 weeks of resistance training, pre-exercise cortisol levels were lower for all groups, whereas post-exercise insulin levels were elevated for treatment groups (Bird et al. 2006b). Body composition increased for all groups as did the cross-sectional area of all muscle fiber types, with the carbohydrate-EAA group having the largest increase in cross-sectional area. However, the carbohydrate-EAA group had the greatest increase in fat free mass and the greatest decrease in fat mass of all groups (Bird et al. 2006b). As for strength changes, all of the groups recorded increases in one-repetition maximums, with the carbohydrate-EAA having larger increases in strength when compared with the placebo group. Finally, all treatment groups displayed increases in strength during all phases of the study, but the placebo group did not display increases in strength during the final four weeks of the study.

As with endurance exercise, the ingestion of a combination of carbohydrate and protein during a resistance-training session, be it an acute bout or prolonged training, may prove beneficial. The results of the research presented above indicate that following such protocols can result in a favorable anabolic environment for the strength and power athlete. Together, the results of the prior sections indicate that during an acute bout of exercise, ingesting a combination of macronutrients before and during exercise will not only result in an anabolic environment from a structural protein standpoint but will result in reduced reliance on glycogen. Regarding long-term benefits, this may translate into better adaptations and recovery from training (i.e., increased muscle mass and strength). In practical terms, the athlete has a better chance at becoming bigger, faster, and stronger.

13.3.4 WHAT TO INGEST DURING EXERCISE

When exercise sessions last longer than 1 hour, it is important for the athlete to consume some source of energy, the preferred source being carbohydrate. The ADA suggests that for events lasting >1 hour, the athlete needs to consume 30–60 g/h (0.5–1 g/min) of carbohydrate or about 0.7 g/kg of body mass to maintain blood glucose levels (Rodriguez et al. 2009). Additionally, 10–15 fluid ounces of liquid should be consumed during the workout (Kerksick et al. 2008). These recommendations can easily be met by consuming sports drinks, which typically provide 6–8% carbohydrate solutions and equates to 6–8 g of carbohydrate/100 ml of fluid (Kerksick et al. 2008). The carbohydrate should be consumed throughout the workout in 15–20-minute intervals and can be in any form, be it solid, gel, or liquid. Lastly, macronutrient combinations are perfectly fine to consume because added protein may provide an added benefit to recovery, as well as possibly enhance the work output during exercise.

13.4 NUTRIENT TIMING FOR OPTIMAL RECOVERY POST-EXERCISE

In the nutrient-timing realm, a great deal of attention has been paid to post-exercise nutrition relative to endurance exercise and strength training. The purported benefits of nutrient timing include better rates of glycogen repletion, greater insulin responses, and greater rates of protein synthesis. With that being said, the integration between the concept of nutrient timing must directly be a major part of a well-designed training table to promote ideal adaptations for athletes.

13.4.1 CARBOHYDRATE CONSUMPTION

13.4.1.1 Endurance Exercise

The idea of post-exercise carbohydrate consumption centers on the enhanced uptake of glucose by skeletal muscle. Glucose uptake immediately after exercise takes place via non-insulin-dependent mechanisms that then switch to an increased sensitivity to insulin (Jentjens and Jeukendrup 2003). As such, timing carbohydrate consumption during the recovery phase is critical for muscle glycogen replenishment (Millard-Stafford et al. 2008). It has been demonstrated that carbohydrate supplementation immediately after exercise results in greater muscle glycogen storage than when that same supplement is delayed by 2 hours (Ivy et al. 1988a).

Additionally, consumption of glucose in higher levels (3 or 1.5 g/kg of body weight) immediately following and at 2 hours after glycogen-depleting exercise results in muscle glycogen storage significantly elevated above basal rates (Ivy et al. 1988b). Further, when carbohydrate supplement is consumed at regular intervals (15–60 minutes) post-exercise, high levels of glycogen replenishment are observed

(Jentjens and Jeukendrup 2003). Carbohydrates in amounts as low as 0.18 g/kg/h can result in an increase in glycogen synthesis (Blom et al. 1987), but greater amounts of glycogen replenishment have been found with larger amounts of the ingestion of glucose from 1.4 to 1.8 g/kg/h (Blom 1989; Casey et al. 1995; Piehl et al. 2000).

13.4.1.2 Strength/Power Exercise

Glucose ingestion following resistance training will not only aid in glycogen synthesis but can also decrease protein breakdown resulting in a positive net protein balance (Roy et al. 1997). In an acute setting, non-resistance-trained men received 1 g/kg of carbohydrate or placebo immediately and 1 hour after completing an intense, high-volume bout of single leg-knee extensor exercise. The results demonstrated that circulating glucose and insulin levels were greater for the carbohydrate group compared with placebo (Roy et al. 1997). Additionally, the researchers concluded that the carbohydrate group also had greater fractional synthesis rates of mixed muscle protein and lower excretion of 3-methylhistidine, which indicates a decreased breakdown of mixed muscle protein. The positive results found from ingestion of carbohydrate post-resistance training are in line with other studies that have reported positive net protein balance (Borsheim et al. 2004a, 2004b). However, the result is not as great as when ingested with amino acids and protein (Borsheim et al. 2004a). Additionally, when consumption of 1.25 g of carbohydrate/kg (from Gatorade) is undertaken in conjunction with 10 weeks of resistance training, improvement in body composition and increase in strength has also been shown (Rankin et al. 2004).

13.4.2 Protein Consumption

13.4.2.1 Strength/Power Exercise

Recall that post-exercise protein consumption enhances the anabolic effect of resistance training (Tipton et al. 2001, 2007). However, it was stated that when the protein source was in the form of free EAA, there was a greater anabolic affect from pre-exercise consumption (Tipton et al. 2001), but if the protein source ingested is intact protein, the anabolic response is similar (Tipton et al. 2007).

Further evidence that post-exercise whole protein ingestion results in an increase in the anabolic effect was also reported comparing the ingestion of casein and whey protein after resistance exercise (Tipton et al. 2004). Compared with a placebo, casein and whey supplements were ingested 1 hour after performing resistance exercises. Both casein and whey resulted in an increase net muscle protein synthesis (Tipton et al. 2004). Despite the different patterns of amino acid response in the blood, which is one of the major differences between casein and whey, there was not a significant difference between the two groups (Tipton et al. 2004). These results indicate that no difference exists in the anabolic response between the two protein sources. Thus, either casein or whey can be used to stimulate an anabolic response after exercise.

It is worth noting, however, that these results differed from previous studies examining the difference between whey and casein. As stated previously, during resting conditions whey protein will result in a faster and more pronounced increase in circulating amino acids than casein because of differences in digestive properties (Boirie et al. 1997; Dangin et al. 2001). It was unclear why the results were different, but the difference may be due to tissue differences because the studies at rest reported whole body responses to casein and whey (Boirie et al. 1997; Dangin et al. 2001), while Tipton et al. (2004) examined skeletal muscle. Another possibility is that muscle protein synthesis stimulated from resistance exercise resulted in an altered response to the digested proteins (Levenhagen et al. 2001; Tipton et al. 2001, 2007).

Whey and casein are commonly utilized proteins that are found in dairy sources. However, for various reasons, not all individuals will chose to regularly consume these proteins. As a result, research that utilizes nondairy protein will also be discussed. For example, the consumption of egg protein is not uncommon amongst athletes. One particular study utilizing egg protein was exceptionally helpful in determining the optimal amount of protein to maximally stimulate protein synthesis following resistance training. Specifically, study participants were given 0, 5, 10, 20, or 40 g of whole egg protein immediately following an acute bout of intense resistance training (Moore et al. 2009). It was discovered that there was an increase in muscle protein synthesis with increasing protein dose. However, it appears muscle protein synthesis was maximized at 20 g. Interestingly, the 40 g dosage did not result in a significant increase in muscle protein above that observed in those consuming 20 g. As a result, the investigators suggest that protein dosages greater than 20 g result in the remainder of the amino acids being irreversibly oxidized (Moore et al. 2009). These findings support previous research reporting similar dose responses at rest and after exercise (Cuthbertson et al. 2005; Tipton et al. 1999). In short, the evidence suggests that there is no anabolic advantage to ingesting a protein dose larger than 20 g in one sitting. What is more, it has been hypothesized that chronic consumption of protein quantities in excess of about 20 g/dose up to six times a day could blunt the anabolic response to dosages under 20 g (Moore et al. 2009).

13.4.3 MACRONUTRIENT COMBINATIONS

13.4.3.1 Endurance Exercise

Like the ingestion of a carbohydrate-protein supplement during endurance exercise, the ingestion of carbohydrate and protein in the early recovery phase of a bout of endurance exercise has also been examined. Compared with carbohydrate alone, adding protein to carbohydrate has been reported to increase glycogen synthesis (Berardi et al. 2006; van Loon et al. 2000; Zawadzki et al. 1992), which is the most significant variable in endurance athletes when discussing recovery nutrition post-exercise. When carbohydrate-protein combinations are compared with carbohydrate alone but are not isocaloric, greater amounts of muscle glycogen resynthesis are found in the carbohydrate-protein group (van Loon et al. 2000; Zawadzki et al. 1992). However, when the supplements are isocaloric, the carbohydrate-protein supplement may not result in greater glycogen resynthesis (Howarth et al. 2009; van Loon et al. 2000).

Only one study has shown greater glycogen resynthesis when the supplements were of equal caloric content (Berardi et al. 2006). However, this study provided a solid meal 4 hours post-exercise and sampled glycogen content via muscle biopsy at 6 hours (Berardi et al. 2006), as compared with the previous two studies sampling within 5 hours via biopsy (van Loon et al. 2000) or using different means of measurement (Howarth et al. 2009). The extended sampling window may have made a difference in resynthesis rates. Thus, adding protein to carbohydrate appears to only be of benefit to glycogen resynthesis during a brief window post-exercise and when inadequate amounts of carbohydrates are provided. This is especially true when the carbohydrate levels are upwards of 1.2 g/kg/h, which has been suggested as the rate to maximize glycogen resynthesis (Ivy 2001; Jentjens et al. 2001). Where the addition of protein to a carbohydrate supplement appears to be beneficial is in improving protein balance (Koopman et al. 2004; Levenhagen et al. 2001; Rowlands et al. 2007) or preventing muscle damage (Saunders et al. 2004), both of which will support the overall recovery from exercise, thus contributing to potential training adaptations.

Other studies have examined the effect of ingesting either a supplement containing carbohydrate, protein, and fat or chocolate milk after a glycogen-depleting bout of endurance exercise (Burke et al. 1995; Pritchett et al. 2009; Tarnopolsky et al. 1997; Thomas et al. 2009). When isoenergetic amounts of carbohydrate and a supplement of carbohydrate-protein-fat were ingested following glycogen-depleting exercises, the carbohydrate group had greater amounts of glycogen replenishment with both groups having greater levels than placebo (Tarnopolsky et al. 1997). Additionally, when trained athletes ingested either a high-glycemic carbohydrate diet, a diet with added fat and protein, or isocaloric-matched diet of only carbohydrate for a 24-hour recovery period, there were no differences in glycogen storage (Burke et al. 1995).

As previously mentioned, chocolate milk has also been studied post-exercise, but glycogen replenishment was not measured in these trials (Pritchett et al. 2009; Thomas et al. 2009). Instead, the authors focused on performance measures during subsequent bouts of exercise and markers of muscle damage when compared with a carbohydrate-replacement drink. One study found no differences in a subsequent performance trial the following day but did find lower levels of creatine kinase following the first bout for the chocolate milk group (Pritchett et al. 2009). The second study found that when chocolate milk or an isocaloric carbohydrate beverage was consumed during four hours of recovery from a glycogen-depleting bout, the chocolate-milk group performed better in the subsequent time to exhaustion trial (Thomas et al. 2009).

Additionally, a study was conducted to determine the effect of cereal and nonfat milk on muscle recovery after exercise (Kammer et al. 2009). The study evaluated acute post-exercise glycogen synthesis rates and phosphorylated states of proteins controlling protein synthesis in trained endurance athletes that consumed a drink providing 78.5 g of carbohydrate or cereal and milk that provided 77 g of carbohydrate, 19.5 g of protein, and 2.7 grams of fat (Kammer et al. 2009). The cereal group had a greater insulin response, lower lactate response, and higher states of phosphorylated mTOR (a marker of protein synthesis) at 1 hour than the carbohydrate-drink group, which could be attributed to the increase in protein. Both groups had increased levels of glycogen and phosphorylated rpS6 (a marker of protein synthesis) at 1 hour post-exercise. Interestingly during that same time, only cereal significantly affected glycogen synthase, Akt, and mTOR (Kammer et al. 2009).

What should be apparent here is that, practically speaking, many different sources of food can be used post-exercise to aid in recovery and adaptation. Although many have been encouraged to consume carbohydrate alone post-exercise, research indicates that advantages can be gained through ingestion of combined macronutrients. This combination can be obtained in whole foods such as milk and cereal, which are relatively easy products to find. Whole foods are adequate choices for ensuring glycogen resynthesis as well as protein synthesis. The practical evidence of this effectiveness can be found in the lower lactate response after an acute bout of exercise (Kammer et al. 2009) and the longer times to exhaustion during subsequent trials that take place on the same day (Thomas et al. 2009).

13.4.3.2 Strength/Power Exercise

Several studies have examined post-exercise ingestion of a mixed macronutrient beverage or meal. Milk or chocolate milk has been shown to be effective at improving strength and body composition (Rankin et al. 2004). Previously untrained men consumed isoenergetic beverages of milk and Gatorade immediately following each resistance-training session for 10 weeks. Gatorade and milk were each provided at 5-kcal/kg of body weight, but Gatorade provided 1.25 g of carbohydrate/kg and electrolytes, whereas milk provided 0.92 g of carbohydrate/kg, 0.21 g of protein/kg, and 0.06 g of fat/kg in addition to the natural vitamins and minerals present in milk.

Although no differences were observed between groups, both groups significantly decreased percent body fat, increased lean mass, and improved muscular strength for all measures (Rankin et al. 2004). Subsequent findings support the notion that improvement in body composition and performance variables can be obtained with mixed macronutrient foods such as milk. Three groups of volunteers ingested either 237 g of fat-free milk, 237 g of whole milk, or 393 g of fat-free milk that was isoenergetic to the whole-milk group so that net muscle protein balance following resistance exercise could be assessed (Elliot et al. 2006). All three groups had an increased net balance for phenylalanine and threonine, which are essential amino acids not oxidized in skeletal muscle (Elliot et al. 2006). Thus, the increased uptake of these amino acids is thought to be indicative of net muscle protein synthesis.

Previous research using the same testing methods revealed that net amino-acid balance was not positive for a placebo (Tipton et al. 2004). Whole milk was reported to result in a greater utilization of amino acids (Elliot et al. 2006). The results of this study are interesting because it is contrary to the common belief that increasing the fat content of a post-exercise meal or supplement may decrease digestive rates and ultimately impede certain aspects of recovery. More research needs to be conducted with varying fat contents of milk before conclusive statements can be made.

However, further evidence that milk effectively supports adaptations and recovery when consumed during the early post-exercise recovery phase can be found in women (Josse et al. 2010). Using young women during a 12-week resistance-training program, the ingestion of milk immediately after and 1 hour after exercise resulted in greater lean-mass gains, greater strength gains for some lifts, and greater fat loss when compared with isocaloric carbohydrate consumption (Josse et al. 2010). However, similar results were not found when yogurt was consumed three times a day with one feeding occurring immediately following training compared with isocaloric protein and carbohydrate (White et al. 2009). These results indicate that perhaps not all dairy products confer the same benefit as milk. However, the results may also be due to differences in research design, because the participants from Josse et al. (2010) not only resistance trained for a longer period of time than did the participants from White et al. (2009), they consumed milk twice after the exercise bout, whereas this was not the case in women consuming yogurt.

The ingestion of a post-exercise meal that contains a combination of macronutrients may provide an added benefit. As has been presented earlier in this section, post-exercise carbohydrate allows for muscle glycogen resynthesis and added protein aids in favorable anabolic conditions for the athlete. Additionally, improvements in performance measures and body composition have been found for men and women. Thus, the positive adaptations that occur from post-exercise nutrient timing are not gender specific.

13.4.4 POST-EXERCISE MEALS AND SNACKS

The post-exercise meal should be geared to aid in recovery. With that in mind, it should contain adequate amounts of fluid and electrolytes to replace what is lost during training (Rodriguez et al. 2009). Additionally, it should consist of enough carbohydrate to facilitate glycogen repletion and moderate amounts of protein to provide sufficient amino acids for tissue repair and to stimulate protein synthesis.

13.4.4.1 What to Eat Minutes after Exercise

It is important to consume a meal or snack within the first 30–45 minutes after the training session. This is especially true regarding carbohydrate intake, which the ADA recommends be between 1.0 and 1.5 g/kg body mass of carbohydrate (Rodriguez et al. 2009). Additionally, the ISSN recommends ingesting protein at a 3:1 ratio of carbohydrate to protein (Kerksick et al. 2008). Table 13.3 provides macronutrient quantities that could be consumed as soon as possible after the workout. Figure 13.4 provides a sample meal plan as well as the amount of each food that should be consumed, the grams of carbohydrate and protein of each food, as well how many kcal each food provides.

13.4.4.2 What to Eat Hours after Exercise

The carbohydrate and protein guidelines should be adhered to for up to three hours post-exercise. Additional carbohydrates should be consumed every 2 hours after the training session for up to six hours. Table 13.4 provides the post-exercise macronutrient quantities for carbohydrate, protein, and the range of calories the pre-exercise meal that should be consumed as soon as possible after the workout. Figure 13.5

TABLE 13.3
Post-exercise Snack

	Carbohydrate	Protein	Calories
Guidelines	1–1.5 g/kg	0.5–0.7 g/kg	300–500
For a 55-kg individual	55–82.5 g	27.5–38.5 g	300–400
For a 70-kg individual	70–105 g	35–49 g	400–500

---

55 kg individual				
ITEM	QUANTITY	CHO (g)	Pro (g)	Kcal
Cottage cheese (1%)	1 cup	6	28	163
Trailmix (with nuts and dried fruit)	1 oz	19	2	115
Sports drink*	16 oz	30	0	100
Substitute 1 medium orange for sports drink if desired.	**TOTALS**	**55**	**30**	**378**
70 kg individual				
ITEM	QUANTITY	CHO (g)	Pro (g)	Kcal
Cottage cheese (1%)	1.5 cup	9	42	245
Trailmix (with nuts and dried fruit)	1 oz	19	2	115
Sports drink*	24 oz	45	0	150
Substitute 2 medium oranges for sports drink if desired.	**TOTALS**	**73**	**44**	**510**

FIGURE 13.4　Example post-exercise snack for 55-kg and 70-kg individuals.

TABLE 13.4
Post-exercise Meal

	Carbohydrate	Protein	Calories
Guidelines	1.2–1.5 g/kg	0.8–1 g/kg	600–900
For a 55-kg individual	66–82.5 g	44–55 g	600–700
For a 70-kg individual	84–105 g	56–70 g	700–900

---

provides a sample meal plan as well as the amount of each food that should be consumed, the grams of carbohydrate and protein of each food, as well how many kcal each food provides. This meal contains foods that could easily be prepared and consumed during a lunch or dinner and that are often found in dining halls.

13.5　MEAL TIMING

It is often advocated that an athlete should consume many (i.e., five or six) small meals per day (i.e., "grazing") rather than two or three larger meals (i.e., "gorging"). One possible reason for this suggestion is the belief that eating smaller, more frequent meals may improve body composition. This widely held belief may be based upon an observed inverse relationship between the frequency of food intake and body weight/body composition in certain animal models (Cohn and Joseph 1959; Cohn et al. 1955; Heggeness 1965) as well as early observational human studies (Fabry et al. 1964; Hejda and Fabry 1964; Metzner et al. 1977). However, the preponderance of studies that control for under-reporting of food intake suggest that meal frequency may not play a significant role in body weight/body composition (Andersson and Rossner 1996; Crawley and Summerbell 1997; Summerbell et al. 1996). Similarly, the preponderance of the research suggests that increased meal frequency does not significantly enhance metabolic rate (Taylor and Garrow 2001; Verboeket-van de Venne and Westerterp 1993; Verboeket-van de Venne et al. 1993).

Although increased meal frequency may not play a major role in weight management or metabolic rate, it may be beneficial in other areas. Athletes, depending on their activity level, may need to consume a greater amount of calories than

55 kg individual				
ITEM	QUANTITY	CHO (g)	Pro (g)	Kcal
Grilled chicken breast (*topped w/ 1 T. BBQ sauce*)	4 oz	7	36	219
Baked potato (*topped w/ 1 t. butter & 1 T. sour cream*)	1 medium	40.5	4.5	221
Dinner roll	1 oz	14	2	84
Steamed green beans	1 cup	8	3	50
Sliced strawberries*	1 cup	10	1	80
*Substitute another fruit for strawberries if desired.	**TOTALS**	79.5	46.5	654
70 kg individual				
ITEM	QUANTITY	CHO (g)	Pro (g)	Kcal
Grilled chicken breast (*topped w/ 1 T. BBQ sauce*)	6 oz	7	54	313
Baked potato (*topped w/ 1 t. butter & 1 T. sour cream*)	1 medium	40.5	4.5	221
Dinner roll	1 oz	14	2	84
Steamed green beans	1.5 cups	12	4.5	75
Sliced strawberries*	1.5 cups	15	1.5	120
*Substitute another fruit for strawberries if desired.	**TOTALS**	88.5	66.5	813

FIGURE 13.5   Example post-exercise meal for 55-kg and 70-kg individuals.

an age-matched sedentary individual because of the increased energy expenditure (Danforth 1985). However, the need to consume more calories, particularly spread over a relatively small number of meals (i.e., two or three), may potentially cause gastric distress in some individuals (Hawley and Burke 1997). As a result, it may be advisable for certain athletes to eat smaller, more frequent meals in order to mitigate the potential issue of gastric discomfort that may occur with eating fewer, larger meals (Hawley and Burke 1997). Certain athletes competing in weight-restricted sports, such as gymnastics and wrestling, may at times need to restrict his or her total daily calories. In these cases, eating more frequently may be advantageous. Specifically, some studies have shown that eating the same total number of daily calories but spread out over more meals per day may decrease feelings of hunger (Smeets and Westerterp-Plantenga 2008; Stote et al. 2007). Theoretically, this may make it easier for some people to adhere to periods of dietary restriction (i.e., dieting).

Lastly, there is scant evidence that suggests eating six versus two meals per day (even when total calories are the same) may help lessen the loss of lean muscle tissue in active individuals during periods of hypocaloric intake (Iwao et al. 1996). Thus, although increasing meal frequency may not be advantageous in athletes attempting to improve body composition, it may be efficacious in those individuals that are dieting or that have issues with gastrointestinal distress when they eat larger meals.

One additional point needs to be made concerning the timing of the last meal of the day. Thus far we have addressed how nutrient timing can optimize adaptation and recovery in regards to glycogen synthesis and protein accretion. However, we would be remiss if we did not briefly address how nutrient timing affects sleep, because sleep is an important aspect of adaptation and recovery. Meals in close proximity to bedtime are associated with sleep disturbances (Dollander 2002). However, certain macronutrients influence sleep via increasing tryptophan, a precursor to serotonin (Hartmann 1982; Hartmann and Spinweber 1979). Examples of this are foods high on the glycemic index, such as mashed potatoes or instant rice (Wurtman et al. 2003). A recent study reported that when the last meal was consumed four hours before bedtime and contained high-glycemic foods, sleep onset was significantly shortened compared with meals containing low-glycemic foods (Afaghi et al. 2007).

13.6 SUMMARY

In the introduction, it was stated that this chapter would provide information to optimize adaptation and recovery with the final result being enhanced performance from chronic, arduous training supplemented by proper nutrition. It is true that a large portion of the research performed in sports nutrition deals with supplementing the diet with products centered on single macronutrients (i.e., whey protein) or a commercial recovery drink containing a combination of macronutrients (i.e., 3–4:1 ratio of carbohydrate to protein). However, what should be clear after reading this chapter is that optimal nutrition, and thus, optimal adaptation and recovery, can be attained from eating whole foods found at the local grocer or in most dining halls. Those foods should:

- Be included in a diet that supplies adequate calories to meet training demands and include carbohydrate in the range of 2.7–4.5 g/lb (6–10 g/kg) of body weight. Protein intake should range from 0.5 to 0.8 g/lb (1.2 to 1.7 g/kg) body weight, and fat intake should range from 20 to 35% of total daily intake (Rodriguez et al. 2009).
- Provide 200–300 g of carbohydrate (Rodriguez et al. 2009) or 1–2 g of carbohydrate/kg of body mass and 0.15–0.25 g of protein/kg of body mass (Kerksick et al. 2008) in the hours before exercise.
- Provide at least 30–60 g/h (0.5–1 g/min) of carbohydrate or about 0.7 g/kg of body mass to maintain blood glucose levels (Rodriguez et al. 2009), 10–15 fluid ounces of liquid (Kerksick et al. 2008), and be consumed in 15–20-minute intervals for exercise longer than 1 hour.
- Provide between 1.0 and 1.5 g/kg body mass of carbohydrate (Rodriguez et al. 2009), as well as a little protein, within 30 minutes of exercise cessation.

Although the majority of the research presented in the chapter concerned prolonged endurance exercise or resistance training, the principles and recommendations provided here can and should be applied to all types of training, from soccer to basketball to swimming to rowing. By following the guidelines set forth and consuming nutrients prior to, during, and after exercise, athletes can enhance their training by optimizing adaptation and ensuring adequate recovery between bouts of exercise.

REFERENCES

Afaghi, A., H. O'Connor, and C. M. Chow. 2007. High-glycemic-index carbohydrate meals shorten sleep onset. *Am J Clin Nutr* 85: 426–430.

Andersson, I., and S. Rossner. 1996. Meal patterns in obese and normal weight men: The "Gustaf" study. *Eur J Clin Nutr* 50: 639–646.

Arnall, D. A., A. G. Nelson, J. Quigley, S. Lex, T. Dehart, and P. Fortune. 2007. Supercompensated glycogen loads persist 5 days in resting trained cyclists. *Eur J Appl Physiol* 99: 251–256.

Berardi, J. M., T. B. Price, E. E. Noreen, and P. W. Lemon. 2006. Postexercise muscle glycogen recovery enhanced with a carbohydrate-protein supplement. *Med Sci Sports Exerc* 38: 1106–1113.

Bergstrom, J., L. Hermansen, E. Hultman, and B. Saltin. 1967. Diet, muscle glycogen and physical performance. *Acta Physiol Scand* 71: 140–150.

Biolo, G., S. P. Maggi, B. D. Williams, K. D. Tipton, and R. R. Wolfe. 1995. Increased rates of muscle protein turnover and amino acid transport after resistance exercise in humans. *Am J Physiol* 268: E514–E520.

Biolo, G., K. D. Tipton, S. Klein, and R. R. Wolfe. 1997. An abundant supply of amino acids enhances the metabolic effect of exercise on muscle protein. *Am J Physiol* 273: E122–E129.

Bird, S. P., K. M. Tarpenning, and F. E. Marino. 2006a. Effects of liquid carbohydrate/essential amino acid ingestion on acute hormonal response during a single bout of resistance exercise in untrained men. *Nutrition* 22: 367–375.

Bird, S. P., K. M. Tarpenning, and F. E. Marino. 2006b. Independent and combined effects of liquid carbohydrate/essential amino acid ingestion on hormonal and muscular adaptations following resistance training in untrained men. *Eur J Appl Physiol* 97: 225–238.

Bird, S. P., K. M. Tarpenning, and F. E. Marino. 2006c. Liquid carbohydrate/essential amino acid ingestion during a short-term bout of resistance exercise suppresses myofibrillar protein degradation. *Metabolism* 55: 570–577.

Blom, C. S. 1989. Post-exercise glucose uptake and glycogen synthesis in human muscle during oral or i.v. glucose intake. *Eur J Appl Physiol Occup Physiol* 59: 327–333.

Blom, P. C., A. T. Hostmark, O. Vaage, K. R. Kardel, and S. Maehlum. 1987. Effect of different post-exercise sugar diets on the rate of muscle glycogen synthesis. *Med Sci Sports Exerc* 19: 491–496.

Boirie, Y., M. Dangin, P. Gachon, M. P. Vasson, J. L. Maubois, and B. Beaufrere. 1997. Slow and fast dietary proteins differently modulate postprandial protein accretion. *Proc Natl Acad Sci USA* 94: 14930–14935.

Borsheim, E., A. Aarsland, and R. R. Wolfe. 2004a. Effect of an amino acid, protein, and carbohydrate mixture on net muscle protein balance after resistance exercise. *Int J Sport Nutr Exerc Metab* 14: 255–271.

Borsheim, E., M. G. Cree, K. D. Tipton, T. A. Elliott, A. Aarsland, and R. R. Wolfe. 2004b. Effect of carbohydrate intake on net muscle protein synthesis during recovery from resistance exercise. *J Appl Physiol* 96: 674–678.

Burk, A., S. Timpmann, L. Medijainen, M. Vahi, and V. Oopik. 2009. Time-divided ingestion pattern of casein-based protein supplement stimulates an increase in fat-free body mass during resistance training in young untrained men. *Nutr Res* 29: 405–413.

Burke, L. M., A. Claassen, J. A. Hawley, and T. D. Noakes. 1998. Carbohydrate intake during prolonged cycling minimizes effect of glycemic index of pre-exercise meal. *J Appl Physiol* 85: 2220–2226.

Burke, L. M., G. R. Collier, S. K. Beasley, P. G. Davis, P. A. Fricker, P. Heeley, K. Walder, and M. Hargreaves. 1995. Effect of coingestion of fat and protein with carbohydrate feedings on muscle glycogen storage. *J Appl Physiol* 78: 2187–2192.

Burke, L. M., J. A. Hawley, E. J. Schabort, A. St Clair Gibson, I. Mujika, and T. D. Noakes. 2000. Carbohydrate loading failed to improve 100-km cycling performance in a placebo-controlled trial. *J Appl Physiol* 88: 1284–1290.

Bussau, V. A., T. J. Fairchild, A. Rao, P. Steele, and P. A. Fournier. 2002. Carbohydrate loading in human muscle: An improved 1 day protocol. *Eur J Appl Physiol* 87: 290–295.

Campbell, C., D. Prince, M. Braun, E. Applegate, and G. A. Casazza. 2008. Carbohydrate-supplement form and exercise performance. *Int J Sport Nutr Exerc Metab* 18: 179–190.

Casey, A., A. H. Short, E. Hultman, and P. L. Greenhaff. 1995. Glycogen resynthesis in human muscle fibre types following exercise-induced glycogen depletion. *J Physiol* 483: 265–271.

Cohn, C., and D. Joseph. 1959. Changes in body composition attendant on force feeding. *Am J Physiol* 196: 965–968.

Cohn, C., E. Shrago, and D. Joseph. 1955. Effect of food administration on weight gains and body composition of normal and adrenalectomized rats. *Am J Physiol* 180: 503–507.

Coyle, E. F., A. R. Coggan, M. K. Hemmert, and J. L. Ivy. 1986. Muscle glycogen utilization during prolonged strenuous exercise when fed carbohydrate. *J Appl Physiol* 61: 165–172.

Coyle, E. F., A. R. Coggan, M. K. Hemmert, R. C. Lowe, and T. J. Walters. 1985. Substrate usage during prolonged exercise following a pre-exercise meal. *J Appl Physiol* 59: 429–433.

Crawley, H., and C. Summerbell. 1997. Feeding frequency and BMI among teenagers aged 16-17 years. *Int J Obes Relat Metab Disord* 21: 159–161.

Creer, A., P. Gallagher, D. Slivka, B. Jemiolo, W. Fink, and S. Trappe. 2005. Influence of muscle glycogen availability on ERK1/2 and Akt signaling after resistance exercise in human skeletal muscle. *J Appl Physiol* 99: 950–956.

Currell, K., and A. E. Jeukendrup. 2008. Superior endurance performance with ingestion of multiple transportable carbohydrates. *Med Sci Sports Exerc* 40: 275–281.

Cuthbertson, D., K. Smith, J. Babraj, G. Leese, T. Waddell, P. Atherton, H. Wackerhage, P. M. Taylor, and M. J. Rennie. 2005. Anabolic signaling deficits underlie amino acid resistance of wasting, aging muscle. *FASEB J* 19: 422–424.

Danforth, E., Jr. 1985. Diet and obesity. *Am J Clin Nutr* 41(5 Suppl): 1132–1145.

Dangin, M., Y. Boirie, C. Garcia-Rodenas, P. Gachon, J. Fauquant, P. Callier, O. Ballevre, and B. Beaufrere. 2001. The digestion rate of protein is an independent regulating factor of postprandial protein retention. *Am J Physiol Endocrinol Metab* 280: E340–E348.

Decombaz, J., M. J. Arnaud, H. Milon, H. Moesch, G. Philippossian, A. L. Thelin, and H. Howald. 1983. Energy metabolism of medium-chain triglycerides versus carbohydrates during exercise. *Eur J Appl Physiol Occup Physiol* 52: 9–14.

DeMarco, H. M., K. P. Sucher, C. J. Cisar, and G. E. Butterfield. 1999. Pre-exercise carbohydrate meals: Application of glycemic index. *Med Sci Sports Exerc* 31: 164–170.

Dollander, M. 2002. [Etiology of adult insomnia]. *Encephale* 28: 493–502.

Earnest, C. P., S. L. Lancaster, C. J. Rasmussen, C. M. Kerksick, A. Lucia, M. C. Greenwood, A. L. Almada, P. A. Cowan, and R. B. Kreider. 2004. Low vs. high glycemic index carbohydrate gel ingestion during simulated 64-km cycling time trial performance. *J Strength Cond Res* 18: 466–472.

Elliot, T. A., M. G. Cree, A. P. Sanford, R. R. Wolfe, and K. D. Tipton. 2006. Milk ingestion stimulates net muscle protein synthesis following resistance exercise. *Med Sci Sports Exerc* 38: 667–674.

Fabry, P., Z. Hejl, J. Fodor, T. Braun, and K. Zvolankova. 1964. The frequency of meals: Its relation to overweight, hypercholesterolemia, and decreased glucose-tolerance. *Lancet* 2: 614–615.

Febbraio, M. A., J. Keenan, D. J. Angus, S. E. Campbell, and A. P. Garnham. 2000. Pre-exercise carbohydrate ingestion, glucose kinetics, and muscle glycogen use: Effect of the glycemic index. *J Appl Physiol* 89: 1845–1851.

Febbraio, M. A., and K. L. Stewart. 1996. CHO feeding before prolonged exercise: Effect of glycemic index on muscle glycogenolysis and exercise performance. *J Appl Physiol* 81: 1115–1120.

Foster, C., D. L. Costill, and W. J. Fink. 1979. Effects of pre-exercise feedings on endurance performance. *Med Sci Sports* 11: 1–5.

Galbo, H., J. J. Holst, and N. J. Christensen. 1979. The effect of different diets and of insulin on the hormonal response to prolonged exercise. *Acta Physiol Scand* 107: 19–32.

Goedecke, J. H., R. Elmer-English, S. C. Dennis, I. Schloss, T. D. Noakes, and C. P. Lambert. 1999. Effects of medium chain triacylglycerol ingested with carbohydrate on metabolism and exercise performance. *Int J Sports Nutr* 9: 35–47.

Goforth, H. W., Jr., D. Laurent, W. K. Prusaczyk, K. E. Schneider, K. F. Petersen, and G. I. Shulman. 2003. Effects of depletion exercise and light training on muscle glycogen supercompensation in men. *Am J Physiol Endocrinol Metab* 285: E1304–E1311.

Haff, G. G., A. J. Koch, J. A. Potteiger, K. E. Kuphal, L. M. Magee, S. B. Green, and J. J. Jakicic. 2000. Carbohydrate supplementation attenuates muscle glycogen loss during acute bouts of resistance exercise. *Int J Sport Nutr Exerc Metab* 10: 326–339.

Hargreaves, M. 2001. Pre-exercise nutritional strategies: Effects on metabolism and performance. *Can J Appl Physiol* 26(Suppl): S64–S70.

Hartmann, E. 1982. Effects of L-tryptophan on sleepiness and on sleep. *J Psychiatr Res* 17: 107–113.

Hartmann, E., and C. L. Spinweber. 1979. Sleep induced by L-tryptophan: Effect of dosages within the normal dietary intake. *J Nerv Ment Dis* 167: 497–499.

Hawley, J. A., and L. M. Burke. 1997. Effect of meal frequency and timing on physical performance. *Br J Nutr* 77(Suppl 1): S91–S103.

Hawley, J. A., G. S. Palmer, and T. D. Noakes. 1997. Effects of 3 days of carbohydrate supplementation on muscle glycogen content and utilization during a 1-h cycling performance. *Eur J Appl Physiol Occup Physiol* 75: 407–412.

Hawley, J. A., E. J. Schabort, T. D. Noakes, and S. C. Dennis. 1997. Carbohydrate-loading and exercise performance: An update. *Sports Med* 24: 73–81.

Hawley, J. A., K. D. Tipton, and M. L. Millard-Stafford. 2006. Promoting training adaptations through nutritional interventions. *J Sports Sci* 24: 709–721.

Heggeness, F. W. 1965. Effect of intermittent food restriction on growth, food utilization and body composition of the rat. *J Nutr* 86: 265–270.

Hejda, S., and P. Fabry. 1964. Frequency of food intake in relation to some parameters of the nutritional status. *Nutr Dieta Eur Rev Nutr Diet* 64: 216–228.

Horowitz, J. F., R. Mora-Rodriguez, L. O. Byerley, and E. F. Coyle. 2000. Pre-exercise medium-chain triglyceride ingestion does not alter muscle glycogen use during exercise. *J Appl Physiol* 88: 219–225.

Howarth, K. R., N. A. Moreau, S. M. Phillips, and M. J. Gibala. 2009. Coingestion of protein with carbohydrate during recovery from endurance exercise stimulates skeletal muscle protein synthesis in humans. *J Appl Physiol* 106: 1394–1402.

Ivy, J. L. 2001. Dietary strategies to promote glycogen synthesis after exercise. *Can J Appl Physiol* 26(Suppl): S236–S245.

Ivy, J. L., D. L. Costill, W. J. Fink, and E. Maglischo. 1980. Contribution of medium and long chain triglyceride intake to energy metabolism during prolonged exercise. *Int J Sport Med* 1: 15–20.

Ivy, J. L., A. L. Katz, C. L. Cutler, W. M. Sherman, and E. F. Coyle. 1988a. Muscle glycogen synthesis after exercise: Effect of time of carbohydrate ingestion. *J Appl Physiol* 64: 1480–1485.

Ivy, J. L., M. C. Lee, J. T. Brozinick, Jr., and M. J. Reed. 1988b. Muscle glycogen storage after different amounts of carbohydrate ingestion. *J Appl Physiol* 65: 2018–2023.

Ivy, J. L., P. T. Res, R. C. Sprague, and M. O. Widzer. 2003. Effect of a carbohydrate-protein supplement on endurance performance during exercise of varying intensity. *Int J Sport Nutr Exerc Metab* 13: 382–395.

Iwao, S., K. Mori, and Y. Sato. 1996. Effects of meal frequency on body composition during weight control in boxers. *Scand J Med Sci Sports* 6: 265–272.

Jentjens, R., and A. Jeukendrup. 2003. Determinants of post-exercise glycogen synthesis during short-term recovery. *Sports Med* 33: 117–144.

Jentjens, R. L., L. Moseley, R. H. Waring, L. K. Harding, and A. E. Jeukendrup. 2004a. Oxidation of combined ingestion of glucose and fructose during exercise. *J Appl Physiol* 96: 1277–1284.

Jentjens, R. L., L. J. van Loon, C. H. Mann, A. J. Wagenmakers, and A. E. Jeukendrup. 2001. Addition of protein and amino acids to carbohydrates does not enhance postexercise muscle glycogen synthesis. *J Appl Physiol* 91: 839–846.

Jentjens, R. L., M. C. Venables, and A. E. Jeukendrup. 2004b. Oxidation of exogenous glucose, sucrose, and maltose during prolonged cycling exercise. *J Appl Physiol* 96: 1285–1291.

Jeukendrup, A. E. 2004. Carbohydrate intake during exercise and performance. *Nutrition* 20: 669–677.

Jeukendrup, A. E., and S. Aldred. 2004. Fat supplementation, health, and endurance performance. *Nutrition* 20: 678–688.

Jeukendrup, A. E., R. L. Jentjens, and L. Moseley. 2005. Nutritional considerations in triathlon. *Sports Med* 35: 163–181.

Jeukendrup, A. E., L. Moseley, G. I. Mainwaring, S. Samuels, S. Perry, and C. H. Mann. 2006. Exogenous carbohydrate oxidation during ultraendurance exercise. *J Appl Physiol* 100: 1134–1141.

Jeukendrup, A. E., W. H. Saris, F. Brouns, D. Halliday, and J. M. Wagenmakers. 1996a. Effects of carbohydrate (CHO) and fat supplementation on CHO metabolism during prolonged exercise. *Metabolism* 45: 915–921.

Jeukendrup, A. E., W. H. Saris, P. Schrauwen, F. Brouns, and A. J. Wagenmakers. 1995. Metabolic availability of medium-chain triglycerides coingested with carbohydrates during prolonged exercise. *J Appl Physiol* 79: 756–762.

Jeukendrup, A. E., W. H. Saris, R. Van Diesen, F. Brouns, and A. J. Wagenmakers. 1996b. Effect of endogenous carbohydrate availability on oral medium-chain triglyceride oxidation during prolonged exercise. *J Appl Physiol* 80: 949–954.

Jeukendrup, A. E., J. J. Thielen, A. J. Wagenmakers, F. Brouns, and W. H. Saris. 1998. Effect of medium-chain triacylglycerol and carbohydrate ingestion during exercise on substrate utilization and subsequent cycling performance. *Am J Clin Nutr* 67: 397–404.

Josse, A. R., J. E. Tang, M. A. Tarnopolsky, and S. M. Phillips. 2010. Body composition and strength changes in women with milk and resistance exercise. *Med Sci Sports Exerc* 42: 1122–1130.

Kammer, L., Z. Ding, B. Wang, D. Hara, Y. H. Liao, and J. L. Ivy. 2009. Cereal and nonfat milk support muscle recovery following exercise. *J Int Soc Sports Nutr* 6: 11.

Kerksick, C., T. Harvey, J. Stout, B. Campbell, C. Wilborn, R. Kreider, D. Kalman, T. Ziegenfuss, H. Lopez, J. Landis, J. L. Ivy, and J. Antonio. 2008. International Society of Sports Nutrition position stand: Nutrient timing. *J Int Soc Sports Nutr* 5: 17.

Kirwan, J. P., D. Cyr-Campbell, W. W. Campbell, J. Scheiber, and W. J. Evans. 2001a. Effects of moderate and high glycemic index meals on metabolism and exercise performance. *Metabolism* 50: 849–855.

Kirwan, J. P., D. J. O'Gorman, D. Cyr-Campbell, W. W. Campbell, K. E. Yarasheski, and W. J. Evans. 2001b. Effects of a moderate glycemic meal on exercise duration and substrate utilization. *Med Sci Sports Exerc* 33: 1517–1523.

Koopman, R., D. L. Pannemans, A. E. Jeukendrup, A. P. Gijsen, J. M. Senden, D. Halliday, W. H. Saris, L. J. van Loon, and A. J. Wagenmakers. 2004. Combined ingestion of protein and carbohydrate improves protein balance during ultra-endurance exercise. *Am J Physiol Endocrinol Metab* 287: E712–E720.

Kuipers, H., E. J. Fransen, and H. A. Keizer. 1999. Pre-exercise ingestion of carbohydrate and transient hypoglycemia during exercise. *Int J Sport Med* 20: 227–231.

Lamb, D. R., A. C. Snyder, and T. S. Baur. 1991. Muscle glycogen loading with a liquid carbohydrate supplement. *Int J Sport Nutr* 1: 52–60.

Lambert, C. P., M. G. Flynn, J. B. Boone, T. J. Michaud, and J. Rodriguez-Zayas. 1991. Effects of carbohydrate feeding on multiple-bout resistance exercise. *J Appl Sport Sci Res* 5: 192–197.

Lambert, G. P., J. Lang, A. Bull, J. Eckerson, S. Lanspa, and J. O'Brien. 2008. Fluid tolerance while running: Effect of repeated trials. *Int J Sports Med* 29: 878–882.

Leatt, P. B., and I. Jacobs. 1989. Effect of glucose polymer ingestion on glycogen depletion during a soccer match. *Can J Sport Sci* 14: 112–116.

Lee, J. K., R. J. Maughan, S. M. Shirreffs, and P. Watson. 2008. Effects of milk ingestion on prolonged exercise capacity in young, healthy men. *Nutrition* 24: 340–347.

Levenhagen, D. K., J. D. Gresham, M. G. Carlson, D. J. Maron, M. J. Borel, and P. J. Flakoll. 2001. Postexercise nutrient intake timing in humans is critical to recovery of leg glucose and protein homeostasis. *Am J Physiol Endocrinol Metab* 280: E982–E993.

MacDougall, J. D., M. J. Gibala, M. A. Tarnopolsky, J. R. MacDonald, S. A. Interisano, and K. E. Yarasheski. 1995. The time course for elevated muscle protein synthesis following heavy resistance exercise. *Can J Appl Physiol* 20: 480–486.

Madsen, K., P. K. Pedersen, P. Rose, and E. A. Richter. 1990. Carbohydrate supercompensation and muscle glycogen utilization during exhaustive running in highly trained athletes. *Eur J Appl Physiol Occup Physiol* 61: 467–472.

Massicotte, D., F. Peronnet, G. R. Brisson, and C. Hillaire-Marcel. 1992. Oxidation of exogenous medium-chain free fatty acids during prolonged exercise: Comparison with glucose. *J Appl Physiol* 73: 1334–1339.

Metzner, H. L., D. E. Lamphiear, N. C. Wheeler, and F. A. Larkin. 1977. The relationship between frequency of eating and adiposity in adult men and women in the Tecumseh Community Health Study. *Am J Clin Nutr* 30: 712–715.

Millard-Stafford, M., W. L. Childers, S. A. Conger, A. J. Kampfer, and J. A. Rahnert. 2008. Recovery nutrition: Timing and composition after endurance exercise. *Curr Sports Med Rep* 7: 193–201.

Miller, S. L., P. C. Gaine, C. M. Maresh, L. E. Armstrong, C. B. Ebbeling, L. S. Lamont, and N. R. Rodriguez. 2007. The effects of nutritional supplementation throughout an endurance run on leucine kinetics during recovery. *Int J Sport Nutr Exerc Metab* 17: 456–467.

Miller, S. L., C. M. Maresh, L. E. Armstrong, C. B. Ebbeling, S. Lennon, and N. R. Rodriguez. 2002. Metabolic response to provision of mixed protein-carbohydrate supplementation during endurance exercise. *Int J Sport Nutr Exerc Metab* 12: 384–397.

Moore, D. R., M. J. Robinson, J. L. Fry, J. E. Tang, E. I. Glover, S. B. Wilkinson, T. Prior, M. A. Tarnopolsky, and S. M. Phillips. 2009. Ingested protein dose response of muscle and albumin protein synthesis after resistance exercise in young men. *Am J Clin Nutr* 89: 161–168.

Moore, L. J., A. W. Midgley, S. Thurlow, G. Thomas, and L. R. Mc Naughton. 2010. Effect of the glycemic index of a pre-exercise meal on metabolism and cycling time trial performance. *J Sci Med Sport* 13: 182–188.

Osterberg, K. L., J. J. Zachwieja, and J. W. Smith. 2008. Carbohydrate and carbohydrate + protein for cycling time-trial performance. *J Sports Sci* 26: 227–233.

Pasin, G., and S. L. Miller. 2000. US Whey proteins and sport nutrition. *Application Monographs of the US Dairy Export Council*, U.S. Dairy Export Council, Arlington, VA, 1–8.

Patterson, S. D., and S. C. Gray. 2007. Carbohydrate-gel supplementation and endurance performance during intermittent high-intensity shuttle running. *Int J Sport Nutr Exerc Metab* 17: 445–455.

Paul, D., K. A. Jacobs, R. J. Geor, and K. W. Hinchcliff. 2003. No effect of pre-exercise meal on substrate metabolism and time trial performance during intense endurance exercise. *Int J Sport Nutr Exerc Metab* 13: 489–503.

Pfeiffer, B., A. Cotterill, D. Grathwohl, T. Stellingwerff, and A. E. Jeukendrup. 2009. The effect of carbohydrate gels on gastrointestinal tolerance during a 16-km run. *Int J Sport Nutr Exerc Metab* 19: 485–503.

Pfeiffer, B., T. Stellingwerff, E. Zaltas, and A. E. Jeukendrup. 2010a. CHO oxidation from a CHO gel compared with a drink during exercise. *Med Sci Sports Exerc* 42: 2038–2045.

Pfeiffer, B., T. Stellingwerff, E. Zaltas, and A. E. Jeukendrup. 2010b. Oxidation of solid versus liquid CHO sources during exercise. *Med Sci Sports Exerc* 42: 2030–2037.

Piehl, A. K., K. Soderlund, and E. Hultman. 2000. Muscle glycogen resynthesis rate in humans after supplentation of drinks containing carbohydrates with low and high molecular masses. *Eur J Appl Physiol* 81: 346–351.

Pritchett, K., P. Bishop, R. Pritchett, M. Green, and C. Katica. 2009. Acute effects of chocolate milk and a commercial recovery beverage on postexercise recovery indices and endurance cycling performance. *Appl Physiol Nutr Metab* 34: 1017–1022.

Rankin, J. W., L. P. Goldman, M. J. Puglisi, S. M. Nickols-Richardson, C. P. Earthman, and F. C. Gwazdauskas. 2004. Effect of post-exercise supplement consumption on adaptations to resistance training. *J Am Coll Nutr* 23: 322–330.

Rauch, L. H., I. Rodger, G. R. Wilson, J. D. Belonje, S. C. Dennis, T. D. Noakes, and J. A. Hawley. 1995. The effects of carbohydrate loading on muscle glycogen content and cycling performance. *Int J Sport Nutr* 5: 25–36.

Rodriguez, N. R., N. M. DiMarco, and S. Langley. 2009. Position of the American Dietetic Association, Dietitians of Canada, and the American College of Sports Medicine: Nutrition and athletic performance. *J Am Diet Assoc* 109: 509–527.

Romano-Ely, B. C., M. K. Todd, M. J. Saunders, and T. S. Laurent. 2006. Effect of an isocaloric carbohydrate-protein-antioxidant drink on cycling performance. *Med Sci Sports Exerc* 38: 1608–1616.

Rowlands, D. S., and W. G. Hopkins. 2002. Effect of high-fat, high-carbohydrate, and high-protein meals on metabolism and performance during endurance cycling. *Int J Sport Nutr Exerc Metab* 12: 318–335.

Rowlands, D. S., R. M. Thorp, K. Rossler, D. F. Graham, and M. J. Rockell. 2007. Effect of protein-rich feeding on recovery after intense exercise. *Int J Sport Nutr Exerc Metab* 17: 521–543.

Roy, B. D., M. A. Tarnopolsky, J. D. MacDougall, J. Fowles, and K. E. Yarasheski. 1997. Effect of glucose supplement timing on protein metabolism after resistance training. *J Appl Physiol* 82: 1882–1888.

Satabin, P., P. Portero, G. Defer, J. Bricout, and C. Y. Guezennec. 1987. Metabolic and hormonal responses to lipid and carbohydrate diets during exercise in man. *Med Sci Sports Exerc* 19: 218–223.

Saunders, M. J., M. D. Kane, and M. K. Todd. 2004. Effects of a carbohydrate-protein beverage on cycling endurance and muscle damage. *Med Sci Sports Exerc* 36: 1233–1238.

Saunders, M. J., N. D. Luden, and J. E. Herrick. 2007. Consumption of an oral carbohydrate-protein gel improves cycling endurance and prevents post-exercise muscle damage. *J Strength Cond Res* 21: 678–684.

Sedlock, D. A. 2008. The latest on carbohydrate loading: A practical approach. *Curr Sports Med Rep* 7: 209–213.

Shelmadine, B., M. Cooke, T. Buford, G. Hudson, L. Redd, B. Leutholtz, and D. S. Willoughby. 2009. Effects of 28 days of resistance exercise and consuming a commercially available pre-workout supplement, NO-Shotgun(R), on body composition, muscle strength and mass, markers of satellite cell activation, and clinical safety markers in males. *J Int Soc Sports Nutr* 6: 16.

Sherman, W. M., D. L. Costill, W. J. Fink, and J. M. Miller. 1981. Effect of exercise-diet manipulation on muscle glycogen and its subsequent utilization during performance. *Int J Sports Med* 2: 114–118.

Smeets, A. J., and M. S. Westerterp-Plantenga. 2008. Acute effects on metabolism and appetite profile of one meal difference in the lower range of meal frequency. *Br J Nutr* 99: 1316–1321.

Sparks, M. J., S. S. Selig, and M. A. Febbraio. 1998. Pre-exercise carbohydrate ingestion: Effect of the glycemic index on endurance exercise performance. *Med Sci Sports Exerc* 30: 844–849.

Stote, K. S., D. J. Baer, K. Spears, D. R. Paul, G. K. Harris, W. V. Rumpler, P. Strycula, S. S. Najjar, L. Ferrucci, D. K. Ingram, D. L. Longo, and M. P. Mattson. 2007. A controlled trial of reduced meal frequency without caloric restriction in healthy, normal-weight, middle-aged adults. *Am J Clin Nutr* 85: 981–988.

Summerbell, C. D., R. C. Moody, J. Shanks, M. J. Stock, and C. Geissler. 1996. Relationship between feeding pattern and body mass index in 220 free-living people in four age groups. *Eur J Clin Nutr* 50: 513–519.

Tarnopolsky, M. A., M. Bosman, J. R. Macdonald, D. Vandeputte, J. Martin, and B. D. Roy. 1997. Postexercise protein-carbohydrate and carbohydrate supplements increase muscle glycogen in men and women. *J Appl Physiol* 83: 1877–1883.

Tarnopolsky, M. A., M. Gibala, A. E. Jeukendrup, and S. M. Phillips. 2005. Nutritional needs of elite endurance athletes: Part I. Carbohydrate and fluid requirements. *Eur J Sport Science* 5: 3–14.

Taylor, M. A., and J. S. Garrow. 2001. Compared with nibbling, neither gorging nor a morning fast affect short-term energy balance in obese patients in a chamber calorimeter. *Int J Obes Relat Metab Disord* 25: 519–528.

Tesch, P. A., and H. E. Berg. 1998. Effects of spaceflight on muscle. *J Gravit Physiol* 5: P19–P22.

Thomas, D. E., J. R. Brotherhood, and J. C. Brand. 1991. Carbohydrate feeding before exercise: Effect of glycemic index. *Int J Sports Med* 12: 180–186.

Thomas, D. E., J. R. Brotherhood, and J. B. Miller. 1994. Plasma glucose levels after prolonged strenuous exercise correlate inversely with glycemic response to food consumed before exercise. *Int J Sport Nutr* 4: 361–373.

Thomas, K., P. Morris, and E. Stevenson. 2009. Improved endurance capacity following chocolate milk consumption compared with 2 commercially available sport drinks. *Appl Physiol Nutr Metab* 34: 78–82.

Tipton, K. D., T. A. Elliott, M. G. Cree, A. A. Aarsland, A. P. Sanford, and R. R. Wolfe. 2007. Stimulation of net muscle protein synthesis by whey protein ingestion before and after exercise. *Am J Physiol Endocrinol Metab* 292: E71–E76.

Tipton, K. D., T. A. Elliott, M. G. Cree, S. E. Wolf, A. P. Sanford, and R. R. Wolfe. 2004. Ingestion of casein and whey proteins result in muscle anabolism after resistance exercise. *Med Sci Sports Exerc* 36: 2073–2081.

Tipton, K. D., T. A. Elliott, A. A. Ferrando, A. A. Aarsland, and R. R. Wolfe. 2009. Stimulation of muscle anabolism by resistance exercise and ingestion of leucine plus protein. *Appl Physiol Nutr Metab* 34: 151–161.

Tipton, K. D., A. A. Ferrando, S. M. Phillips, D. Doyle, Jr., and R. R. Wolfe. 1999. Postexercise net protein synthesis in human muscle from orally administered amino acids. *Am J Physiol* 276: E628–E634.

Tipton, K. D., B. B. Rasmussen, S. L. Miller, S. E. Wolf, S. K. Owens-Stovall, B. E. Petrini, and R. R. Wolfe. 2001. Timing of amino acid-carbohydrate ingestion alters anabolic response of muscle to resistance exercise. *Am J Physiol Endocrinol Metab* 281: E197–E206.

Tipton, K. D., and R. R. Wolfe. 1998. Exercise-induced changes in protein metabolism. *Acta Physiol Scand* 162: 377–387.

Tokmakidis, S. P., and I. A. Karamanolis. 2008. Effects of carbohydrate ingestion 15 min before exercise on endurance running capacity. *Appl Physiol Nutr Metab* 33: 441–449.

Toone, R. J., and J. A. Betts. 2010. Isocaloric carbohydrate versus carbohydrate-protein ingestion and cycling time-trial performance. *Int J Sport Nutr Exerc Metab* 20: 34–43.

Valentine, R. J., M. J. Saunders, M. K. Todd, and T. G. St. Laurent. 2008. Influence of carbohydrate-protein beverage on cycling endurance and indices of muscle disruption. *Int J Sport Nutr Exerc Metab* 18: 363–378.

van Essen, M., and M. J. Gibala. 2006. Failure of protein to improve time trial performance when added to a sports drink. *Med Sci Sports Exerc* 38: 1476–1483.

van Loon, L. J., W. H. Saris, M. Kruijshoop, and A. J. Wagenmakers. 2000. Maximizing postexercise muscle glycogen synthesis: Carbohydrate supplementation and the application of amino acid or protein hydrolysate mixtures. *Am J Clin Nutr* 72: 106–111.

Van Zyl, C. G., E. V. Lambert, J. A. Hawley, T. D. Noakes, and S. C. Dennis. 1996. Effects of medium-chain triglyceride ingestion on fuel metabolism and cycling performance. *J Appl Physiol* 80: 2217–2225.

Verboeket-van de Venne, W. P., and K. R. Westerterp. 1993. Frequency of feeding, weight reduction and energy metabolism. *Int J Obes Relat Metab Disord* 17: 31–36.

Verboeket-van de Venne, W. P., K. R. Westerterp, and A. D. Kester. 1993. Effect of the pattern of food intake on human energy metabolism. *Br J Nutr* 70: 103–115.

Vistisen, B., L. Nybo, X. Xu, C. E. Hoy, and B. Kiens. 2003. Minor amounts of plasma medium-chain fatty acids and no improved time trial performance after consuming lipids. *J Appl Physiol* 95: 2434–2443.

Wallis, G. A., D. S. Rowlands, C. Shaw, R. L. Jentjens, and A. E. Jeukendrup. 2005. Oxidation of combined ingestion of maltodextrins and fructose during exercise. *Med Sci Sports Exerc* 37: 426–432.

Wee, S. L., C. Williams, S. Gray, and J. Horabin. 1999. Influence of high and low glycemic index meals on endurance running capacity. *Med Sci Sports Exerc* 31: 393–399.

White, K. M., S. J. Bauer, K. K. Hartz, and M. Baldridge. 2009. Changes in body composition with yogurt consumption during resistance training in women. *Int J Sport Nutr Exerc Metab* 19: 18–33.

Wong, S. H., P. M. Siu, A. Lok, Y. J. Chen, J. Morris, and C. W. Lam. 2008. Effect of the glycemic index of pre-exercise carbohydrate meals on running performance. *Eur J Sport Sci* 8: 23–33.

Wu, C. L., and C. Williams. 2006. A low glycemic index meal before exercise improves endurance running capacity in men. *Int J Sport Nutr Exerc Metabol* 16: 1854–1859.

Wurtman, R. J., J. J. Wurtman, M. M. Regan, J. M. McDermott, R. H. Tsay, and J. J. Breu. 2003. Effects of normal meals rich in carbohydrates or proteins on plasma tryptophan and tyrosine ratios. *Am J Clin Nutr* 77: 128–132.

Zawadzki, K. M., B. B. Yaspelkis, 3rd, and J. L. Ivy. 1992. Carbohydrate-protein complex increases the rate of muscle glycogen storage after exercise. *J Appl Physiol* 72: 1854–1859.

Zehnder, M., E. R. Christ, M. Ith, K. J. Acheson, E. Pouteau, R. Kreis, R. Trepp, P. Diem, C. Boesch, and J. Decombaz. 2006. Intramyocellular lipid stores increase markedly in athletes after 1.5 days lipid supplementation and are utilized during exercise in proportion to their content. *Eur J Appl Physiol* 98: 341–354.

14 Carbohydrates
What We Know about Low versus High Levels for Athletes

Abbie E. Smith, Jose Antonio,
and David H. Fukuda

CONTENTS

14.1 INTRODUCTION

As discussed previously in detail (Chapter 7), carbohydrates hold various physiological roles in both brain and muscle function, and they contribute to muscle and liver glycogen-storage content. An interest in carbohydrate, as a key nutritional component, stems from original research in the 1960s (Bergstrom et al. 1967) and has become the stronghold for diet manipulation with the goal of maximizing its importance in muscle. Coaches, athletes, and researchers often disregard the role of carbohydrate in tissues other than muscle, as well as the partnership of high-carbohydrate ingestion and low-fat diets. The majority of available literature evaluates the effects of a high-carbohydrate diet (70-15-15; carbohydrates, fat, protein) or a low-carbohydrate diet, i.e., a high-fat diet (40-50-10), on performance, failing to realize the other key macronutrient in exercise metabolism: protein. Additionally, although there are three important macronutrients to consider with diet manipulation, storage of protein and carbohydrate cannot be substantially enhanced, whereas fat stores, or adipose tissue, reflect an increased consumption or decreased oxidation of all the nutrients (Graham and Adamo 1999).

Carbohydrate consumption is frequently associated with muscle metabolism, energy, and a delay in fatigue. Although the liver and skeletal muscle house almost all of the body's carbohydrate stores, blood glucose homeostasis is primarily regulated by liver glycogen (Hultman et al. 1971). Hultman and colleagues (1971) demonstrated that after a 24-hour fast, liver glycogen is almost completely depleted, and even an overnight fast severely reduced liver glycogen stores, creating a need for gluconeogenesis to maintain blood glucose levels. In addition, these large diurnal variations in liver glycogen levels create an environment highly sensitive to dietary carbohydrate consumption (i.e., breakfast, post-exercise). In contrast, whereas skeletal muscle contains about 80% of the body's carbohydrate stores, with low levels of variation throughout the day, dietary intake of carbohydrate only slightly influences muscle glycogen levels.

Carbohydrate availability and, specifically, low levels of muscle glycogen, are repeatedly linked to fatigue and reduced exercise performance. Although this theory has stimulated a carbohydrate "frenzy," the mechanisms linking carbohydrate to fatigue are disputable. Norman and colleagues (1988) suggest that glycogen depletion reduces the rate of adenosine triphosphate (ATP) regeneration, subsequently hindering energy availability and therefore causing fatigue. At high levels of exercise (60–85% VO_{2max}), muscle glycogen levels are nearly depleted at the time of fatigue (Saltin and Karlsson 1972). Additionally, the ATP efficiency is higher for glycogen than for fat or glucose (Connett and Sahlin 1996). A more sound theory of fatigue is related to factors other than glycogen depletion; instead, there is an accumulation of various metabolic by-products such as inorganic phosphate, hydrogen ions, magnesium, lactate, and/or an ionic balance (Allen et al. 2008; Robergs et al. 2004). Although prolonged moderate- to high-intensity exercise coincides with muscle glycogen depletion (Costill and Hargreaves 1992), excessive amounts of carbohydrate may not be the solution. Small amounts of carbohydrate, ingested during exercise, have been shown to decrease rates of glycogen depletion, while also reducing endogenous carbohydrate oxidation (Bosch et al. 1993; Coggan and Coyle 1987; Costill and Hargreaves 1992). Consuming about 0.5–1 g/min of a 4–8% carbohydrate solution (profile of today's common sports drink) during activities lasting more than an hour may be beneficial for an athlete to maintain and replenish muscle glycogen stores (Campbell et al. 2008; Coyle et al. 1991).

According to the position of the American Dietetic Association (ADA) and the American College of Sports Medicine (ACSM), carbohydrate recommendations range from 6 to 10 g/kg of body weight/day (2.7–4.5 g/pounds) (Rodriguez et al. 2009a, 2009b). An important emphasis on post-exercise carbohydrate consumption of 1.0–1.5 g/kg of body weight within the first 30 minutes, and again every 2 hours for 4–6 hours, in order to replace glycogen stores, is recommended. However, even the ADA and ACSM issue caution for a high-carbohydrate diet; with higher calorie needs and a greater consumption of calories, athletes can overconsume carbohydrate, leading to weight gain. Among all the hype of low-carb and carbohydrate loading, rarely are those practices defined. Identifying characteristics of common practices and evaluating evidence for or against each category will help shed light on the various physiological and metabolic adaptations.

14.1.1 HIGH CARBOHYDRATE

High carbohydrate (60–70%; 300–400 g; 5–7 g/kg) consumption is widely recommended to athletes, on the belief that this practice maximizes muscle glycogen stores and delays the onset of fatigue (Bergstrom et al. 1967; Costill et al. 1981; Coyle et al. 1986) (see Figure 14.2A). Typical recommendations for carbohydrate consumption suggest that athletes engaged in moderate intensity training consume 7–10 g/kg to maximize muscle glycogen stores (Lambert and Goedecke 2003; Sherman et al. 1981). However, a series of studies have found ingestion of a carbohydrate-loading diet does not spare muscle glycogen during exercise (Bosch et al. 1993), instead this strategy attenuates fat oxidation (Gollnick et al. 1972; Hawley et al. 1997; Rauch et al. 1995; Sherman et al. 1981) and has no sparing effect on liver glycogen (Bosch et al. 1993; Weltan et al. 1998a, 1998b). Interestingly, carbohydrate ingestion during exercise yields a muscle glycogen sparing effect only under a non-carbohydrate-loading state, with no effects on carbohydrate saturation (Bosch et al. 1996). Specifically, 50–60% of the energy required for continuous exercise lasting up to 4 hours at 70% of maximal intensity is derived from carbohydrates, with 40–50% coming from free fatty acids (Coyle et al. 1997). Also, as the result of an increase in cardiovascular fitness, the proportion of energy derived from fat increases, while carbohydrate use decreases (Coyle et al. 1997; Mougios 2006; Turcotte 1999). Also, as the relative intensity of exercise decreases, the contribution of carbohydrate to energy production decreases in the trained muscle (Figure 14.1).

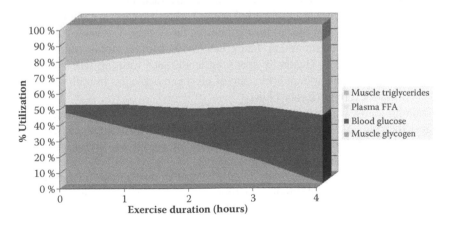

FIGURE 14.1 Fuel utilization during exercise. Initially, glycogen utilization may be very high, but as the duration of the exercise bout is extended, the reliance on glycogen begins to decline, and the utilization of fat as a fuel becomes more prevalent (Costill et al. 1971). FFA, free fatty acid.

14.1.2 Moderate Carbohydrate

In active muscle tissue, carbohydrate and fat oxidation can be balanced at the appropriate ratio, limiting adipose storage (Schrauwen et al. 1997). Specifically, when consuming a mixed meal (i.e., not low-fat) following exercise, fat oxidation increases to match intake, whereas the exercised muscle consumes the majority of the ingested carbohydrate, replenishing glycogen levels. The Zone diet is a common moderate carbohydrate (40–50%; 200–250 g; 3.25–4 g/kg) diet, with adequate amounts of fat and protein (Figure 14.2B). One study has evaluated the effects of this dietary manipulation on performance, demonstrating a slight decline (9%) in time to exhaustion at 80% VO_{2max}. Although the decrease in performance is not something to neglect, total caloric consumption was reduced by 320 calories, which may have been the primary influence on the decrease in performance time (Jarvis et al. 2002). Van Zant et al. (2002) demonstrated that a moderate carbohydrate and fat (42-40-18) diet did not differ from a high-carbohydrate (62-20-18) diet on peak power, total work production, One repetition max (1RM) upper-body strength, and/or repetitions to fatigue. Furthermore, 7 days of a moderate carbohydrate diet (40%) was no different than a high-carbohydrate diet (70%) in time to exhaustion at 80 or 90% VO_{2max} exercise trials, lasting up to 30 minutes. The higher-carbohydrate diet led to higher levels of blood lactate and a higher respiratory quotient, indicating higher rates of carbohydrate oxidation and reduced fat utilization (Pitsiladis et al. 1996; Pitsiladis and Maughan 1999).

Of further consideration, when evaluating and implementing specific macronutrients, is training status. Trained individuals have a more rapid uptake of dietary glucose, enhancing muscle glycogen stores, while increasing fat oxidation (Hamilton et al. 1996; Liu et al. 1996) and therefore potentially reducing their need for large amounts of carbohydrate consumption to saturate muscle glycogen stores. Calles-Escandon et al. (1996) evaluated three treatments by: 1) overfeeding a group of men by 50% caloric intake; 2) feeding to equal energy balance; or 3) exercising to a 50% caloric deficit. The nonexercised/overfed group had an increase in carbohydrate oxidation and decrease in fat oxidation, augmenting fat storage. The exercising groups, regardless of caloric consumption, had greater carbohydrate storage and enhanced fat oxidation/utilization. Generally speaking, endurance training will augment fat utilization, with a concomitant lower rate of glycogen depletion in both intermittent and continuous exercise (Essen 1978).

Training status can play an important role in macronutrient recommendations, because they become more efficient at utilizing fat for fuel. Another consideration is timing of fuel and exercise. For example, if an athlete goes to bed and skips breakfast prior to practice or competition, his pre-exercise liver glycogen levels are decreased by 50%. During prolonged exercise, liver glycogen stores become further depleted, requiring fuel from muscle tissue creating a hypoglycemic-sensitive environment (Graham and Adamo 1999; Nilsson and Hultman 1973, 1974). A trained athlete will adapt and more rapidly store a greater amount of liver glycogen with reduced carbohydrate influx. A moderate carbohydrate diet may be more suitable for a trained individual, in order to maximize fat oxidation and prevent weight gain from excess carbohydrate storage.

14.1.3   Low-CHO and Very-Low-Carbohydrate Ketogenic Diets

Low (20–30%; 100–150 g; 1.75–2.5 g/kg) carbohydrate (Low-CHO) and very-low (~10% <50 g/day, 0.75 g/kg) carbohydrate ketogenic diets (VLCKD) have a poor reputation (Figure 14.2, C and D), because of high levels of ketone formation. In reality, ketones are efficient fuel sources, yielding 25% more ATP than glucose or fatty acids

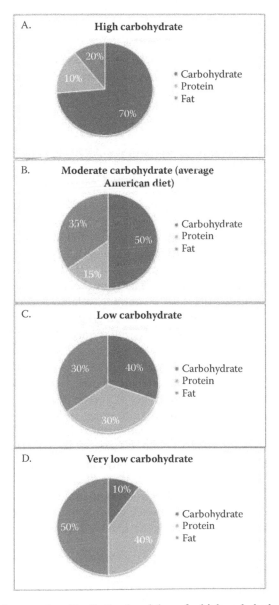

FIGURE 14.2   Macronutrient distribution breakdown for high-carbohydrate (A), moderate-carbohydrate (B), low-carbohydrate (C), and very-low-carbohydrate (D) diets.

(Cahill and Veech 2003). Under periods of carbohydrate restriction, lipid oxidation rates increase accelerating enzymes and substrates involved in lipid metabolism and ultimately spare carbohydrate use. Additionally, the metabolic and body-composition adaptations may be advantageous for a clinical population or possibly for an athlete striving for body-composition changes during an off-season. VLCKDs have been shown to decrease blood triglyceride, total cholesterol and low-density lipoprotein (LDL) levels, while augmenting the utilization of fat. Furthermore, the use of VLCKDs for body composition have demonstrated a significant reduction in body fat tissue while preserving lean mass, in comparison with a high-carbohydrate, low-fat diet (Volek et al. 2002b, 2004a; Volek and Westman 2002a). However, for athletes, muscle glycogen depletion followed by a period of low carbohydrate ingestion is likely to impair high-intensity exercise performance (Lima-Silva et al. 2009). A VLCKD should not be practiced during the competition season but may be useful for its weight-loss potential in the off-season.

14.2 THE OLD-SCHOOL BASICS ON CARBOHYDRATES

14.2.1 CARBOHYDRATE-LOADING AND HIGH-CARBOHYDRATE DIETS

The practice of carbohydrate loading dates back to the 1960s when Scandinavian researchers began 3–6 days of diet manipulation (Bergstrom et al. 1967). The protocol was initiated by glycogen-depleting exercise followed by 3–6 days of high-carbohydrate consumption and no training. Carbohydrate loading has demonstrated increases in muscle glycogen stores by up to 300%, therefore suggesting longer times to fatigue and prevention of "bonking." The typical carbohydrate-loading protocol consists of a simultaneous decrease in training volume and intensity, combined with 3 days of high-carbohydrate feeding (7–10 g/kg/body mass [BM]; 70–85% of energy) to successfully induce muscle glycogen storage (Table 14.1).

Although this idea of carbohydrate loading has led to significant increases in muscle glycogen concentration, this strategy is not optimal (Sedlock 2008). A carbohydrate-depletion phase may interfere with normal training, possibly leading to hypoglycemia and decreased mental acuity (Lamb et al. 1991). Also, refeeding to stimulate glycogen saturation may result in bloating, weight gain, and gastrointestinal distress. Burke et al. (2000) examined the effects of two separate carbohydrate feeding strategies with well-trained cyclists. Participants completed a 100-km time trial (~2.5 hours) either after 3 days of carbohydrate (CHO) loading (9 g of CHO/kg of BM/day) or after a moderate-carbohydrate diet (6 g of CHO/kg of BM/day), while consuming 1 g of CHO/kg of BM/hour. Both protocols resulted in significant increases in muscle glycogen content while yielding no differences in cycling trial performance times, thus demonstrating the ineffectiveness of carbohydrate loading in real-life competitions.

Another popular strategy initiated in the 1980s and still used today has been demonstrated to double or "supercompensate" muscle glycogen levels, starting a week out from competition (Sherman et al. 1981). Supercompensation strategy starts with a 3-day training taper while consuming a moderate-carbohydrate diet (50% CHO), followed by 3 days of high-carbohydrate consumption (70%) with 20 minutes

TABLE 14.1
Carbohydrate-Loading Strategies

Traditional method (Berstrom et al. 1967)

1. Deplete muscle glycogen stores with exercise.
2. Maintain low glycogen concentration by consuming a CHO-free, high-fat diet for 3 days.
3. Follow with a second glycogen-depletion exercise bout and a 3-day high-CHO diet.
4. Increases muscle glycogen two-fold.

Newer methods

Sherman et al. (1981)

1. Lower muscle glycogen stores with an intense training session.
2. During subsequent 3 days, consume a mixed diet of 45–50% CHO, with a natural training taper.
3. On days 4–6, continue training taper, while increasing CHO consumption to 70%.
4. Increases muscle glycogen 200 $\mu mol \cdot g^{-1}$ (similar to Bergstrom).

Goforth et al. (1997)

1. Three-day depletion phase with intense exercise.
2. Maintain low-CHO (12%), high-protein (41%), high-fat (49%) diet.
3. Three-day depletion phase with no exercise and high-CHO (83%), low-fat (8%) diet.
4. Increases muscle glycogen ~250 $\mu mol \cdot g^{-1}$.

Bussau et al. (2002)

1. Deplete muscle glycogen stores with exercise.
2. Within 24 hours, ingest 10 g of CHO·kg⁻¹ of body weight.
3. Increases muscle glycogen ~180 $\mu mol \cdot g^{-1}$.

of low-intensity exercise, resting on the last day. More recently, athletes and scientists have demonstrated increases in muscle glycogen stores after 1 day of high-carbohydrate consumption (10 g/kg/day of high–glycemic-index foods) (Fairchild et al. 2002). Bussau et al. (2002) demonstrated that 1 day yielded a 90% increase in muscle glycogen stores, while maintaining normal training regimens (Table 14.1).

14.2.1.1 High Carbohydrates: Effects on Performance

The strategy of carbohydrate loading generally elicits an increase in muscle glycogen stores but may not always be effective in women (Tarnopolsky et al. 1995), and the effects on performance in men and women are unequivocal (Andrews et al. 2003; Sedlock 2008; Tarnopolsky et al. 1995). Although the importance of carbohydrates in endurance performance is fundamental for metabolism, a chronic high carbohydrate diet may not be the only strategy to maximize muscle glycogen and performance. Comparing a high-carbohydrate (75% CHO), moderate-carbohydrate (50%), and placebo supplementation revealed that there was no advantage to carbohydrate supplementation for a 24.2-km endurance run (Andrews et al. 2003). Moreover, this protocol yielded higher rates of carbohydrate oxidation during exercise, when compared to placebo.

Although this seems advantageous, normal adaptations to aerobic training results in more efficient fat utilization and therefore a reduced reliance upon muscle glycogen stores for energy. The enhanced ability to utilize fat for energy may yield greater body composition adaptations and may also increase time to exhaustion, lengthening time to fatigue and available glycogen for fuel. There are various studies comparing high carbohydrate diets to low carbohydrate consumption on performance, with higher carbohydrate yielding more consistent results. Chronic endurance training of 2 hours daily, combined with a 40% CHO diet, yielded a decline in muscle glycogen content but a reduced lactate accumulation, as well as increasing fat mobilization (Costill et al. 1971), which may be more beneficial adaptations to chronic training and body composition. Costill et al. (1981) examined the effects of an isocaloric diet (3000 kcal) on glycogen resynthesis after a 16.1-km run, in trained individuals, with a low carbohydrate (20% CHO), mixed/moderate carbohydrate meal (50% CHO), high carbohydrate (70%) in seven meals, or high carbohydrate (70%) in two meals. Results demonstrated that the amount of carbohydrates consumed post-glycogen depletion is directly proportionate to glycogen resynthesis, with the mixed meal increasing glycogen content by 51% and the high carbohydrate meal (two meals) increasing glycogen content by 127%. This study reveals that timing of carbohydrate consumption may be important directly post-workout, but also that a moderate carbohydrate diet increases glycogen content to near baseline levels.

Evaluation of higher-intensity, shorter-duration activities may also be of interest. Hatfield and associates (2006) demonstrated that a high-carbohydrate consumption (~80%, 6.5 g/kg) was no different than a moderate-carbohydrate consumption (~50%; 4.4 g/kg) on repeated anaerobic jump squats, supported by previous research demonstrating no effects of carbohydrate ingestion on repeated short-duration maximal effort exercise lasting less than 5 minutes (Haub et al. 2003; MacDougall et al. 1977; Medbo 1993). A new study out of Brazil evaluated the effects of a high-carbohydrate diet compared with a control group on high-intensity intermittent running over a 9-day period (de Sousa et al. 2010), demonstrating that a higher consumption of carbohydrates with intense training may stimulate a greater increase in testosterone (~6%) and cortisol (8% greater than controls). Despite the small changes in hormones, there were no differences in performance of 10 sets of 800-m intervals or multiple 1000-m time trials.

14.2.1.2   High Carbohydrates: Effects on Body Composition

Carbohydrate loading studies typically focus on the elite endurance athlete, although numerous moderately active individuals follow the old adage. Muscle makes up about 40–45% of our body tissue and has a major role in carbohydrate regulation and the management of fat tissue. Carbohydrate-loading strategies are often centered around a period of reduced/no training, stimulating a reduction in carbohydrate oxidation but concomitantly increasing fat storage. An increase in dietary carbohydrate consumption has been shown to lead to a significant increase in carbohydrate oxidation, with a subsequent drop in fat oxidation (Schwarz et al. 1995). In a practical sense, although the use of carbohydrate for fuel is enhanced and fat for fuel drops, adipose stores increase. Increases in fat tissue after high carbohydrate consumption have been shown after one (Abbott et al. 1988), two (Tremblay et al. 1991), and seven days.

Every gram of carbohydrate is concomitantly stored with 3 grams of water, equaling about 500 g for 2,000 kcal. The increase in water from carbohydrate overconsumption is accompanied by an increase in body weight, of approximately 2 kg for

500 g. Acheson et al. (1988) demonstrated the effects of a carbohydrate-loading strategy on body composition; following a muscle glycogen depletion phase there was a 0.8-kg (1.75-pound) loss in body weight, followed by a phase of high-carbohydrate intake to 83% of the diet for 7 days. The refeeding phase led to a 4.6-kg (10-pound) increase in weight, with 0.7 kg (1.5 pounds) attributed to an increase in carbohydrate storage, 1.1 kg (2.4 pounds) attributed to fat storage, and the remaining 2.8 kg (6.2 pounds) attributed to water. In a two-month observation, individuals about doubled their caloric intake, with the majority of the calories coming from carbohydrates. On average there was a 17-kg (37-pound) increase in body weight, with 24–28 pounds reported as fat tissue (Pasquet et al. 1992). It has been suggested that long-term dietary adaptations to excessive carbohydrate intake are dominated by adipose tissue enhancing the storage of triglycerides (Aarsland et al. 1997) and low-density lipoproteins (Acheson et al. 1988) and reducing insulin sensitivity (Laybutt et al. 1997).

14.3 HIGHER PROTEIN CONSUMPTION: MACRONUTRIENT MANIPULATION

The fad of a low-carbohydrate, high-protein diet for weight loss has become increasingly popular. However, the majority of research has focused on a reduction in carbohydrate consumption with a subsequent increase in fat intake, yielding a misinterpretation of a "low-carbohydrate" diet. The true question should evaluate the effects of manipulating protein and carbohydrate, while maintaining fat consumption. Unfortunately, the available research on these manipulations is minimal. In some instances, high-protein diets have reported decreased endurance performance as a result of glycogen depletion in both fast- and slow-twitch muscle fibers (Jarvis et al. 2002; Macdermid and Stannard 2006; Tesch et al. 1978). A decrease in muscle glycogen is often associated with an early onset of fatigue; however, little research exists on the actual effects of higher-protein, lower-carbohydrate intake on anaerobic and aerobic performance.

For optimal athletic performance, gaining lean body mass (i.e., primarily skeletal muscle mass) and losing fat mass is the ideal outcome when combining training, nutrition, and supplementation. Endurance athletes typically have very little body fat with varying levels of lean body mass. For instance, distance runners tend to carry the least amount of body fat, whereas rowers tend to be more muscular compared with other endurance athletes (Kerr et al. 2007). Nevertheless, maximizing fat loss while maintaining or perhaps gaining lean body mass is an ideal strategy for athletes, including endurance athletes. It is our contention that the consumption of a high-carbohydrate diet is not the best nutritional approach for endurance athletes. In fact, the isocaloric replacement of carbohydrate with protein and unsaturated fat is an effective way to promote the loss of fat mass while sparing lean body mass. Furthermore, there is no evidence that the substitution of carbohydrate with protein or fat has long-term deleterious effects (Foster et al. 2010).

14.3.1 MACRONUTRIENT MANIPULATION: PERFORMANCE

Investigators examined the effects of a low-, medium-, and high-fat isocaloric diet on performance and metabolism in runners. A group of male and female runners

(42 miles/week) consumed diets of 16% (low) and 31% (moderate) fat for 4 weeks. Six males and six females increased their fat intakes to a 44% high-fat diet (HFD). Endurance and VO_{2max} were tested at the end of each diet. Runners on the low-fat diet ate 19% fewer calories than on the medium- or high-fat diets. However, body weight, percent body fat (males = 71 kg, 16% body fat; females = 57 kg, 19% body fat), VO_{2max}, and anaerobic power were not affected by the level of dietary fat. In contrast, endurance time increased for the low-fat to medium-fat diet by 14%. No differences were seen in plasma lactate, glucose, glycerol, triglycerides, or fatty-acid levels when comparing the low-fat versus the medium-fat diet.

Subjects who increased dietary fat to the HFD had higher plasma pyruvate (46%) and lower lactate levels (39%) after the endurance run. These results suggest that runners on a low-fat diet consume fewer calories and have reduced endurance performance than on a medium- or high-fat diet. A high-fat diet, providing sufficient total calories, does not compromise anaerobic power (Horvath et al. 2000a) and in fact may be superior to a higher carbohydrate, low-fat diet. Another investigation suggested that endurance runners may not be consuming enough calories on a low-fat diet and that increasing dietary fat sufficiently increases energy consumption. On the low-fat diet, essential fatty acids and some minerals (especially zinc) may be too low. Thus, a low-fat (i.e., high-carbohydrate) diet could negatively impact performance (Horvath et al. 2000a).

Endurance cyclists who consumed an HFD for 15 days did not experience any negative performance effects. Sixteen endurance-trained cyclists were assigned randomly to a control group, who consumed their habitual diet (30 ± 8% fat), or an HFD group, who consumed a high-fat isocaloric diet (69 ± 1% fat). They discovered that athletes consuming an HFD had an enhanced ability to oxidize fat during submaximal exercise with no negative effects on 40-km time-trial performance (Goedecke et al. 1999). Thus, an HFD and the traditional higher carbohydrate diet produced equivocal performance results. Interestingly, an additional study has suggested that skeletal muscle glycogen concentrations may not be a reliable predictor of performance. Nine trained male cyclists were studied during 75 seconds of all-out exercise on an air-braked cycle ergometer following muscle glycogen-lowering exercise and consumption of isocaloric diets that were either high (80% CHO) or low (25% CHO) in carbohydrate content. The exercise-diet regimen was successful in producing differences in pre-exercise muscle glycogen contents; that is, the high-carbohydrate condition produced much higher concentrations of skeletal muscle glycogen. Despite the greater skeletal muscle glycogen availability, there were no differences between performance trials for peak power, mean power, and maximal accumulated oxygen deficit. The authors of this study suggested that increased muscle glycogen availability has no direct effect on performance during all-out high-intensity exercise (Hargreaves et al. 1997).

Furthermore, the effects of nine days of a high-carbohydrate diet (80% of calories as CHO, 80% CHO diet) versus a moderate-carbohydrate diet (43% of calories as CHO, 43% CHO diet) found no diet effects on mean swim velocities for any interval distance, and mean velocities for all swims were identical for both diets. Thus, in this scenario an 80% CHO diet provided no advantage over a 43% CHO diet for maintaining interval-swim-training intensity (Lamb et al. 1990). In comparing a high-protein versus a high-CHO diet on performance and physiological responses during an ultraendurance climbing race at moderate altitude, investigators found no differences in mental or physical performance (Bourrilhon et al.). On the other hand, 2 weeks of a high-fat (70% fat, 7% CHO) compared with a high-carbohydrate (74% CHO, 12% fat) diet found enhanced endurance after the high-fat diet. This was associated with a lower respiratory exchange ratio and a decreased rate of carbohydrate oxidation (Lambert et al. 1994).

Does consuming less carbohydrate and more protein hamper the acute response to heavy resistance training? Scientists investigated the effects of an isocaloric high-protein diet on upper- and lower-limb strength and fatigue during high-intensity resistance exercise. Ten recreationally active women, aged 25–40 years, followed a control diet (55%, 15%, and 30% of energy from carbohydrate, protein, and fat, respectively) and a high-protein diet (respective values: 30%, 40%, and 30%) for 7 days each in a random counterbalanced design. No differences were found between diets in any of the strength performance parameters (handgrip strength, handgrip endurance, peak torque, total work, and fatigue) or the responses of heart rate, systolic and diastolic arterial pressure, blood lactate, and blood glucose to exercise. Thus, women on a short-term isocaloric high-protein, moderate-fat diet maintained muscular strength and endurance of upper and lower limbs during high-intensity resistance exercise without experiencing fatigue earlier compared with a control diet (Dipla et al. 2008).

14.3.2 MACRONUTRIENT MANIPULATION: BODY COMPOSITION AND HEALTH

Alterations in the percentage of calories from carbohydrate, protein, and fat (while maintaining isocaloric status) can significantly impact body composition. In fact, it is our contention that high-carbohydrate diets (i.e., 60% or higher in calories) are deleterious with respect to optimizing body composition (i.e., maintain or gain lean body mass (LBM) while promoting a decrease in fat mass). Furthermore, the notion that consuming protein or fat as an isocaloric replacement for carbohydrate is deleterious to one's health is unsupported in the scientific literature (Foster et al. 2010). For instance, the long-term weight loss and cardio-metabolic effects of a very-low-carbohydrate, high-saturated-fat diet (LC) and a high-carbohydrate, low-fat diet (LF) were evaluated under isocaloric conditions. Men and women with abdominal obesity and at least one additional metabolic syndrome risk factor were randomly assigned to either an energy-restricted (approximately 6–7 MJ) LC diet (4%, 35%, and 61% of energy as carbohydrate, protein, and fat, respectively) or an isocaloric LF diet (46%, 24%, and 30% of energy as carbohydrate, protein, and fat, respectively) for 1 year. Both dietary patterns resulted in similar weight loss and changes in body composition. However, the LC diet may offer clinical benefits to obese persons with insulin resistance (Brinkworth et al. 2009).

In contrast, an energy-restricted, high-protein, low-fat diet was found to provide nutritional and metabolic benefits that were equal to and sometimes greater than those observed with a high-carbohydrate diet (Noakes et al. 2005). In fact, a cursory examination of the literature shows that lower carbohydrate diets (whether it is an isoenergetic replacement of carbohydrate with fat or protein) are either the same or better with respect to alterations in body composition and various health indices. Recently, scientists compared the effects of isocaloric, energy-restricted VLCKD and LF diets on weight loss, body composition, trunk fat mass, and resting energy expenditure (REE) in overweight/obese men and women. Subjects were prescribed two energy-restricted (–500 kcal/day) diets: a VLCK diet with a goal to decrease carbohydrate levels below 10% of energy and induce ketosis and an LF diet with a goal similar to national recommendations (% carbohydrate:fat:protein = ~60:25:15%). Both between and within group comparisons revealed a distinct advantage of a VLCKD over an LF diet for weight loss, total fat loss, and trunk fat loss for men (despite significantly greater energy intake). The majority of women also responded more favorably to the VLCKD, especially in terms of trunk fat loss. Absolute REE (kcal/day) was decreased with both diets as expected, but REE expressed relative to body mass (kcal/kg), was better maintained on the VLCKD for men only. Therefore, it is apparent that a VLCKD may be superior to a traditional LF diet for short-term body weight and fat loss, especially in men (Volek et al. 2004a). Other results support the use of dietary carbohydrate restriction as an effective approach to improve features of metabolic syndrome and cardiovascular risk (Volek et al. 2009).

Another study compared changes in body weight and composition, as well as blood lipids, after short-term weight loss (4 months) followed by weight maintenance (8 months) using moderate protein (PRO) or conventional high-carbohydrate diets. At 4 months, the PRO group had lost 22% more fat mass (–5.6 kg) than the high-carbohydrate group (–4.6 kg), but weight loss did not differ between groups (–8.2 kg vs. -7.0 kg). At 12 months, the PRO group had more participants complete the study (64% versus 45%) with greater improvement in body composition; however, weight loss did not differ between groups (–10.4 kg versus –8.4 kg). The high-carbohydrate diet reduced serum cholesterol and LDL cholesterol compared with PRO at 4 months, but the effect did not remain at 12 months. PRO had sustained favorable effects on serum triacylglycerol, high-density lipoprotein (HDL) cholesterol, and TAG:HDL-C compared with CHO at 4 and 12 months. Thus, the PRO diet was more effective for fat-mass loss and body-composition improvement during initial weight loss and long-term maintenance and produced sustained reductions in triacylglycerol and increases in HDL cholesterol compared with the CHO diet (Layman et al. 2009).

In a study that examined two diets (high-protein, lower-carbohydrate versus low-protein, higher-carbohydrate) with exercise, scientists found that subjects in the protein-only and protein-plus exercise groups lost more total weight and fat mass and tended to lose less lean mass than the higher-carbohydrate and higher-carbohydrate plus-exercise groups. This study demonstrated that a diet with higher protein and reduced carbohydrates, combined with exercise, additively improved body composition during weight loss, whereas the effects on blood lipids differed between diet treatments (Layman et al. 2005). Another investigation demonstrated that increasing the proportion of protein to carbohydrate in the diet of adult women has positive effects on body composition, blood lipids, glucose homeostasis, and satiety during weight loss (Layman et al. 2003). Furthermore, the data suggest that higher protein intake promotes satiety in overweight and obese men (Leidy et al. 2010).

14.4 CARBOHYDRATE MANIPULATION FOR SPORT

The reduction of dietary carbohydrate with a concurrent increase or maintenance of lean dietary protein is an appealing strategy often used by weight-class athletes to maintain muscle mass during brief or extended periods of weight loss. Lower carbohydrate intake yields increased lipid oxidation and gluconeogenesis, but protein oxidation is also enhanced. Therefore, protein intake is crucial to maintain lean muscle mass, and when consumed in lean meat sources with unsaturated fat, can be used to avoid drastic drops in total calories while maximizing the use of the greater energy density of fat. Protein also provides an increased feeling of satiety that is of benefit to athletes under caloric restriction. Regulations for weight loss have been put into place for high-school and collegiate wrestlers in the United States, with the specific intention of the discontinuation of the practice of rapid and severe dehydration, prompting the need for the development of alternate weight-loss strategies. Subsequent wrestling research has shown that caloric restriction with a decreased carbohydrate intake and increased protein consumption leads to gradual weight loss without decrements in strength or aerobic and anaerobic performance (Mourier et al. 1997). Therefore, adjusting relative macronutrient levels through a planned diet without extreme dehydration may serve as an appropriate method for weight-class athletes.

A recent case study by Morton et al. (2010) highlights the effectiveness of a moderate-carbohydrate, high-protein diet during the 12-week training camp leading up to a major boxing bout. The authors noted that the diet employed (caloric intake equivalent to resting metabolic rate; 40% carbohydrate, 38% protein, 22% protein) was a major modification from the boxer's traditional weight-cutting strategy, which included relative starvation and dehydration methods. The nutritional intervention lead to a decrease in body weight of 9.4 kg at a rate of approximately 0.9 kg/week with no intentional method of dehydration. Bone mineral density was not affected by the weight loss, but lean mass decreased by approximately 3 kg.

A common practice that was also followed by the boxing athlete was a substantial increase in interim carbohydrate consumption between the weigh-in and competition. According to follow-up commentary by the author, a subsequent training camp using an altered strategy that included a slightly higher daily caloric intake and acute dehydration the day before weigh-in resulted in an additional 1–2 kg of lean mass and increased strength gains throughout the process. The details of this case study represent a positive step forward in the preparation process of weight-class athletes, both in terms of health and the incorporation of the concepts presented in this chapter.

This gradual change in macronutrient distribution with an increasing emphasis on protein consumption during the lead up to competition has even begun to be adopted by younger athletes. Boisseau et al. (2005) noted a change in dietary habits in adolescent female judo athletes between three weeks and one week prior to competition. The altered diet, including a significant increase in protein-intake percentage and a nonsignificant decrease in carbohydrate-intake percentage, resulted in a significant decrease in body weight of approximately 2%. The authors did show concerns with the possibility of this strategy being coupled with dehydration techniques, and as noted previously, this practice may be avoidable. Another issue commonly discussed with regard to rapid weight loss before competition is the possibility of altered antioxidant status caused by changes in macronutrient distribution and limitation in total caloric intake. However, a separate study noted that a simulated judo competition yielded similar levels of oxidative stress with or without dietary carbohydrate reduction during the weight-cutting process the week prior to competition (Finaud et al. 2006).

Research involving weight-class athletes has shown that a majority of these individuals may have adapted to repeated weight-cutting and may exhibit fewer adverse effects on performance because of both carbohydrate and total calorie restriction during rapid weight loss. Specifically, Artioli et al. (2010) examined experienced weight-cycling judo athletes conducting a self-selected weight-cutting regimen, generally employing a low-carbohydrate diet (approximately 50% compared with non-weight-cycling controls) while reducing body weight by 5% over a period of 5 days. After weighing in, the athletes were allotted 4 hours for recovery, during which a self-selected diet that tended to be carbohydrate-rich was selected, and the weight-cycling group regained 50% of the weight lost. Judo-related performance, including match-time analysis (effort times, recovery times, methods of combat) and repeated upper-body Wingate tests, revealed no difference between groups despite significantly lower resting glucose levels in the weight-cycling groups. Interestingly, no differences between groups were observed in plasma-lactate concentrations at rest or throughout the testing protocols. The authors concluded that a 5% body-weight reduction in experienced weight-cycling athletes had limited impact on judo-related performance.

The use of specific diets to maintain lean muscle mass while decreasing body fat percentage is not novel. Bodybuilders and physique competitors have traditionally employed low-carbohydrate diets to decrease fat mass prior to competitions. Gymnasts generally follow a similar meal plan to maximize lean body mass in order to perform techniques with maximum explosiveness and efficiency (Nova et al. 2001). Athletes with intentions of altering body composition in the off-season may adopt a similar dietary regimen. Lightweight rowers demonstrate seasonal changes in macronutrient distribution with decreased carbohydrate intake during the postseason and preseason and a gradual increase throughout the competition season (Morris and Payne 1996). Many athletes set goals for the off-season that include alterations in body composition, specifically general weight-loss and increased lean muscle mass, that may be realized through appropriate training and a low- to moderate-carbohydrate diet.

14.5   CONCLUSIONS AND RECOMMENDATIONS

- Carbohydrates are not an essential nutrient. Unlike fats and proteins, which are essential, your body can manufacture glucose.
- The carbohydrate portion of the typical American diet (i.e., 60%) is much too high for an average person and high for an athlete.
- A more appropriate range would be 45–55% carbohydrates.
- A more moderate consumption of carbohydrates leads to a greater efficiency of fat utilization.

- Carbohydrate recommendations are specific to the athlete. A more highly trained athlete may require less carbohydrate because of their enhanced ability to utilize fat and a greater training efficiency.
- High-carbohydrate diets (i.e., 60% or higher in calories) are deleterious with respect to optimizing body composition (i.e., maintain or gain lean body mass while promoting a decrease in fat mass).
- Isocaloric replacement of carbohydrate with protein and unsaturated fat is an effective way to promote the loss of fat mass while sparing lean body mass. Furthermore, there is no evidence that the substitution of carbohydrate with protein or fat has long-term deleterious effects (see Topic Box 14.1).
- Timing of carbohydrates is the most important. If you eat simple/high–glycemic-index carbohydrates, consume them within 30 minutes after exercise.
- Carbohydrates can be anabolic, when combined with amino acids, post-workout.
- In exercising muscle, the metabolic response to carbohydrate consumption is enhanced. In trained muscle, the efficiency of muscle glycogen is augmented, requiring a reduced influx of exogenous carbohydrate ingestion.
- A lower carbohydrate consumption provides a weight-loss method that maintains lean muscle mass and performance in weight-class athletes. This unique distribution of macronutrients may also be utilized by athletes during their competitive season or as a tool used to accomplish off-season body composition goals. See Topic Boxes 14.2 and 14.3 for practical applications.

TOPIC BOX 14.1   OVERFEEDING ON FAT AND PROTEIN VERSUS CARBOHYDRATE

In an intriguing study, scientists examined the effects of snacking based on fast-acting carbohydrates (candy) or fat and protein (peanuts) in a prospective randomized, parallel intervention study. Basal metabolic rate and cardiovascular risk factors were measured before and after hyperalimentation by the addition of 20 kcal/kg (84 kJ/kg) body weight of either candy or roasted peanuts, to the regular caloric intake, for 2 weeks in healthy subjects. This amounts to an additional ~1363 extra calories for a 150-pound individual. They discovered that energy intake increased similarly in the groups. Body weight and waist circumference increased significantly only in the candy group, thus suggesting body-fat gains. At the end of the study, LDL cholesterol and ApoB/ApoA-1-ratio were higher in the candy group than in the peanut group. On the other hand, basal metabolic rate increased only in the peanut group. Thus, two weeks of overfeeding on fat and protein (i.e., peanuts) does not cause deleterious changes in health or body composition whereas high-glycemic carbohydrate results in a body-weight and waist-circumference increases, as well as harmful alterations in LDL cholesterol (Claesson et al. 2009). In fact, the adaptive response to fat-protein overfeeding is an elevation of resting metabolic rate.

TOPIC BOX 14.2   JOSE ANTONIO: CONFESSIONS OF A COMPETITIVE OUTRIGGER PADDLER

Outrigger-canoe paddling is a very popular competitive sport in the Hawaiian Islands and Polynesia. Additionally, the sport is growing rapidly in Australia and the mainland United States including California and Florida (Haley and Nichols 2009). As a recreational "paddler" (note that the term "paddling" refers to those who paddle on outrigger canoes; do not use the term "rower" to describe a paddler; rowers row backwards on flat water; outrigger canoes are built for the open ocean, and paddlers face forward), I compete in races that cover ~10–16 miles, often taking approximately 2–2.5 hours to complete. Thus, it is an endurance sport in the sense that you are exercising for a pro-longed period of time. However, because you alternate right and left sides while paddling (thus, there is a built-in rest interval), it is a bit different than traditional endurance sports such as running or swimming in which your extremities are always moving and as such, they do not have a rest interval. One might describe paddling as a strength-endurance sport. A premium is placed on a high-power output per unit body mass. Thus, it is not a hindrance to carry additional lean body mass on a canoe and explains why elite male paddlers can easily outrace elite female paddlers.

However, as far as nutrition and supplementation, I do not follow a tradi-tional high-carbohydrate diet. A cursory examination of my diet reveals an intake of ~45% carbohydrate, with the remainder split between fat and protein. I contend that anytime one increases training volume, it is best to increase the intake of fat, protein, and carbohydrate, not just carbohydrate. It is nonsensical for "nutritionists" to recommend an increased intake of carbohydrate second-ary to increases in training. First of all, you need the extra protein to help repair skeletal muscle tissue, as well as extra fat to meet the caloric needs of enhanced training volume. Your body has a very limited capacity to store glycogen. Hence, there is no compelling need to consume a high-carbohydrate diet. Also, it should be noted that protein and fat are the only essential macronutrients.

Regarding supplementation, I consume 2000–6000 IUs of vitamin D daily, a multi-vitamin, caffeine (200–400 mg) pre-workout, and a protein shake post-workout (40 g of whey, 5 of g creatine, 1–2 g of beta-alanine). I have found from simple trial-and-error that fatigue in training or during a race is often a function of "brain" or central fatigue. If my head doesn't fatigue, I can force myself to paddle regardless of the muscle pain I might feel. Thus, what often works best for me during training is consuming a sports drink spiked with branched-chain amino acids and caffeine. Sports nutrition is part science, part art. I realize that there will not be any studies on outrigger pad-dlers. Furthermore, the needs of this particular sport differ from traditional endurance events in that the upper body is the primary musculature used, and muscle power output per unit of body weight is critical for optimal perfor-mance. Would carbohydrate loading help this sport? I seriously doubt it.

TOPIC BOX 14.3   ABBIE SMITH: COMPETITIVE TRIATHLETE

As a collegiate cross-country and track athlete and current triathlete, I have heard carbohydrates described as the essential component of training and performance for as long as I can remember. Half of my teammates went out for the sport for the pasta parties. I often wonder if my adversaries ever picked up a research article or questioned the carb-frenzy environment. In their defense, every textbook explains carbohydrates as the quintessential component of performance, recovery, and injury prevention. Why is it that there is this norm of high-carbohydrate recommendations when it may not influence performance? In fact, high-carbohydrate consumption may lead to weight gain, poor glucose regulation, and a poor grasp on healthy eating. Is it because everyone is too lazy to dig beyond the surface of our carb-centered society? Or is it because no one has enough guts to defy the old wives' tale that carbs are safe, delicious, and essential for muscle glycogen?

Fortunately, my innate aversion for carbohydrates has left me with a leaner physique and more race hardware than I know what to do with. Even more, I am grateful for the ability to synthesize literature for what it is, not what the book chapters lead you to believe. And of course, personal trial and error has taught me what to eat and what not to eat. Although diet is going to be a little bit different for everyone, here's some insight into my world of high intensity training.

- First rule of thumb: whenever you eat, whether it's a snack or a meal, ALWAYS include some form of protein. For example: almonds and raisins; celery and natural peanut butter; turkey breast on whole-wheat bread; milk. Combine protein WITH your carbohydrates.
- Eating carbohydrates is important, but make sure the bulk of them come from fruits, vegetables, and milk. If you have a sweet tooth, take advantage of your body's needs and eat sugared items immediately post-workout.
- Don't be fat-phobic. Healthy fats are essential for any athlete, including endurance athletes. In fact, most athletes have a hard time consuming enough calories to offset their energy expenditure: fat is energy dense, providing a bigger bang for your calorie buck.
- Consuming a moderate amount of carbohydrates (3–4 g/kg/day) will stimulate a greater reliance upon fat for fuel and a decreased demand for muscle glycogen.
- To maintain lean body mass and muscle glycogen stores, timing is everything. Consumption of a combination of carbohydrates and protein before and after exercise is crucial.
- Personally speaking, during normal training shoot for a 40-30-30 ratio of carbs-protein-fat. During higher-volume, high-intensity periods, a 50-30-20 strategy might be more ideal.

Supplement Strategy

I've never figured out why supplements have such a bad rap. I must admit though, as a former college athlete, even I thought supplement use was like "cheating" or somehow shouldn't be a part of my training. If only I knew then what I know now, I could have prevented the nine stress fractures that I ran through, despite having a bone density of "The Hulk," and I could have avoided sleeping through my 4 years of undergrad, due to overtraining and fatigue. Who would have thought that a female distance runner could benefit from supplements? Turns out a few supplements, combined with some healthy training, have kept me injury free and stronger than ever. What a beautiful thing, to train less, work more, and still flaunt a leaner physique, run faster, and lift more.

I will admit that hard work goes a long way, but incorporating some key supplements in your diet can make you happier, healthier, and stronger than ever before. While my daily concoction of some morning java, omegas, vitamin D, whey protein, combined with a steady dosing of beta-alanine and branched-chain amino acids throughout the day and during workouts, topped off with some creatine monohydrate as my afternoon wake-me-up, work as a nice little mental and physical booster, the key to supplementing is just that, "supplementing" your diet with components that you're lacking. Amino acids help build lean body mass and aid in recovery. Creatine and beta-alanine also augment recovery while delaying fatigue. Omega-3 and vitamin D have a powerful mental and physical influence, and whey protein is an easily digested form of protein that helps maximize your nutrient timing window. Above all else, a well-rounded diet of protein, fats, and a moderate amount of carbohydrate is the place to start.

REFERENCES

Aarsland, A., D. Chinkes, and R. R. Wolfe. 1997. Hepatic and whole-body fat synthesis in humans during carbohydrate overfeeding. *Am J Clin Nutr* 65: 1774–1782.

Abbott, W. G., B. V. Howard, L. Christin, D. Freymond, S. Lillioja, V. L. Boyce, T. E. Anderson, C. Bogardus, and E. Ravussin. 1988. Short-term energy balance: Relationship with protein, carbohydrate, and fat balances. *Am J Physiol* 255: E332–E337.

Acheson, K. J., Y. Schutz, T. Bessard, K. Anantharaman, J. P. Flatt, and E. Jequier. 1988. Glycogen storage capacity and de novo lipogenesis during massive carbohydrate overfeeding in man. *Am J Clin Nutr* 48: 240–247.

Allen, D. G., G. D. Lamb, and H. Westerblad. 2008. Skeletal muscle fatigue: Cellular mechanisms. *Physiol Rev* 88: 287–332.

Andrews, J. L., D. A. Sedlock, M. G. Flynn, J. W. Navalta, and H. Ji. 2003. Carbohydrate loading and supplementation in endurance-trained women runners. *J Appl Physiol* 95: 584–590.

Artioli, G. G., R. T. Iglesias, E. Franchini, B. Gualano, D. B. Kashiwagura, M. Y. Solis, F. B. Benatti, M. Fuchs, and A. H. Lancha. 2010. Rapid weight loss followed by recovery time does not affect judo-related performance. *J Sports Sci* 28: 21–32.

Bergstrom, J., L. Hermansen, E. Hultman, and B. Saltin. 1967. Diet, muscle glycogen and physical performance. *Acta Physiol Scand* 71: 140–150.

Boisseau, N., S. Vera-Perez, and J. Poortmans. 2005. Food and fluid intake in adolescent female judo athletes before competition. *Pediatr Exerc Sci* 17: 62–71.

Bosch, A. N., S. C. Dennis, and T. D. Noakes. 1993. Influence of carbohydrate loading on fuel substrate turnover and oxidation during prolonged exercise. *J Appl Physiol* 74: 1921–1927.

Bosch, A. N., S. M. Weltan, S. C. Dennis, and T. D. Noakes. 1996. Fuel substrate turnover and oxidation and glycogen sparing with carbohydrate ingestion in non-carbohydrate-loaded cyclists. *Pflugers Arch* 432: 1003–1010.

Bourrilhon, C., R. Lepers, M. Philippe, P. V. Beers, M. Chennaoui, C. Drogou, M. C. Beauvieux, P. Burnat, C. Y. Guezennec, and D. Gomez-Merino. Influence of protein-versus carbohydrate-enriched feedings on physiological responses during an ultraendurance climbing race. *Horm Metab Res* 42: 31–37.

Brinkworth, G. D., M. Noakes, J. D. Buckley, J. B. Keogh, and P. M. Clifton. 2009. Long-term effects of a very-low-carbohydrate weight loss diet compared with an isocaloric low-fat diet after 12 mo. *Am J Clin Nutr* 90: 23–32.

Burke, L. M., J. A. Hawley, E. J. Schabort, A. St Clair Gibson, I. Mujika, and T. D. Noakes. 2000. Carbohydrate loading failed to improve 100-km cycling performance in a placebo-controlled trial. *J Appl Physiol* 88: 1284–1290.

Bussau, V. A., T. J. Fairchild, A. Rao, P. Steele, and P. A. Fournier. 2002. Carbohydrate loading in human muscle: An improved 1 day protocol. *Eur J Appl Physiol* 87: 290–295.

Cahill, G. F., Jr., and R. L. Veech. 2003. Ketoacids? Good medicine? *Trans Am Clin Climatol Assoc* 114: 149–163.

Calles-Escandon, J., M. I. Goran, M. O'Connell, K. S. Nair, and E. Danforth, Jr. 1996. Exercise increases fat oxidation at rest unrelated to changes in energy balance or lipolysis. *Am J Physiol* 270: E1009–E1014.

Campbell, C., D. Prince, M. Braun, E. Applegate, and G. A. Casazza. 2008. Carbohydrate-supplement form and exercise performance. *Int J Sport Nutr Exerc Metab* 18: 179–190.

Claesson, A. L., G. Holm, A. Ernersson, T. Lindstrom, and F. H. Nystrom. 2009. Two weeks of overfeeding with candy, but not peanuts, increases insulin levels and body weight. *Scand J Clin Lab Invest* 69: 598–605.

Coggan, A. R., and E. F. Coyle. 1987. Reversal of fatigue during prolonged exercise by carbohydrate infusion or ingestion. *J Appl Physiol* 63: 2388–2395.

Connett, R.J., and K. Sahlin, eds. 1996. Control of glycolysis and glycogen metabolism. In *Handbook of Physiology: Section 12: Regulation and Integration of Multiple Systems*, edited by L. B. Rowell and J. T. Shepherd. New York: Oxford Press.

Costill, D. L., R. Bowers, G. Branam, and K. Sparks. 1971. Muscle glycogen utilization during prolonged exercise on successive days. *J Appl Physiol* 31: 834–838.

Costill, D. L., and M. Hargreaves. 1992. Carbohydrate nutrition and fatigue. *Sports Med* 13: 86–92.

Costill, D. L., W. M. Sherman, W. J. Fink, C. Maresh, M. Witten, and J. M. Miller. 1981. The role of dietary carbohydrates in muscle glycogen resynthesis after strenuous running. *Am J Clin Nutr* 34: 1831–1836.

Coyle, E. F., A. R. Coggan, M. K. Hemmert, and J. L. Ivy. 1986. Muscle glycogen utilization during prolonged strenuous exercise when fed carbohydrate. *J Appl Physiol* 61: 165–172.

Coyle, E. F., M. T. Hamilton, J. G. Alonso, S. J. Montain, and J. L. Ivy. 1991. Carbohydrate metabolism during intense exercise when hyperglycemic. *J Appl Physiol* 70: 834–840.

Coyle, E. F., A. E. Jeukendrup, A. J. Wagenmakers, and W. H. Saris. 1997. Fatty acid oxidation is directly regulated by carbohydrate metabolism during exercise. *Am J Physiol* 273: E268–E275.

de Sousa, M. V., K. Madsen, H. G. Simoes, R. M. Pereira, C. E. Negrao, R. Z. Mendonca, L. Takayama, R. Fukui, and M. E. da Silva. 2010. Effects of carbohydrate supplementation on competitive runners undergoing overload training followed by a session of intermittent exercise. *Eur J Appl Physiol* 109: 507–516.

Dipla, K., M. Makri, A. Zafeiridis, D. Soulas, S. Tsalouhidou, V. Mougios, and S. Kellis. 2008. An isoenergetic high-protein, moderate-fat diet does not compromise strength and fatigue during resistance exercise in women. *Br J Nutr* 100: 283–286.

Essen, B. 1978. Studies on the regulation of metabolism in human skeletal muscle using intermittent exercise as an experimental model. *Acta Physiol Scand Suppl* 454: 1–32.

Fairchild, T. J., S. Fletcher, P. Steele, C. Goodman, B. Dawson, and P. A. Fournier. 2002. Rapid carbohydrate loading after a short bout of near maximal-intensity exercise. *Med Sci Sports Exerc* 34: 980–986.

Finaud, J., F. Degoutte, V. Scislowski, M. Rouveix, D. Durand, and E. Filaire. 2006. Competition and food restriction effects on oxidative stress in judo. *Int J Sports Med* 27: 834–841.

Foster, G. D., H. R. Wyatt, J. O. Hill, A. P. Makris, D. L. Rosenbaum, C. Brill, R. I. Stein, B. S. Mohammed, B. Miller, D. J. Rader, B. Zemel, T. A. Wadden, T. Tenhave, C. W. Newcomb, and S. Klein. 2010. Weight and metabolic outcomes after 2 years on a low-carbohydrate versus low-fat diet: A randomized trial. *Ann Intern Med* 153: 147–157.

Goedecke, J. H., C. Christie, G. Wilson, S. C. Dennis, T. D. Noakes, W. G. Hopkins, and E. V. Lambert. 1999. Metabolic adaptations to a high-fat diet in endurance cyclists. *Metabolism* 48: 1509–1517.

Gollnick, P. D., K. Piehl, C. W. Saubert, R. B. Armstrong, and B. Saltin. 1972. Diet, exercise, and glycogen changes in human muscle fibers. *J Appl Physiol* 33: 421–425.

Graham, T. E., and K. B. Adamo. 1999. Dietary carbohydrate and its effects on metabolism and substrate stores in sedentary and active individuals. *Can J Appl Physiol* 24: 393–415.

Haley, A., and A. Nichols. 2009. A survey of injuries and medical conditions affecting competitive adult outrigger canoe paddlers on O'ahu. *Hawaii Med J* 68: 162–165.

Hamilton, K. S., F. K. Gibbons, D. P. Bracy, D. B. Lacy, A. D. Cherrington, and D. H. Wasserman. 1996. Effect of prior exercise on the partitioning of an intestinal glucose load between splanchnic bed and skeletal muscle. *J Clin Invest* 98: 125–135.

Hargreaves, M., J. P. Finn, R. T. Withers, J. A. Halbert, G. C. Scroop, M. Mackay, R. J. Snow, and M. F. Carey. 1997. Effect of muscle glycogen availability on maximal exercise performance. *Eur J Appl Physiol Occup Physiol* 75: 188–192.

Hatfield, D. L., W. J. Kraemer, J. S. Volek, M. R. Rubin, B. Grebien, A. L. Gomez, D. N. French, T. P. Scheett, N. A. Ratamess, M. J. Sharman, M. R. McGuigan, R. U. Newton, and K. Hakkinen. 2006. The effects of carbohydrate loading on repetitive jump squat power performance. *J Strength Cond Res* 20: 167–171.

Haub, M. D., G. G. Haff, and J. A. Potteiger. 2003. The effect of liquid carbohydrate ingestion on repeated maximal effort exercise in competitive cyclists. *J Strength Cond Res* 17: 20–25.

Hawley, J. A., G. S. Palmer, and T. D. Noakes. 1997. Effects of 3 days of carbohydrate supplementation on muscle glycogen content and utilisation during a 1-h cycling performance. *Eur J Appl Physiol Occup Physiol* 75: 407–412.

Horvath, P. J., C. K. Eagen, N. M. Fisher, J. J. Leddy, and D. R. Pendergast. 2000a. The effects of varying dietary fat on performance and metabolism in trained male and female runners. *J Am Coll Nutr* 19: 52–60.

Horvath, P. J., C. K. Eagen, S. D. Ryer-Calvin, and D. R. Pendergast. 2000b. The effects of varying dietary fat on the nutrient intake in male and female runners. *J Am Coll Nutr* 19: 42–51.

Hultman, E., J. Bergstrom, and A. E. Roch-Norlan. 1971. Glycogen storage in human skeletal muscle. *Acta Med Scand* 182: 274–276.

Jarvis, M., L. McNaughton, A. Seddon, and D. Thompson. 2002. The acute 1-week effects of the Zone diet on body composition, blood lipid levels, and performance in recreational endurance athletes. *J Strength Cond Res* 16: 50–57.

Kerr, D. A., W. D. Ross, K. Norton, P. Hume, M. Kagawa, and T. R. Ackland. 2007. Olympic lightweight and open-class rowers possess distinctive physical and proportionality characteristics. *J Sports Sci* 25: 43–53.

Lamb, D. R., K. F. Rinehardt, R. L. Bartels, W. M. Sherman, and J. T. Snook. 1990. Dietary carbohydrate and intensity of interval swim training. *Am J Clin Nutr* 52: 1058–1063.

Lamb, D. R., A. C. Snyder, and T. S. Baur. 1991. Muscle glycogen loading with a liquid carbohydrate supplement. *Int J Sport Nutr* 1: 52–60.

Lambert, E. V., and J. H. Goedecke. 2003. The role of dietary macronutrients in optimizing endurance performance. *Curr Sports Med Rep* 2: 194–201.

Lambert, E. V., D. P. Speechly, S. C. Dennis, and T. D. Noakes. 1994. Enhanced endurance in trained cyclists during moderate intensity exercise following 2 weeks adaptation to a high fat diet. *Eur J Appl Physiol Occup Physiol* 69: 287–293.

Laybutt, D. R., D. J. Chisholm, and E. W. Kraegen. 1997. Specific adaptations in muscle and adipose tissue in response to chronic systemic glucose oversupply in rats. *Am J Physiol* 273: E1–E9.

Layman, D. K., R. A. Boileau, D. J. Erickson, J. E. Painter, H. Shiue, C. Sather, and D. D. Christou. 2003. A reduced ratio of dietary carbohydrate to protein improves body composition and blood lipid profiles during weight loss in adult women. *J Nutr* 133: 411–417.

Layman, D. K., E. Evans, J. I. Baum, J. Seyler, D. J. Erickson, and R. A. Boileau. 2005. Dietary protein and exercise have additive effects on body composition during weight loss in adult women. *J Nutr* 135: 1903–1910.

Layman, D. K., E. M. Evans, D. Erickson, J. Seyler, J. Weber, D. Bagshaw, A. Griel, T. Psota, and P. Kris-Etherton. 2009. A moderate-protein diet produces sustained weight loss and long-term changes in body composition and blood lipids in obese adults. *J Nutr* 139: 514–521.

Leidy, H. J., C. L. Armstrong, M. Tang, R. D. Mattes, and W. W. Campbell. 2010. The influence of higher protein intake and greater eating frequency on appetite control in overweight and obese men. *Obesity* 18: 1725–1732.

Lima-Silva, A. E., F. R. De-Oliveira, F. Y. Nakamura, and M. S. Gevaerd. 2009. Effect of carbohydrate availability on time to exhaustion in exercise performed at two different intensities. *Braz J Med Biol Res* 42: 404–412.

Liu, S., V. E. Baracos, H. A. Quinney, and M. T. Clandinin. 1996. Dietary fat modifies exercise-dependent glucose transport in skeletal muscle. *J Appl Physiol* 80: 1219–1224.

Macdermid, P. W., and S. R. Stannard. 2006. A whey-supplemented, high-protein diet versus a high-carbohydrate diet: Effects on endurance cycling performance. *Int J Sport Nutr Exerc Metab* 16: 65–77.

MacDougall, J. D., G. R. Ward, and J. R. Sutton. 1977. Muscle glycogen repletion after high-intensity intermittent exercise. *J Appl Physiol* 42: 129–132.

Medbo, J. I. 1993. Glycogen breakdown and lactate accumulation during high-intensity cycling. *Acta Physiol Scand* 149: 85–89.

Morris, F. L., and W. R. Payne. 1996. Seasonal variations in the body composition of lightweight rowers. *Br J Sports Med* 30: 301–304.

Morton, J. P., C. Robertson, L. Sutton, and D. P. MacLaren. 2010. Making the weight: A case study from professional boxing. *Int J Sport Nutr Exerc Metab* 20: 80–85.

Mougios, V. 2006. *Exercise Biochemistry*. Champaign, IL: Human Kinetics.

Mourier, A., A. X. Bigard, E. de Kerviler, B. Roger, H. Legrand, and C. Y. Guezennec. 1997. Combined effects of caloric restriction and branched-chain amino acid supplementation on body composition and exercise performance in elite wrestlers. *Int J Sports Med* 18: 47–55.

Nilsson, L. H., and E. Hultman. 1973. Liver glycogen in man: The effect of total starvation or a carbohydrate-poor diet followed by carbohydrate refeeding. *Scand J Clin Lab Invest* 32: 325–330.

Nilsson, L. H., and E. Hultman. 1974. Liver and muscle glycogen in man after glucose and fructose infusion. *Scand J Clin Lab Invest* 33: 5–10.

Noakes, M., J. B. Keogh, P. R. Foster, and P. M. Clifton. 2005. Effect of an energy-restricted, high-protein, low-fat diet relative to a conventional high-carbohydrate, low-fat diet on weight loss, body composition, nutritional status, and markers of cardiovascular health in obese women. *Am J Clin Nutr* 81: 1298–1306.

Norman, B., A. Sollevi, and E. Jansson. 1988. Increased IMP content in glycogen-depleted muscle fibres during submaximal exercise in man. *Acta Physiol Scand* 133: 97–100.

Nova, E., A. Montero, S. Lopez-Varela, and A. Marcos. 2001. Are elite gymnasts really malnourished? Evaluation of diet, anthropometry and immunocompetence. *Nutr Res* 21: 15–29.

Pasquet, P., L. Brigant, A. Froment, G. A. Koppert, D. Bard, I. de Garine, and M. Apfelbaum. 1992. Massive overfeeding and energy balance in men: The Guru Walla model. *Am J Clin Nutr* 56: 483–490.

Pitsiladis, Y. P., and R. J. Maughan. 1999. The effects of alterations in dietary carbohydrate intake on the performance of high-intensity exercise in trained individuals. *Eur J Appl Physiol Occup Physiol* 79: 433–442.

Pitsiladis, Y. P., C. Duignan, and R. J. Maughan. 1996. Effects of alterations in dietary carbohydrate intake on running performance during a 10 km treadmill time trial. *Br J Sports Med* 30: 226–231.

Rauch, L. H., A. N. Bosch, T. D. Noakes, S. C. Dennis, and J. A. Hawley. 1995. Fuel utilisation during prolonged low-to-moderate intensity exercise when ingesting water or carbohydrate. *Pflugers Arch* 430: 971–977.

Robergs, R. A., F. Ghiasvand, and D. Parker. 2004. Biochemistry of exercise-induced metabolic acidosis. *Am J Physiol Regul Integr Comp Physiol* 287: R502–R516.

Rodriguez, N. R., N. M. Di Marco, and S. Langley. 2009a. American College of Sports Medicine position stand: Nutrition and athletic performance. *Med Sci Sports Exerc* 41: 709–731.

Rodriguez, N. R., N. M. DiMarco, and S. Langley. 2009b. Position of the American Dietetic Association, Dietitians of Canada, and the American College of Sports Medicine: Nutrition and athletic performance. *J Am Diet Assoc* 109: 509–527.

Saltin, B., and J. Karlsson, eds. 1972. Muscle glycogen utilisation during work of different intensities. *Muscle Metabolism during Exericse*, edited by B. Pernow and B. Saltin. New York: Plenum Press.

Schrauwen, P., W. D. van Marken Lichtenbelt, W. H. Saris, and K. R. Westerterp. 1997. Role of glycogen-lowering exercise in the change of fat oxidation in response to a high-fat diet. *Am J Physiol* 273: E623–E629.

Schwarz, J. M., R. A. Neese, S. Turner, D. Dare, and M. K. Hellerstein. 1995. Short-term alterations in carbohydrate energy intake in humans: Striking effects on hepatic glucose production, de novo lipogenesis, lipolysis, and whole-body fuel selection. *J Clin Invest* 96: 2735–2743.

Sedlock, D. A. 2008. The latest on carbohydrate loading: A practical approach. *Curr Sports Med Rep* 7: 209–213.

Sherman, W. M., D. L. Costill, W. J. Fink, and J. M. Miller. 1981. Effect of exercise-diet manipulation on muscle glycogen and its subsequent utilization during performance. *Int J Sports Med* 2: 114–118.

Tarnopolsky, M. A., S. A. Atkinson, S. M. Phillips, and J. D. MacDougall. 1995. Carbohydrate loading and metabolism during exercise in men and women. *J Appl Physiol* 78: 1360–1368.

Tesch, P., L. Larsson, A. Eriksson, and J. Karlsson. 1978. Muscle glycogen depletion and lactate concentration during downhill skiing. *Med Sci Sports* 10: 85–90.

Tremblay, A., N. Lavallee, N. Almeras, L. Allard, J. P. Despres, and C. Bouchard. 1991. Nutritional determinants of the increase in energy intake associated with a high-fat diet. *Am J Clin Nutr* 53: 1134–1137.

Turcotte, L. P. 1999. Role of fats in exercise. Types and quality. *Clin Sports Med* 18: 485–498.

Van Zant, R. S., J. M. Conway, and J. L. Seale. 2002. A moderate carbohydrate and fat diet does not impair strength performance in moderately trained males. *J Sports Med Phys Fitness* 42: 31–37.

Volek, J. S., S. D. Phinney, C. E. Forsythe, E. F. Quann, R. J. Wood, M. J. Puglisi, W. J. Kraemer, D. M. Bibus, M. L. Fernandez, and R. D. Feinman. 2009. Carbohydrate restriction has a more favorable impact on the metabolic syndrome than a low fat diet. *Lipids* 44: 297–309.

Volek, J. S., N. A. Ratamess, M. R. Rubin, A. L. Gomez, D. N. French, M. M. McGuigan, T. P. Scheett, M. J. Sharman, K. Hakkinen, and W. J. Kraemer. 2004a. The effects of creatine supplementation on muscular performance and body composition responses to short-term resistance training overreaching. *Eur J Appl Physiol* 91: 628–637.

Volek, J. S., M. J. Sharman, A. L. Gomez, C. DiPasquale, M. Roti, A. Pumerantz, and W. J. Kraemer. 2004b. Comparison of a very low-carbohydrate and low-fat diet on fasting lipids, LDL subclasses, insulin resistance, and postprandial lipemic responses in overweight women. *J Am Coll Nutr* 23: 177–184.

Volek, J. S., M. J. Sharman, D. M. Love, N. G. Avery, A. L. Gomez, T. P. Scheett, and W. J. Kraemer. 2002b. Body composition and hormonal responses to a carbohydrate-restricted diet. *Metabolism* 51: 864–870.

Volek, J. S., and E. C. Westman. 2002a. Very-low-carbohydrate weight-loss diets revisited. *Cleve Clin J Med* 69: 849, 853, 856–858 passim.

Weltan, S. M., A. N. Bosch, S. C. Dennis, and T. D. Noakes. 1998a. Influence of muscle glycogen content on metabolic regulation. *Am J Physiol* 274: E72–E82.

Weltan, S. M., A. N. Bosch, S. C. Dennis, and T. D. Noakes. 1998b. Preexercise muscle glycogen content affects metabolism during exercise despite maintenance of hyperglycemia. *Am J Physiol* 274: E83–E88.

15 Nutrition for the Aging Athlete

*Thomas W. Buford, Matthew B. Cooke,
and Jean L. Gutierrez*

CONTENTS

15.1 INTRODUCTION

The "aging athlete" is a broad term comprising a quite heterogeneous population of individuals. In its own right, the term "aging" is almost superfluous because all individuals are aging chronologically. For the purposes of this chapter, we will define aging athletes as those who are 50 years of age or older. "Athlete" can refer to a wide range of individuals from weekend warriors to master athletes: the most active of older individuals. Across this spectrum of athletes, a parallel spectrum of nutritional needs exists. As is true for all athletes, a "cookie cutter" approach should not be taken to designing a nutritional program for physically active older adults. Each individual's nutritional program should be individualized to account for differences in age, size, gender, training regimen, and bioenergetic demands of the activity or sport. Fortunately, older athletes can use simple guidelines to maximize performance and maintain health. Furthermore, older athletes can use nutrition to maximize training benefits by understanding how the physiological changes that accompany aging change nutrient needs.

15.1.1 AGING-RELATED CHANGES IN PERFORMANCE

Aging is a slow and continuous process that modulates the function of various organs and organ systems. A single book chapter allows for only a cursory discussion of these changes as volumes have been written on the etiologies of aging (Bengston et al. 2009; Ekerdt 2002; Masoro and Austad 2006). Innumerable biological changes, including declines in the production of sex hormones (O'Donnell et al. 2006), cellular metabolic efficiency (Epel 2009), the number of motor neurons innervating skeletal muscle fibers (Faulkner et al. 2007, 2008), and the number of muscle fibers themselves (Faulkner et al. 2007), contribute to age-related declines in performance, regardless of activity level.

For most sports, athletes' performance initially declines in their early 30s (Faulkner et al. 2008). Although highly gifted athletes may still outperform younger counterparts, these athletes still demonstrate declines from their own peak levels. Despite decades of regular training, master athletes experience age-related declines in both muscle force production and power that parallel sedentary controls (Pearson et al. 2002). Though trained older people are significantly stronger than their sedentary peers, the rate of strength loss is not significantly different between the two groups. These data demonstrate that, to maintain optimal performance, older athletes must consider all factors that influence performance, including nutrient intake and training technique.

15.1.2 AGE-RELATED CHANGES IN NUTRIENT ABSORPTION

All athletes should consume a varied and balanced diet; however, several physiological changes in older adulthood can result in age-related nutritional deficiencies. Therefore, older athletes need to be aware of these potential deficiencies and strategies to reduce the likelihood of nutrient deficiency-related performance decrements. Specific nutrients of which older athletes need increased intake are discussed later in the chapter. Prior to discussing age-related changes in nutrient needs, we present first some major physiological changes that may contribute to age-related nutrient deficiency.

15.2 PHYSIOLOGIC AND PHARMACOLOGIC CAUSES OF AGE-RELATED NUTRIENT DEFICIENCY

15.2.1 DYSPHAGIA

Approximately 15% of individuals older than 60 years develop dysphagia (Brady 2008). Dysphagia is characterized by difficulty controlling food in the mouth and swallowing. This chronic problem typically follows a stroke, neurological abnormalities, and many other conditions. The most disconcerting consequence of dysphasia is the increased risk for aspiration. Aspiration is the accidental sucking in of food particles or fluids into the lungs, and patients with undiagnosed dysphasia are at increased of aspiration pneumonia. Typically speaking, people with dysphasia have more difficulty swallowing solid, as compared to liquid, foods. In the context of physically active older people, even mild dysphasia may result in inadequate food and beverage swallowing during exercise. Older people with a history of stroke may benefit from only eating or drinking during rest periods during training sessions. Furthermore, a liquid post-exercise nutrient supplement may be tolerated better than solid foods in some older people. Exercise physiologists and nutritionists should contact a dysphasic individual's speech pathologist to ensure that the correct food consistency is recommended for pre- and post-exercise meals.

15.2.2 CHANGES IN SECRETION OF GASTRIC ACID

A physiological change that may impact absorption of some nutrients is a 40% decrease in gastric pepsin output (Feldman et al. 1996). After stomach (gastric) acid denatures the three-dimensional structure of the proteins, the peptide bonds are more vulnerable to proteolysis by gastric pepsin, produced by the chief cells of the stomach. Conceivably, this significant reduction in pepsin output may inhibit rapid protein absorption in physically active older people. Older athletes *may* benefit from a partially hydrolyzed protein supplement or elemental essential amino acids (Volpi et al. 2003), as compared to food, to stimulate protein anabolism after training.

15.2.3 PHARMACEUTICAL–NUTRIENT AND NUTRACEUTICAL–NUTRIENT INTERACTIONS

Many (if not most) older adults, including master athletes, consume a number of drugs, herbs, or nutritional supplements in addition to their regular diet. All of these pharmaceuticals/nutraceuticals interact within the human body, potentially with unexpected or undesirable results. A comprehensive discussion of the infinite interactions that these drugs or supplements can have with nutrient intake is far beyond the scope of this chapter, but readers can consult Tables 15.1, 15.2, and 15.3 for information regarding common drug-nutrient and herb-nutrient interactions.

TABLE 15.1

Common Age-Related Dietary Symptoms: Potential Drug Causes

Nutrient-Related Symptoms	Drugs
Decrease appetite	Antibiotics: amphotercin B, gentamicin, metronidazole, and zidovudine (AZT)
	Carbonic anhydrase inhibitors: acetazolamide, diclorphenamide
	Digitalis
	Methylphenidate (Ritalin)
Stimulate appetite	Antidepressants
	Antihistamines: astemizole, cyproheptadine
	Tranquilizers: lithium carbonate, diazepam, pranepam, chlorpromazine, promethazine
	Steroids: anabolic steroids, glucocorticoids
Generally reduces absorptions of nutrients	Astemizole, azithromycin, digoxin, levodopa, penicillins, tetracyclines

TABLE 15.2

Potential Interactions of Commonly Used Drugs with Nutrient Absorption and Utilization

Drug[a]	Condition Treated	Nutrient Interaction
Antacids	Stomach ache	Decreases iron absorption secondary to increased gastric pH
Aspirin	Pain, inflammation, and blood thinning	Increased excretion of vitamin C, iron deficiency secondary to GI tract blood loss
Carbonic anhydrase inhibitors	Edema, mountain sickness, duodenal ulcers	High blood glucose and increased excretion of potassium
Corticosteroids		Increased protein catabolism, decreased protein synthesis, high blood glucose, increase serum lipids, decreased absorption of calcium, phosphorus, potassium, and increased requirements for zinc and vitamins C, B_6, D, and folate
Diazoxide	High blood pressure	High blood glucose
Hydralazine	High blood pressure	Increased excretion of vitamin B_6
Neomycin		Decreased absorption of fat lactose, protein, calcium, iron, potassium, and vitamins A, D, K, and B_{12}
Nitroprusside	High blood pressure	Decrease serum B_{12}
Primidone	Seizures	Decreased absorption of calcium

[a] Selected from Mosby's Pocket Guide Series: Nutritional Care

TABLE 15.3
Potential Interactions of Common Herbal Supplements with Nutrient Absorption and Utilization

Herb[a]	Condition Treated	Nutrient Interaction or Side Effect
Black cohash	Menopausal symptoms	Liver failure (site of bile production and vitamin activation)
Ephedra	Colds, fever, flu, headaches, asthma, wheezing, and nasal congestion	Increase in blood pressure
Flaxseed	Constipation	May lower the body's ability to absorb medications or other supplements that are taken by mouth
Kava	Anxiety, insomnia, and menopausal symptoms	Liver damage
Licorice root	Hepatitis C	High blood pressure, salt and water retention, and low potassium levels
St. John's wort	Mild to moderate depression	Interacts with several drugs, including: antidepressants, birth control pills, cyclosporine, digoxin, indinavir, irinotecan, warfarin
Yohimbe		Increased blood pressure and heart rate; severe stomach pain

[a] Selected from National Center for Complementary and Alternative Medicine "Herbs at a Glance" (http://nccam.nih.gov/health/herbsataglance.htm).

15.3 DIETARY NEEDS OF OLDER ADULTS

15.3.1 FLUIDS

One of the most important aspects of nutrition, regardless of age and activity level, is fluid intake. Indeed, the human body is approximately 60% water and even slight dehydration (<2%) can negatively affect performance in athletes of any age (Barr 1999). Older athletes are at an increased risk of dehydration because of a number of age-related changes including decreased renal function (Rolls and Phillips 1990), decreased thirst sensitivity (Kenney and Chiu 2001), and reduced ability to dissipate heat (Kenney et al. 1990). Subsequently, older athletes may intake insufficient fluids to meet the demands of exercise. Insufficient fluid intake is not only detrimental to performance but also poses serious risk of heat-related illness.

As with all aspects of nutrition, the best approach to combating inadequate thirst mechanisms is to have a plan. To that end, older athletes should be intentional about consuming adequate fluids prior to, during, and following exercise. Athletes should consume plenty of fluids in the 24 hours prior to exercise, which for most athletes is daily (American College of Sports Medicine et al. 2007). In the 2–3 hours preceding exercise, approximately 14–22 oz of fluid should be consumed, followed by approximately 6–12 oz every 15–20 minutes during a training session. Furthermore, in cases where the duration of aerobic exercise exceeds 60 minutes, water may alone be inadequate to optimally rehydrate the athlete. Commercial sports drinks are useful for supplying glucose and electrolytes that are lost during extended activity. Finally, athletes should also record their body weight prior to and following exercise and, upon completion of exercise, ingest 16–24 oz of fluid for every pound of body weight lost.

15.3.2 ENERGY

Consuming an adequate number of calories is important for all athletes because insufficient caloric intake will likely result in muscle and bone catabolism as well as increased risk of fatigue, injury, and/or illness (Campbell and Geik 2004). Energy requirements for older adults are typically lower than for younger people, partially as a consequence of decreased metabolic rate secondary to age-related muscle loss. On the other hand, older athletes need to match energy intake to their level of physical activity. Consequently, the energy needs of older athletes are probably lower than younger athletes but higher than older sedentary people. Some athletes may choose to consult with a dietitian or sports nutritionist to determine specific energy requirements, whereas others may prefer to monitor body weight, body composition, and quality of training bouts as a gauge of energy needs.

15.3.3 CARBOHYDRATES

Carbohydrates are important for all athletes to provide energy throughout the body, including exercising muscles and the brain. Furthermore, carbohydrates maintain blood glucose during exercise and restore muscle glycogen during recovery from exercise. A general recommendation for athletes is to consume between 6 and 10 g/kg/day, depending on the type, volume, and intensity of exercise, in addition to interpersonal factors (e.g., body weight and gender) and environmental conditions (American College of Sports Medicine, American Dietetic Association, and Dietitians of Canada 2000). For endurance sports, carbohydrate intake should be increased in the days prior to competition to "load" muscle with glycogen as higher glycogen concentrations are associated with improved times to exhaustion and performance. This recommendation seems pertinent to older adults because they appear to maintain the capacity to store muscle glycogen (Campbell and Geik 2004); however, no study has formally examined a carbohydrate-loading protocol in older adults.

15.3.4 PROTEIN

In recent years, experts have increasingly recognized the importance of dietary protein for maintenance of muscle mass in aging people, gaining muscle mass in conjunction with resistance training, and maintaining musculoskeletal integrity following prolonged endurance exercise. Furthermore, adequate protein intake is also critical for maintaining proper immune function during periods of intense training (Calder 2006).

In the post-absorptive state, mixed muscle protein synthesis rates do not appear to differ between young and old adults (Volpi et al. 2001). Similarly, reports indicate that aging does not reduce muscle protein synthesis in response to a high-protein (25–30 g) meal (Paddon-Jones and Rasmussen 2009; Volpi et al. 2001). However, protein synthesis declines in older adults when meals contain minimal amino acids or the amino acids are ingested in conjunction with carbohydrates (Guillet et al. 2004; Volpi et al. 2000). Researchers have attributed this defect to an age-related state of insulin resistance (Guillet et al. 2004) and to reduced or slowed responsiveness of the aged muscle to amino acids (Drummond et al. 2008; Wolfe 2006).

Additionally, low-grade chronic inflammation, which is common among older persons, may also directly impair protein synthesis (Balage et al. 2009). Evidence also exists suggesting that these impairments in amino-acid accumulation may be at least partially ablated by intake of essential amino acids (i.e., leucine, isoleucine, and valine) (Dillon et al. 2009; Henderson et al. 2009). Most notably, a number of studies suggest that leucine may be the most critical amino acid for stimulation of muscle protein synthesis (Anthony et al. 2002; Combaret et al. 2005; Holecek et al. 2001; Katsanos et al. 2006). However, further study is needed to confirm this hypothesis.

During the aging process, adequate protein intake is necessary to combat the age-related loss of skeletal muscle, a process known as sarcopenia. A recent study indicated that over the course of three years, older adults who consumed more than the recommended dietary allowance (RDA) for protein of 0.8 g/kg/day experienced the smallest losses of lean mass (Houston et al. 2008). In contrast, persons who experienced the most significant muscle atrophy consumed protein in quantities either at or below the RDA. This study is significant because it adds to a growing body of literature suggesting that the current RDA for protein intake may not be adequate to maintain optimal skeletal muscle health in older adults (Evans et al. 2008; Look AHEAD Research Group et al. 2007; Morais et al. 2006; Sood et al. 2008). Paddon-Jones and Rasmussen (2009) have also suggested that a good protein source should be ingested with each meal.

Consequently, the RDA is likely insufficient for older athletes, particularly those engaging in resistance training. Older individuals who consume inadequate amounts of protein are unlikely to gain muscle mass and strength while engaging in resistance training (Rolland et al. 2008). This problem can lead to significant impairments in performance for athletes participating in sports that require significant muscle strength and/or power. Studies by Campbell and colleagues (Campbell et al. 1999a; Campbell and Leidy 2007) demonstrate that older athletes performing regular resistance exercise should ensure that their dietary protein intake is between 1.0 and 1.2 g/kg/day and that the sources of protein are primarily those with complete amino acid profiles such as eggs, milk, beef, and fish.

No study to date has evaluated the protein requirements of older endurance athletes; however, data suggest that top endurance athletes in younger age groups require dietary protein up to 1.6 or 1.7 g/kg/day. Tarnopolsky (2008) stated that it would be "nearly impossible" for older endurance athletes to maintain a training volume that would warrant such a high protein intake and suggests that 1.0–1.2 g/kg/day is likely sufficient for these athletes as well.

15.3.5 Fat

No evidence exists to suggest that the dietary need for fat differs significantly between younger and older athletes. However, older people should consider the type and quantity of dietary fats to prevent disease, but these choices have little relevance to sport performance (Campbell and Geik 2004). All people should strive to obtain approximately 20–35% of total energy from fat sources, and this recommendation allows for significant variability in eating styles. Specific recommendations exist for polyunsaturated intakes for older men and older women. Omega-6 fatty acids (linoleic) should be consumed at a rate of 14 g/day for older men and 11 g/day for older women, whereas omega-3 fatty acids (linolenic) should be consumed at a rate of 1.6 g/day for men and 1.1 g/day for women (Campbell and Geik, 2004). These recommendations are suitable for older athletes as well.

15.3.6 MICRONUTRIENTS

Regular training, especially intense exercise, may increase an athlete's requirement for vitamins and minerals above recommended levels as a result of increased metabolism, biochemical adaptations associated with training, increased concentrations of mitochondrial enzymes that require a nutrient as a cofactor, and the need for tissue maintenance and repair (Manore 2000). Sedentary individuals may not notice the effects of marginal micronutrient deficiencies. However, inadequate micronutrient intakes by athletes may adversely affect performance because of small impairments in exercise capacity (Maughan 1999). Older athletes, because of factors discussed earlier in the chapter, may be at a greater risk of micronutrient deficiencies than younger athletes (Table 15.4). Furthermore, deficiencies are most likely to occur in those athletes who restrict calorie intake, leave out one or numerous food groups from their dietary intake, practice severe methods of weight loss, or consume "empty-calorie" foods and/or beverages in place of foods and beverages that are more nutrient-dense (American Dietetic Association et al. 2009).

Vitamin and mineral supplementation is appropriate when scientific evidence supports safety and efficacy. Because some groups of physically active people may be at increased risk of nutrient depletion, the use of a vitamin and mineral supplement, not exceeding the dietary reference intake (DRI) may be consumed as a preventive measure (Rodriguez et al. 2009). Regarding the DRI, the Institute of Medicine of the U.S. National Academy of Sciences makes micronutrient recommendations based on the culmination of scientific evidence and uses four values to define adequate vitamin and mineral intake in the human diet:

- Estimated average requirement: the amount of a nutrient deemed sufficient to meet the needs of approximately 50% of healthy people in the United States in a given age and gender group.
- Recommended dietary allowance: the amount of a nutrient that is considered to be adequate to meet the needs of 97.5% of the healthy United States population in each age and gender group. The RDA recommendations are typically used in planning the diets of individuals or making individual nutrient recommendations.
- Adequate intake (AI): When there is insufficient evidence to determine an RDA, an AI is set based the on typical nutrient intake of people in a given age and gender group. This value is used *in place* of the RDA for planning and evaluating individual diets. No nutrient has both an RDA and an AI.

TABLE 15.4
Micronutrients of Special Concern for Older Athletes

Micronutrient	Function	DRI	UL	Rationale for use in older adults	Recommendations
Vitamin A	Important to maintain normal vision, for cell differentiation, efficient immune function, and genetic expression	Women 50–70 years: 700 μg >70 years: 700 μg Men 50–70 years: 900 μg >70 years: 900 μg	3000 mg	Some researchers have recommended that current recommendations be set at lower levels because although the vitamin A intake for many older adults is below current recommendations, their vitamin A levels remain normal.	Current DRIs for retinol may be too high; older athletes should focus on consuming vitamin A precursors, the carotenoids.
Riboflavin	Coenzyme in energy metabolism	Women 50–70 years: 1.1 mg >70 years: 1.1 mg Men 50–70 years: 1.3 mg >70 years: 1.3 mg	ND	Riboflavin requirements were increased in endurance-trained older women (50–67 years).	Russell and Suter (1993) suggested increasing to 1.3 and 1.7 mg/day for women and men, respectively; a high-carbohydrate intake may enhance bacterial synthesis of riboflavin and thus decrease dietary riboflavin needs.
Vitamin B₆	Coenzyme in the metabolism of amino acids and glycogen	Women 50–70 years: 1.5 mg >70 years: 1.5 mg Men 50–70 years:1.7 mg >70 years: 1.7 mg	100 mg	It is not completely understood why age affects vitamin B₆ requirements, but some studies have increased needs and shown compromised immunity with inadequate B₆.	Sacheck and Roubenoff (1999) suggested an increase to 2.0 mg/day for women and men.
Folate	Coenzyme in the metabolism of amino acids and nucleic acids and red blood cell formation; prevents megaloblastic anemia	Women 50–70 years: 400 μg >70 years: 400 μg Men 50–70 years: 400 μg >70 years: 400 μg	1000 μg	Decreases in stomach acid because of atrophic gastritis can lead to decrease absorption of folate and hence increase the risk of anemia.	The latest DRI (1998) for folate was increased from the 1989 RDA of 180 μg/day for women and 200 μg/day for men.

continued

TABLE 15.4   (CONTINUED)
Micronutrients of Special Concern for Older Athletes

Micronutrient	Function		DRI	UL	Rationale for use in older adults	Recommendations
Vitamin B$_{12}$	Coenzyme in the metabolism of nucleic acids; prevents megaloblastic anemia; required for red blood cell production	Women 50–70 years: 2.4 µg >70 years: 2.4 µg Men 50–70 years: 2.4 µg >70 years: 2.4 µg		ND	Atrophic gastritis, not uncommon in older individuals, decreases stomach acid and intrinsic factor secretion, which can lead to malabsorption of vitamin B$_{12}$ and risk of anemia.	Sacheck and Roubenoff (1999) suggested an increase to 2.8 µg/day for women and men, particularly for vegetarian athletes.
Vitamin C	Antioxidant; protects body tissues from oxidative damage; enhances iron absorption	Women 50–70 years: 75 mg >70 years: 75 mg Men 50–70 years: 90 mg >70 years: 90 mg		2000mg	Supplementation may offer protection against health problems typically encountered as one ages. There is no clear consensus as to whether extra vitamin C is necessary or beneficial for intense training.	The latest DRI for vitamin C (2000) was increased from 1989 RDA of 60 mg for men and women.
Vitamin D	Promotes growth and mineralization of bones by maintaining calcium and phosphorus homeostasis; enhances absorption of calcium; modulates phagocyte and lymphocyte immune cells	Women 50–70 years: 10 µg >70 years: 15 µg Men 50–70 years: 10 µg >70 years: 15 µg		50 µg	The skin of an older person is less able to synthesize vitamin D; less exposure to sunlight due to clothing, northern latitude, and indoor training may further compromise vitamin D status.	Vitamin D requirements for adults >70 years were increased from 10 µg in 1987 to 15 µg in 1997.
Vitamin E	Antioxidant; protects body tissues from increased oxidative damage	Women 50–70 years: 15 mg >70 years: 15 mg Men 50–70 years: 15 mg >70 years: 15 mg		1000 µg	Supplementation may offer protection against health problems typically encountered as one ages. There is no clear consensus as to whether extra vitamin E is necessary or beneficial for intense training.	The latest DRI for vitamin E (2000) was increased from 1989 RDA of 8 mg for women and 10 mg for men. Endurance trained athletes may consider a daily supplement of 100–200 mg.

Nutrient	Function	RDA/AI	UL	Comments	
Calcium	Required for blood clotting, muscle contraction, nerve transmission, and bone health	Women 50–70 years: 1200 mg >70 years: 1200 mg Men 50–70 years: 1200 mg >70 years: 1200 mg	2500 mg	Older athletes whose bone density and/or dietary intakes are low are at particular risk of stress fractures, especially with high impact, repetitive sport activities. Atrophic gastritis negatively affects calcium bioavailability. Low vitamin D intake also hinders calcium absorption; calcium is lost by sweat.	If an older athlete is unable to consume adequate dietary calcium, then a supplement is warranted.
Iron	Required as a component of hemoglobin and myoglobin and for enzyme transportation within blood and muscle tissue; prevents microsytic hypochromitic anemia	Women 50–70 years: 8 mg >70 years: 8 mg Men 50–70 years: 8 mg >70 years: 8 mg	45 mg	Because iron stores tend to increase with age, older individuals have less need for dietary iron.	Sacheck and Roubenoff (1999) suggested that older women and vegetarian athletes who partake in endurance training in temperature extremes consume up to 15 mg/day.
Magnesium	Involved in more than 300 enzymatic reactions including glycolysis, fat and protein metabolism, adenosine triphosphate hydrolysis, and the second-messenger system	Women 50–70 years: 320 mg >70 years: 320 mg Men 50–70 years: 420 mg >70 years: 420 mg	ND	Intakes of magnesium in elderly people may be marginal, but even in individuals with atrophic gastritis, there does not appear to be any interference with magnesium absorption.	There is no indication that elderly adults have needs different from younger adults.
Zinc	Required for the structure and activity of more than 300 enzymes nucleic acid, protein synthesis, cellular differentiation and replication, and glucose use and insulin secretion	Women 50–70 years: 11 mg >70 years: 11 mg Men 50–70 years: 8 mg >70 years: 8 mg	40 mg	Zinc requirements may be increased for older power, team players, or endurance athletes undertaking high-intensity training.	Pregnant and lactating women may need to increase to 11 and 12 mg/day, respectively. Vegetarian athletes may need to take in a two-fold greater intake compared with those who eat meat.

Source: Adapted from Campbell, W. W., and R. A. Geik. 2004. Nutritional considerations for the older athlete. *Nutrition* 20: 603–608.

- Tolerable upper intake level (UL): The UL is the maximum amount of a given nutrient that may be consumed without toxicity symptoms. Only nutrients with distinct toxicity symptoms have a UL.

In summary, in this chapter, we will use either the RDA or the AI components of the DRI to describe the nutrient needs of older people. The American College of Sports Medicine, American Dietetic Association, and Dietitians of Canada encourage athletes to strive to consume diets that provide at least the DRI for all micronutrients from food (American Dietetic Association et al. 2009). Older competitive athletes should consult a registered dietitian to evaluate the adequacy of their nutrient intakes prior to micronutrient supplementation. Deficiencies in vitamins B_{12} and D, as well as calcium, are among the most common micronutrient deficiencies observed in older athletes. We will discuss the age-related challenges in consuming adequate amounts of these nutrients here. Information regarding other age-sensitive micronutrients can be found in Table 15.4.

15.3.6.1   Vitamin B_{12}

Vitamin B_{12}, or cobalamin, is essential for DNA synthesis, neural health, and cell division. Cobalamin is required for DNA synthesis and cell division. This is especially relevant for the aging athlete because red blood cells turn over every 2–3 months, and these cells are required for oxygen transport. Impairments in red–blood-cell production are likely to have serious consequences on exercise performance and overall health.

One common cause of cobalamin deficiency in older adults is a reduced intake of meat. Often meat intake may decrease because of the expense, chewing difficulty, or physician recommendation in response to elevated blood lipids (Chernoff 2005). Even if cobalamin intake is maintained at previously sufficient levels, cobalamin status may become insufficient because of digestive changes associated with aging. Absorption of the nutrient is largely dependent upon endogenously secreted intrinsic factor (IF), which is synthesized in the gastric parietal cells. Although IF is released in the stomach, it binds to cobalamin in the small intestine and enables absorption of the vitamin. In older age, the parietal cells may fail to secrete IF, which results in a functional vitamin B_{12} deficiency despite adequate B_{12} intake.

As a consequence, older athletes are at increased risk of pernicious anemia, which is characterized by a megaloblastic anemia, similar to that observed in a folic-acid deficiency. Red blood cells in a person with pernicious anemia are unusually large and have an irregular and globular shape, resulting in reduced oxygen-carrying capacity. Cobalamin deficiency is also associated with elevated blood homocysteine, an important mediator in the development of cardiovascular disease (Humphrey et al. 2008). If deficiency persists, older adults may also experience neurological symptoms including permanent nerve damage.

Scientists have suggested that the DRI for vitamin B_{12} should be increased in older people undertaking regular exercise, particularly those who are vegetarians or have atrophic gastritis (Sacheck and Roubenoff 1999). Others have recommended an increase in intake to 150% of the current U.S. DRI recommendations (2.4 µg/day) or between 2.8 and 3.6 µg/day of B_{12} to prevent deficiency symptoms (Russell and Suter 1993). Older athletes may meet these needs by consuming cobalamin-rich foods such as liver meats, fish and shellfish, beef, pork, poultry, eggs, milk, and milk products or a vitamin supplement. Notably, vegetarian athletes should pay special attention to intake of cobalamin through supplements because no known vegetarian sources exist.

15.3.6.2 Vitamin D

The primary function of vitamin D is to regulate the calcium status of the blood, but it is also an essential nutrient in maintaining immune function (Marian and Sacks 2009). The majority of people meet their vitamin D needs through endogenous production in sun-exposed skin cells (Holick 1995), which permits the conversion of a cholesterol precursor to previtamin D. There are, however, some food sources of this vitamin, including fish, beef liver, cheese, and egg yolks, and milk is usually fortified with vitamin D. Both dietary and endogenously produced vitamin D are activated by two hydroxylations, one each in the liver and kidney. This active form of vitamin D enhances the absorption of calcium from the small intestine and stimulates the osteoclasts to release bone calcium in order to prevent hypocalcemic tetany (DeLuca 1988).

Chronic vitamin D deficiency places older people at greater risk of developing osteomalacia, which is a softening of the bones that may result in susceptibility to bone fractures, muscle weakness, and extensive bone pain. Additionally, research indicates that a chronic deficiency of vitamin D may increase one's risk of developing hypertension and type 1 diabetes mellitus (Holick 1995). Older people are at greater risk of vitamin D deficiency because of decreased sun exposure, decreased ability to endogenously produce vitamin D, and impaired activation of the vitamin in the kidney (Gloth et al. 1995a, 1995b; Gloth and Tobin 1995).

A large proportion of Americans over 50 years of age are deficient in vitamin D; thus, the DRI was increased in 1997 to 10 µg/day in males and females over 51 years of age and 15 µg/day in those individuals over 70 years of age (Institute of Medicine 1997). Vitamin D supplementation may be needed in older persons, including older athletes who have difficulty meeting recommendations by dietary means, little exposure to sunlight, or dark skin. Moreover, severe deficiencies may require high-dose supplements prescribed by a physician.

15.3.6.3 Calcium

Calcium is an essential mineral that many older athletes, especially women, consume in inadequate amounts. Calcium is essential for neuromuscular transmission, blood coagulation, muscular contraction, and bone health. This mineral is particularly important for athletes (McArdle et al. 2008). Both males and females experience greater rates of bone resorption, as compared to bone formation, in older age; therefore, adequate dietary calcium intake is especially important in older people (Lewis and Modlesky 1998). Chronic calcium deficiency places older people at greater risk of developing osteoporosis, a significant loss of bone mass that predisposes older adults to fractures and falls. Although lifelong habits of weight-bearing activity may stave off osteoporosis to some extent, older athletes who have low bone density and poor dietary intakes of calcium are at high risk of stress fractures during activities requiring repetitive impact (Heaney and Bachmann 2005). Moreover, such repetitive impact activities (e.g., running), particularly in a hot or humid environment, may lead to significant calcium loss via sweating (Bullen et al. 1999).

Calcium needs are 200 mg/day higher for older people than younger people (1200 and 1000 mg/day, respectively). However, calcium-balance studies have supported intakes as high as 1500 mg/day for older females (Dawson-Hughes et al. 1990). Calcium recommendations may be met fairly easily given wide availability of dietary and supplemental sources; dairy foods and fortified products such as soymilk, orange juice, and breakfast cereals are all rich in calcium. Despite fortification of common products, research has consistently shown that a large percentage of older males and females from industrialized countries have calcium intakes below the DRI (Bates et al. 2002). Therefore, calcium supplements may be warranted, especially in those people who are lactose intolerant, dislike milk and dairy products, are allergic to milk, or cannot meet these calcium requirements through other dietary means. Supplements of calcium citrate malate are better absorbed than calcium-carbonate supplements in postmenopausal women with low dietary intakes of calcium and may more effectively reduce bone demineralization and fractures (Dawson-Hughes et al. 1990).

15.4 NUTRITIONAL SUPPLEMENTATION FOR THE OLDER ATHLETE

Older competitors are increasing interested in nutritional strategies designed to: 1) maximize resistance and/or endurance performance, 2) enhance adaptations from exercise, and 3) quicken recovery post-exercise. The scientific evidence for the efficacy of such strategies in older athletes is growing in parallel. For the sake of simplicity, exercise modalities will be divided into two general categories: resistance exercise (e.g., weight training, high intensity/power sports) and endurance exercise (e.g., running, cycling, cross-country skiing). The primary outcome measures for resistance training studies are gains in fat-free mass, strength, and functional capacity. The primary outcome measures for endurance exercise training programs are increases in aerobic capacity (VO_{2max}/VO_{2peak}) and changes in body composition (i.e., decreased body fat). Ergogenic aids that have yielded significant improvements in measurable outcome variables in controlled research studies are included in this book chapter.

15.4.1 PROTEIN AND AMINO-ACID SUPPLEMENTATION

Adequate dietary protein intake is essential to maintain skeletal muscle mass; protein intake may also be a treatment of sarcopenia, which is the age-related loss of skeletal muscle mass and quality (Dreyer and Volpi 2005). The RDA for protein is 0.8 g/kg/day for all men and women aged 19 years and above, independent of physical activity status (Institute of Medicine of National Academies 2002/2005). The American College of Sports Medicine, American Dietetic Association, and Dietitians of Canada joint position statement on nutrition and athletic performance for younger adults indicates that athletes may require 50–100% more protein for exercise-related energy production, exercise-induced muscle damage repair, and muscle hypertrophy (American College of Sports Medicine, American Dietetic Association, and Dietitians of Canada 2000).

In a recent review, Campbell and Leidy (2007) performed a retrospective assessment of resistance training study data to determine whether the level of protein intake, in conjunction with resistance training, influences fat-free mass accretion, muscle morphology, and strength in older people. The data were compiled from 106 men and women aged 50–80 years who participated in diet and resistance training studies conducted by Campbell and colleagues over a 15-year period (Campbell et al. 1995, 1999a, 1999b, 2002a, 2002b; Iglay et al. 2007). Taken together, these studies suggest that resistance training-induced changes in muscle strength and size were not enhanced when older people increased their protein intake either by increasing the ingestion of higher-protein foods or consuming protein-enriched nutritional supplements.

The timing of protein supplementation or feeding may have limited the effect of the treatment on the adaptive response to long-term resistance training in these studies, however. Esmarck et al. (2001) reported that the timing of protein intake after resistance exercise influences the potential for skeletal muscle hypertrophy following exercise training in older people. In one study, older men who consumed a milk and soy-based protein supplement (10 g of protein, 100 kcal of energy) immediately after resistance exercise experienced increases in whole body fat-free mass (1.8%), cross-sectional area of the quadriceps femoris muscle group (7%), and mean fiber area of the vastus lateralis (24%) in response to a 12-week period of resistance training. Meanwhile, men who consumed the same supplement 2 hours after exercising experienced blunted responses (−1.5% fat-free mass, 0.2% quadriceps femoris cross-sectional area, −4.9% muscle vastus lateralis mean fiber area). In contrast, results from several other studies (Andrews et al. 2006; Candow et al. 2008; Carter et al. 2005) suggest that the ingestion of protein-containing supplements soon after resistance exercise sessions do not influence muscle hypertrophy and increased fat-free mass responses to training.

An explanation for the lack of effect of timed protein intake pre- and/or post-exercise could be total protein intake ingested by participants. Recently, Verdijk et al. (2009) examined timed protein supplementation immediately before and after each exercise session (3 sessions/week, 20 g of protein/session) for 12 weeks in 26 healthy older men who habitually consumed adequate amounts of dietary protein. Muscle hypertrophy was assessed at the whole-body (dual-energy x-ray absorptiometry), limb (computed tomography), and muscle-fiber (biopsy) level. Despite overall significant increases in 1RM strength, leg muscle mass, and type II fiber area, there was no difference between the groups.

The results suggested that resistance-training–induced improvements in muscle mass and strength are not enhanced when older people who consume adequate amounts of dietary protein (in excess of the RDA) further increase their protein intake. Taken together, the results from Campbell's lab and others suggest that protein-enriched nutritional supplements, whether consumed immediately after or separate from the exercise sessions, do not significantly enhance the resistance-training–induced strength, body composition, muscle hypertrophy, and physical function, especially when older adults are ingesting their dietary protein intake over 0.8

g/kg/day (more appropriately between 1.0 and 1.2 g/kg/day). However, Paddon-Jones and Rasmussen (2009) have suggested that each bolus of protein intake should be >25 g for adequate protein synthesis, so the individual boluses of protein given during these studies may have been insufficient. Future studies are needed to determine whether a larger amount of protein intake at each meal would lead to differing results.

15.4.2 CREATINE MONOHYDRATE

Creatine monohydrate (CrM) has been studied extensively over the past 20 years as a nutritional supplement and ergogenic aid for athletes (Kreider 2003; Rawson and Volek 2003; Williams and Branch 1998). Investigations into creatine's role in energy (adenosine triphosphate) production can be found as early as 1914 (Denis and Folin 1914), when consumption of CrM (20 g/day for 5–6 days) increased muscle creatine (Cr) concentrations (by ~25 mmol/kg of dry mass). However, despite several problems with the study (i.e., no standardization of dosage based on subjects body weight, age of subjects varied from 20–62 years, and both males and females were used), it was the first study to demonstrate increased creatine content of muscle following this supplementation protocol. Numerous studies since have consistently reported that ingestion of CrM at a rate of 20–30 g/day for 5–6 days increases total muscle creatine concentration (TCr) in both human and animal models by 15–40%. Furthermore, an expert committee from the American College of Sports Medicine Roundtable meeting suggested a subsequent daily maintenance dosage of 2 g/day to sufficiently maintain these elevated TCr stores (Terjung et al. 2000).

Because low initial intramuscular creatine levels respond better to CrM supplementation than higher resting creatine levels, researchers have suggested that older individuals who have lower resting creatine concentrations may show greater increases in intramuscular creatine levels following CrM supplementation and thus respond better to supplementation than young people (Tarnopolsky 2008). However, the data are inconsistent with regard to this issue (Conley et al. 2000; McCully et al. 1991), since a previous study indicates that Cr content in muscles from older people is higher than in younger people (Rawson et al. 2002).

To date, available evidence regarding the effects of CrM supplementation in older adults is equivocal because numerous studies have reported both improvements and/or no change in numerous measures of body composition and muscle performance. One possible explanation for these interstudy differences in observed outcomes may be interindividual responses to CrM supplementation. Three types of response to creatine have been described, including responders or individuals who experience a >20 mmol·kg^{-1} per day increase in TCr; quasiresponders or individuals who experience a 10–20 mmol·kg^{-1} per day increase in TCr; and nonresponders or individuals who experience <10 mmol·kg^{-1} dw increase in total creatine (Greenhaff et al. 1994; Syrotuik and Bell 2004). Those that are considered "responders" normally show benefits in body composition and athletic performance.

Despite equivocal findings, well-designed studies have reported CrM supplementation to safely enhance muscle strength (Chrusch et al. 2001; Gotshalk et al. 2002, 2008) and hypertrophy (Brose et al. 2003; Candow et al. 2008; Gotshalk et al. 2002), in older adults. Of equal interest, such results have been observed in response to relatively short interventions (5–7 days of creatine supplementation). Therefore, creatine supplementation should be considered a safe, inexpensive, and often effective nutritional intervention to potentially help slow the rate of muscle wasting with age, particularly when consumed in conjunction with a resistance-training regimen.

15.4.3 B-Hydroxy-b-methyl Butyrate

b-Hydroxy-b-methyl butyrate (HMB), a downstream metabolite of leucine, has been studied for its purported ability to act as an anti-catabolic, lipolytic dietary supplement leading to gains in strength, muscle size, recovery, fat oxidation, and fat loss in humans when used in conjunction with a resistance training program (Rowlands and Thomson 2009). With some evidential support, HMB has become a popular nutritional supplement for strength and body-building athletes looking to improve strength and muscle size (Kreider 1999; Nissen and Sharp 2003). Several mechanisms of action of HMB have been proposed, largely on the basis of extrapolation from early research on animal carcasses and deduction from indirect measures in humans (Nissen et al. 1996; Slater and Jenkins 2000). Supplementation with HMB may attenuate training-induced proteolysis in the muscle via down-regulation of proteolytic pathways (Nissen et al. 1996; Slater and Jenkins 2000; Smith et al. 2005) and may also stimulate protein synthesis similarly to leucine (Smith et al. 2005).

In the sarcoplasm, HMB is thought to be metabolized to b-hydroxy-b-methyl-glutaryl-coenzyme A, providing a readily available carbon source for cholesterol synthesis, which in turn provides material for muscle cell growth (Nissen et al. 1996). Also, HMB may undergo polymerization and be used as a structural component of the cell membrane, leading to enhanced stability. Additionally, HMB has been proposed to increase muscle cell fatty-acid oxidation capacity. One study has reported that 8 weeks of resistance training in conjunction with 3 g/day of HMB significantly reduced body fat and tended to increase lean muscle mass in older adults (approximately 70 years of age) as compared to a placebo rice flour (Vukovich et al. 2001). Because the fat-free mass gains in this study only manifested as a trend, and given there was no change in strength and that no subsequent studies have been completed in older adults, the use of HMB cannot be recommended for this population until further research is conducted.

15.4.4 Caffeine

Caffeine (1,3,7-trimethylxanthine) is not only a component of common drinks including coffee, tea, and soda but is also a potential ergogenic aid for endurance athletes. The mechanism most often noted for the ergogenic effects of caffeine is its ability to stimulate the central nervous system (CNS). CNS effects are then transferred through the neuromuscular system to the skeletal muscle, thereby altering metabolic priorities of the muscle (Spriet 1995). Caffeine appears to act largely by decreasing reliance on glycogen utilization and increasing dependence on free fatty acid mobilization (Erickson et al. 1987; Ivy et al. 1979). Essig and Van Handel (1980) reported a significant increase in intramuscular fat oxidation during leg ergometer cycling when subjects consumed caffeine at an approximate dose of

5 mg/kg. Additionally, Spriet et al. (1992) demonstrated reduced net glycogenolysis at the beginning of exercise (cycling to exhaustion at 80% VO_{2max}), following ingestion of a high dose of caffeine (9 mg/kg). Consequently, performance was significantly improved, suggesting an enhanced reliance on both intra- and extramuscular fat oxidation.

Caffeine ingestion of approximately 6 mg/kg increases the endurance of young people exercising at 60–85% of their maximal oxygen uptake. It also seems to improve endurance as measured by repeated submaximal isometric contraction and decreases in the rate of perceived exertion during exercise. Despite these observations from young persons, only one study has examined its ergogenic effects in the elderly (Norager et al. 2005). The randomized, double-blind, placebo-controlled, crossover study was conducted in 15 men and 15 women recruited by their general practitioner. Participants abstained from caffeine for 48 h and were randomized to receive one capsule of placebo and then caffeine (6 mg/kg) or caffeine and then placebo with 1 week in between. One hour after intervention, reaction and movement times, postural stability, walking speed, cycling at 65% of expected maximal heart rate, perceived effort during cycling, maximal isometric arm flexion strength, and endurance were measured. Caffeine increased cycling endurance by 25% and isometric arm flexion endurance by 54%. Caffeine also reduced the rating of perceived exertion after 5 minutes of cycling by 11% and postural stability with eyes open by 25%. Caffeine ingestion did not affect muscle strength, walking speed, reaction, and movement times. These authors later reported caffeine-induced increases in plasma epinephrine and norepinephrine (Norager et al. 2006), possibly explaining the beneficial effects on performance. These results at least suggest that caffeine ingestion elicits a metabolic response in elderly participants (~70 years) similar to that seen in younger subjects.

15.5 TRAINING TABLE: SUGGESTIONS FOR OLDER ATHLETES

Listed here are a few basic nutritional guidelines for older athletes based on the principals described in this chapter:

- Consume fluid liberally prior to exercise and 6–12 oz every 15–20 minutes during exercise if tolerable.
- Consume 16–24 oz of fluid for every pound of body weight lost during training sessions or competitions.
- Consume ≥0.8 g/kg of dietary protein/day, including a protein source at every meal.
- Follow traditional recommendations for carbohydrate intake (i.e., 6–10 g/kg/day).
- Use of a multi-vitamin supplement will likely prove beneficial; however, an awareness of adequate intakes is necessary.
- Be aware that many medications can have interactions with each other and different foods. Consulting a physician and possibly a sports nutritionist is recommended when multiple interactions may be present or when the athlete wishes to add a new nutritional supplement to his/her diet.

15.6 CONCLUSION

A physically active lifestyle is widely accepted as a critical component of preventing chronic disease, especially in advanced age. Older adults who continue to perform regular exercise are a small minority and among the healthiest of older persons. Still, several physiologic changes create nutritional challenges for physically active and competitive older people. Moreover, their high activity levels and subsequent increased energy expenditure and micronutrient turnover may create nutritional challenges not experienced by their sedentary counterparts. These older athletes should be strongly encouraged to continue their active lifestyles but should also be encouraged to match nutrient intake to activity to avoid nutrient deficiencies and dehydration. This proactive approach may help prevent health complications associated with nutrient deficiency and maximize performance for older people who engage in formal competition. Knowledge of safe, potentially efficacious nutritional supplement strategies may also give these competitors a leg up on their competition. An effective nutritional plan for these athletes should start with self-education supplemented by sound advice from physicians, trainers, dietitians, and/or sports nutritionists.

REFERENCES

American College of Sports Medicine, American Dietetic Association, and Dieticians of Canada. 2000. Joint position statement: Nutrition and athletic performance. *Med Sci Sports Exerc* 32: 2130–2145.

American College of Sports Medicine, M. N. Sawka, L. M. Burke, E. R. Eichner, R. J. Maughan, S. J. Montain, and N. S. Stachenfeld. 2007. American College of Sports medicine position stand: Exercise and fluid replacement. *Med Sci Sports Exerc* 39: 377–390.

American Dietetic Association, Dieticians of Canada, American College of Sports Medicine, N. R. Rodriguez, N. M. Di Marco, and S. Langley. 2009. *Med Sci Sports Exerc* 41: 709–731.

Andrews, R. D., D. A. MacLean, and S. E. Riechman. 2006. Protein intake for skeletal muscle hypertrophy with resistance training in seniors. *Int J Sport Nutr Exerc Metabol* 16: 362–372.

Anthony, J. C., A. K. Reiter, T. G. Anthony, S. J. Crozier, C. H. Lang, D. A. MacLean, S. R. Kimball, and L. S. Jefferson. 2002. Orally administered leucine enhances protein synthesis in skeletal muscle of diabetic rats in the absence of increases in 4E-BP1 or S6K1 phosphorylation. *Diabetes* 51: 928–936.

Balage, M., J. Averous, D. Remond, C. Bos, E. Pujos-Guillot, I. Papet, L. Mosoni, L. Combaret, and D. Dardevet. 2009. Presence of low-grade inflammation impaired postprandial stimulation of muscle protein synthesis in old rats. *J Nutr Biochem* 2010 21(4): 325–331.

Barr, S. I. 1999. Effects of dehydration on exercise performance. *Can J Appl Physiol* 24: 164–172.

Bates, C. J., D. Benton, H. K. Biesalski, H. B. Staehelin, W. van Staveren, P. Stehle, P. M. Suter, and G. Wolfram. 2002. Nutrition and aging: A consensus statement. *J Nutr Health Aging* 6: 103–116.

Bengston, V. L., D. Gans, N. M. Putney, and M. Silverstein. 2009. *Handbook of Theories of Aging*, 2nd Ed. New York: Springer.

Brady, A. 2008. Managing the patient with dysphagia. *Home Healthcare Nurse* 26: 41, 46; quiz 47–48.

Brose, A., G. Parise, and M. A. Tarnopolsky. 2003. Creatine supplementation enhances isometric strength and body composition improvements following strength exercise training in older adults. *J Gerontol Series A Biol Sci Med Sci* 58: 11–19.

Bullen, D. B., M. L. O'Toole, and K. C. Johnson. 1999. Calcium losses resulting from an acute bout of moderate-intensity exercise. *Int J Sport Nutr* 9: 275–284.

Calder, P. C. 2006. Branched-chain amino acids and immunity. *J Nutr* 136(1 Suppl): 288S–293S.

Campbell, W. W., M. L. Barton, Jr., D. Cyr-Campbell, S. L. Davey, J. L. Beard, G. Parise, and W. J. Evans. 1999a. Effects of an omnivorous diet compared with a lacto-ovo-vegetarian diet on resistance-training-induced changes in body composition and skeletal muscle in older men. *Am J Clin Nutr* 70: 1032–1039.

Campbell, W. W., M. C. Crim, V. R. Young, L. J. Joseph, and W. J. Evans. 1995. Effects of resistance training and dietary protein intake on protein metabolism in older adults. *Am J Physiol* 268: E1143–E1153.

Campbell, W. W., and R. A. Geik. 2004. Nutritional considerations for the older athlete. *Nutrition* 20: 603–608.

Campbell, W. W., L. J. Joseph, R. A. Anderson, S. L. Davey, J. Hinton, and W. J. Evans. 2002a. Effects of resistive training and chromium picolinate on body composition and skeletal muscle size in older women. *Int J Sport Nutr Exerc Metabol* 12: 125–135.

Campbell, W. W., and H. J. Leidy. 2007. Dietary protein and resistance training effects on muscle and body composition in older persons. *J Am Col Nutr* 26: 696S–703S.

Campbell, W. W., T. A. Trappe, A. C. Jozsi, L. J. Kruskall, R. R. Wolfe, and W. J. Evans. 2002b. Dietary protein adequacy and lower body versus whole body resistive training in older humans. *J Physiol* 542: 631–642.

Candow, D. G., J. P. Little, P. D. Chilibeck, S. Abeysekara, G. A. Zello, M. Kazachkov, S. M. Cornish, and P. H. Yu. 2008. Low-dose creatine combined with protein during resistance training in older men. *Med Sci Sports Exerc* 40: 1645–1652.

Carter, J. M., D. A. Bemben, A. W. Knehans, M. G. Bemben, and M. S. Witten. 2005. Does nutritional supplementation influence adaptability of muscle to resistance training in men aged 48 to 72 years. *J Geriatric Physical Ther* 28: 40–47.

Chernoff, R. 2005. Micronutrient requirements in older women. *Am J Clin Nutr* 81: 1240S–125S.

Chrusch, M. J., P. D. Chilibeck, K. E. Chad, K. S. Davison, and D. G. Burke. 2001. Creatine supplementation combined with resistance training in older men. *Med Sci Sports Exerc* 33: 2111–2117.

Combaret, L., D. Dardevet, I. Rieu, M. N. Pouch, D. Bechet, D. Taillandier, J. Grizard, and D. Attaix. 2005. A leucine-supplemented diet restores the defective postprandial inhibition of proteasome-dependent proteolysis in aged rat skeletal muscle. *J Physiol* 569: 489–499.

Conley, K. E., S. A. Jubrias, and P. C. Esselman. 2000. Oxidative capacity and ageing in human muscle. *J Physiol* 526: 203–210.

Dawson-Hughes, B., G. E. Dallal, E. A. Krall, L. Sadowski, N. Sahyoun, and S. Tannenbaum. 1990. A controlled trial of the effect of calcium supplementation on bone density in postmenopausal women. *New Eng J Med* 323: 878–883.

DeLuca, H. F. 1988. The vitamin D story: A collaborative effort of basic science and clinical medicine. *FASEB J* 2: 224–236.

Denis, W., and O. Folin. 1914. Protein metabolism from standpoint of blood and tissue analysis: An interpretation of creatine and creatinine in relation to animal metabolism. *J Biol Chem* 17: 493–502.

Dillon, E. L., M. Sheffield-Moore, D. Paddon-Jones, C. Gilkison, A. P. Sanford, S. L. Casperson, J. Jiang, D. L. Chinkes, and R. J. Urban. 2009. Amino acid supplementation increases lean body mass, basal muscle protein synthesis, and insulin-like growth factor-I expression in older women. *J Clin Endocrin Metabol* 94: 1630–1637.

Dreyer, H. C., and E. Volpi. 2005. Role of protein and amino acids in the pathophysiology and treatment of sarcopenia. *J Am Col Nutr* 24: 140S–145S.

Drummond, M. J., H. C. Dreyer, B. Pennings, C. S. Fry, S. Dhanani, E. L. Dillon, M. Sheffield-Moore, E. Volpi, and B. B. Rasmussen. 2008. Skeletal muscle protein anabolic response to resistance exercise and essential amino acids is delayed with aging. *J Appl Physiol* 104: 1452–1461.

Ekerdt, D. J. 2002. *The Macmillan Encyclopedia of Aging.* New York: Macmillan Reference USA.

Epel, E. S. 2009. Psychological and metabolic stress: A recipe for accelerated cellular aging? *Hormones* 8: 7–22.

Erickson, M. A., R. J. Schwarzkopf, and R. D. McKenzie. 1987. Effects of caffeine, fructose, and glucose ingestion on muscle glycogen utilization during exercise. *Med Sci Sports Exerc* 19: 579–583.

Esmarck, B., J. L. Andersen, S. Olsen, E. A. Richter, M. Mizuno, and M. Kjaer. 2001. Timing of post-exercise protein intake is important for muscle hypertrophy with resistance training in elderly humans. *J Physiol* 535: 301–311.

Essig, D. A., and P. J. Van Handel. 1980. Effects of caffeine ingestion on utilization of muscle glycogen and lipid during leg ergometer exercise. *Int J Sports Med* 1: 86–90.

Evans, M. D., R. Singh, V. Mistry, K. Sandhu, P. B. Farmer, and M. S. Cooke. 2008. Analysis of urinary 8-oxo-7,8-dihydro-purine-2'-deoxyribonucleosides by LC-MS/MS and improved ELISA. *Free Radical Res* 42: 831–840.

Faulkner, J. A., C. S. Davis, C. L. Mendias, and S. V. Brooks. 2008. The aging of elite male athletes: Age-related changes in performance and skeletal muscle structure and function. *Clin J Sport Med* 18: 501–507.

Faulkner, J. A., L. M. Larkin, D. R. Claflin, and S. V. Brooks. 2007. Age-related changes in the structure and function of skeletal muscles. *Clin Exper Pharmacol Physiol* 34: 1091–1096.

Feldman, M., B. Cryer, K. E. McArthur, B. A. Huet, and E. Lee. 1996. Effects of aging and gastritis on gastric acid and pepsin secretion in humans: A prospective study. *Gastroenterology* 110: 1043–1052.

Gloth, F. M., 3rd, C. M. Gundberg, B. W. Hollis, J. G. Haddad, Jr., and J. D. Tobin. 1995a. Vitamin D deficiency in homebound elderly persons. *JAMA* 274: 1683–1686.

Gloth, F. M., 3rd, C. E. Smith, B. W. Hollis, and J. D. Tobin. 1995b. Functional improvement with vitamin D replenishment in a cohort of frail, vitamin D-deficient older people. *J Am Geriat Soc* 43: 1269–1271.

Gloth, F. M., 3rd, and J. D. Tobin. 1995. Vitamin D deficiency in older people. *J Am Geriat Soc* 43: 822–828.

Gotshalk, L. A., W. J. Kraemer, M. A. Mendonca, J. L. Vingren, A. M. Kenny, B. A. Spiering, D. L. Hatfield, M. S. Fragala, and J. S. Volek. 2008. Creatine supplementation improves muscular performance in older women. *Euro J Appl Physiol* 102: 223–231.

Gotshalk, L. A., J. S. Volek, R. S. Staron, C. R. Denegar, F. C. Hagerman, and W. J. Kraemer. 2002. Creatine supplementation improves muscular performance in older men. *Med Sci Sports Exerc* 34: 537–543.

Greenhaff, P. L., K. Bodin, K. Soderlund, and E. Hultman. 1994. Effect of oral creatine supplementation on skeletal muscle phosphocreatine resynthesis. *Am J Physiol* 266: E725–E730.

Guillet, C., M. Prod'homme, M. Balage, P. Gachon, C. Giraudet, L. Morin, J. Grizard, and Y. Boirie. 2004. Impaired anabolic response of muscle protein synthesis is associated with S6K1 dysregulation in elderly humans. *FASEB J* 18: 1586–1587.

Heaney, R. P., and G. A. Bachmann. 2005. Interpreting studies of nutritional prevention: A perspective using calcium as a model. *J Women's Health (2002)* 14: 889–897.

Henderson, G. C., B. A. Irving, and K. S. Nair. 2009. Potential application of essential amino acid supplementation to treat sarcopenia in elderly people. *J Clin Endocrinol Metabol* 94: 1524–1526.

Holecek, M., L. Sprongl, I. Tilser, and M. Tichy. 2001. Leucine and protein metabolism in rats with chronic renal insufficiency. *Exper Toxicol Pathol* 53: 71–76.

Holick, M. F. 1995. Environmental factors that influence the cutaneous production of vitamin D. *Am J Clin Nutr* 61(3 Suppl): 638S–645S.

Houston, D. K., B. J. Nicklas, J. Ding, T. B. Harris, F. A. Tylavsky, A. B. Newman, J. S. Lee, N. R. Sahyoun, M. Visser, and S. B. Kritchevsky. 2008. Dietary protein intake is associated with lean mass change in older, community-dwelling adults: The health, aging, and body composition (health ABC) study. *Am J Clin Nutr* 87: 150–155.

Humphrey, L. L., R. Fu, K. Rogers, M. Freeman, and M. Helfand. 2008. Homocysteine level and coronary heart disease incidence: A systematic review and meta-analysis. *Mayo Clinic Proc* 83: 1203–1212.

Iglay, H. B., J. P. Thyfault, J. W. Apolzan, and W. W. Campbell. 2007. Resistance training and dietary protein: Effects on glucose tolerance and contents of skeletal muscle insulin signaling proteins in older persons. *Am J Clin Nutr* 85: 1005–1013.

Institute of Medicine. 1997. *Dietary reference intakes for calcium, phosphorous, magnesium, vitamin D, and fluoride.* Washington, D.C.: National Academies Press.

Institute of Medicine of National Academies. 2002/2005. *Dietary reference intakes for energy, carbohydrates, fiber, fat, protein, and amino acids (macronutrients).* Washington, D.C.: The National Academies Press.

Ivy, J. L., D. L. Costill, W. J. Fink, and R. W. Lower. 1979. Influence of caffeine and carbohydrate feedings on endurance performance. *Med Sci Sports Exerc* 11: 6–11.

Katsanos, C. S., H. Kobayashi, M. Sheffield-Moore, A. Aarsland, and R. R. Wolfe. 2006. A high proportion of leucine is required for optimal stimulation of the rate of muscle protein synthesis by essential amino acids in the elderly. *Am J Physiol Endocrinol Metab* 291: E381–E387.

Kenney, W. L., and P. Chiu. 2001. Influence of age on thirst and fluid intake. *Med Sci Sports Exerc* 33: 1524–1532.

Kenney, W. L., C. G. Tankersley, D. L. Newswanger, D. E. Hyde, S. M. Puhl, and N. L. Turner. 1990. Age and hypohydration independently influence the peripheral vascular response to heat stress. *J Appl Physiol* 68: 1902–1908.

Kreider, R. B. 2003. Effects of creatine supplementation on performance and training adaptations. *Mol Cell Biochem* 244: 89–94.

Kreider R. B., M. Ferreira, M. Wilson, and A. L. Almada. 1999. Effects of calcium beta-hydroxy-beta-methylbutyrate (HMB) supplementation during resistance-training on markers of catabolism, body composition, and strength. *Int J Sports Med* Nov; 20(8): 503–509.

Lewis, R. D., and C. M. Modlesky. 1998. Nutrition, physical activity, and bone health in women. *Int J Sport Nutr* 8: 250–284.

Look AHEAD Research Group, X. Pi-Sunyer, G. Blackburn, F. L. Brancati, G. A. Bray, R. Bright, J. M. Clark, et al. 2007. Reduction in weight and cardiovascular disease risk factors in individuals with type 2 diabetes: One-year results of the look AHEAD trial. *Diabetes Care* 30: 1374–1383.

Manore, M. M. 2000. Effect of physical activity on thiamine, riboflavin, and vitamin B-6 requirements. *Am J Clin Nutr* 72(2 Suppl): 598S–606S.

Marian, M., and G. Sacks. 2009. Micronutrients and older adults. *Nutr Clin Prac* 24: 179–195.

Maughan, R. J. 1999. Role of micronutrients in sport and physical activity. *Brit Med Bull* 55: 683–690.

Masoro, E. J., and S. N. Austad. 2006. *Handbook of the Biology of Aging,* 6th Ed. San Diego: Academic Press.

McArdle, W. D., F. I. Katch, and V. L. Katch. 2008. *Sport and exercise nutrition,* 3rd Ed. New York: Lippincott Williams Wilkins.

McCully, K. K., M. A. Forciea, L. M. Hack, E. Donlon, R. W. Wheatley, C. A. Oatis, T. Goldberg, and B. Chance. 1991. Muscle metabolism in older subjects using 31P magnetic resonance spectroscopy. *Can J Physiol Pharmacol* 69: 576–580.

Morais, J. A., S. Chevalier, and R. Gougeon. 2006. Protein turnover and requirements in the healthy and frail elderly. *J Nutr Health Aging* 10: 272–283.

Nissen, S. L., and R. L. Sharp. 2003. Effect of dietary supplements on lean mass and strength gains with resistance exercise: A meta-analysis. *J Appl Physiol* 94: 651–659.

Nissen, S., R. Sharp, M. Ray, J. A. Rathmacher, D. Rice, J. C. Fuller, Jr., A. S. Connelly, and N. Abumrad. 1996. Effect of leucine metabolite beta-hydroxy-beta-methylbutyrate on muscle metabolism during resistance-exercise training. *J Appl Physiol* 81: 2095–2104.

Norager, C. B., M. B. Jensen, M. R. Madsen, and S. Laurberg. 2005. Caffeine improves endurance in 75-yr-old citizens: A randomized, double-blind, placebo-controlled, crossover study. *J Appl Physiol* 99: 2302–2306.

Norager, C. B., M. B. Jensen, A. Weimann, and M. R. Madsen. 2006. Metabolic effects of caffeine ingestion and physical work in 75-year-old citizens. A randomized, double-blind, placebo-controlled, cross-over study. *Clin Endocrinol* 65: 223–228.

O'Donnell, A. B., T. G. Travison, S. S. Harris, J. L. Tenover, and J. B. McKinlay. 2006. Testosterone, dehydroepiandrosterone, and physical performance in older men: Results from the Massachusetts male aging study. *J Clin Endocrinol Metabol* 91: 425–431.

Paddon-Jones, D., and B. B. Rasmussen. 2009. Dietary protein recommendations and the prevention of sarcopenia. *Curr Opinion Clin Nutr Metabolic Care* 12: 86–90.

Pearson, S. J., A. Young, A. Macaluso, G. Devito, M. A. Nimmo, M. Cobbold, and S. D. Harridge. 2002. Muscle function in elite master weightlifters. *Med Sci Sports Exerc* 34: 1199–1206.

Rawson, E. S., P. M. Clarkson, T. B. Price, and M. P. Miles. 2002. Differential response of muscle phosphocreatine to creatine supplementation in young and old subjects. *Acta Physiol Scand* 174: 57–65.

Rawson, E. S., and J. S. Volek. 2003. Effects of creatine supplementation and resistance training on muscle strength and weightlifting performance. *J Strength Cond Res* 17: 822–831.

Rodriguez, N. R., N. M. DiMarco, S. Langley, American Dietetic Association, Dietitians of Canada, and American College of Sports Medicine. 2009. Position of the American Dietetic Association, Dieticians of Canada, and the American College of Sports Medicine: Nutrition and athletic performance. *J Am Dietetic Assoc* 109: 509–527.

Rolland, Y., S. Czerwinski, G. Abellan Van Kan, J. E. Morley, M. Cesari, G. Onder, J. Woo, et al. 2008. Sarcopenia: Its assessment, etiology, pathogenesis, consequences and future perspectives. *J Nutr Health Aging* 12: 433–450.

Rolls, B. J., and P. A. Phillips. 1990. Aging and disturbances of thirst and fluid balance. *Nutrition Reviews* 48: 137–144.

Rowlands, D. S., and J. S. Thomson. 2009. Effects of beta-hydroxy-beta-methylbutyrate supplementation during resistance training on strength, body composition, and muscle damage in trained and untrained young men: A meta-analysis. *J Strength Cond Res* 23: 836–846.

Russell, R. M., and P. M. Suter. 1993. Vitamin requirements of elderly people: An update. *Am J Clin Nutr* 58: 4–14.

Sacheck, J. M., and R. Roubenoff. 1999. Nutrition in the exercising elderly. *Clinics Sports Med* 18: 565–584.

Slater, G. J., and D. Jenkins. 2000. Beta-hydroxy-beta-methylbutyrate (HMB) supplementation and the promotion of muscle growth and strength. *Sports Med* 30: 105–116.

Smith, H. J., P. Mukerji, and M. J. Tisdale. 2005. Attenuation of proteasome-induced proteolysis in skeletal muscle by {beta}-hydroxy-{beta}-methylbutyrate in cancer-induced muscle loss. *Cancer Res* 65: 277–283.

Sood, N., W. L. Baker, and C. I. Coleman. 2008. Effect of glucomannan on plasma lipid and glucose concentrations, body weight, and blood pressure: Systematic review and meta-analysis. *Am J Clin Nutr* 88: 1167–1175.

Spriet, L. L. 1995. Caffeine and performance. *Int J Sport Nutr* 5(Suppl): S84–S99.

Spriet, L. L., D. A. MacLean, D. J. Dyck, E. Hultman, G. Cederblad, and T. E. Graham. 1992. Caffeine ingestion and muscle metabolism during prolonged exercise in humans. *Am J Physiol* 262: E891–E898.

Syrotuik, D. G., and G. J. Bell. 2004. Acute creatine monohydrate supplementation: A descriptive physiological profile of responders vs. non-responders. *J Strength Cond Res* 18: 610–617.

Tarnopolsky, M. A. 2008. Nutritional consideration in the aging athlete. *Clin J Sport Med* 18: 531–538.

Terjung, R. L., P. Clarkson, E. R. Eichner, P. L. Greenhaff, P. J. Hespel, R. G. Israel, W. J. Kraemer, et al. 2000. American College of Sports Medicine roundtable: The physiological and health effects of oral creatine supplementation. *Med Sci Sports Exerc* 32: 706–717.

Verdijk, L. B., R. A. Jonkers, B. G. Gleeson, M. Beelen, K. Meijer, H. H. Savelberg, W. K. Wodzig, P. Dendale, and L. J. van Loon. 2009. Protein supplementation before and after exercise does not further augment skeletal muscle hypertrophy after resistance training in elderly men. *Am J Clin Nutr* 89: 608–616.

Volpi, E., H. Kobayashi, M. Sheffield-Moore, B. Mittendorfer, and R. R. Wolfe. 2003. Essential amino acids are primarily responsible for the amino acid stimulation of muscle protein anabolism in healthy elderly adults. *Am J Clin Nutr* 78: 250–258.

Volpi, E., B. Mittendorfer, B. B. Rasmussen, and R. R. Wolfe. 2000. The response of muscle protein anabolism to combined hyperaminoacidemia and glucose-induced hyperinsulinemia is impaired in the elderly. *J Clin Endocrinol Metabol* 85: 4481–4490.

Volpi, E., M. Sheffield-Moore, B. B. Rasmussen, and R. R. Wolfe. 2001. Basal muscle amino acid kinetics and protein synthesis in healthy young and older men. *JAMA* 286: 1206–1212.

Vukovich, M. D., N. B. Stubbs, and R. M. Bohlken. 2001. Body composition in 70-year-old adults responds to dietary beta-hydroxy-beta-methylbutyrate similarly to that of young adults. *J Nutr* 131: 2049–2052.

Williams, M. H., and J. D. Branch. 1998. Creatine supplementation and exercise performance: An update. *J Am Col Nutr* 17: 216–234.

Wolfe, R. R. 2006. Skeletal muscle protein metabolism and resistance exercise. *J Nutr* 136: 525S–528S.

Index

Milton Keynes UK
Ingram Content Group UK Ltd.
UKHW020315111024
449327UK00040B/1254